Wellness Architecture and Urban Design

Wellness is a contemporary concept with deep ancient roots promoting preventative and holistic activities, lifestyle choices, and salient architecture and urban design practices. *Wellness Architecture and Urban Design* presents definitions, an analysis of the wellness literature, and a brief history of the wellness movement. Specific planning and design strategies are presented citing examples worldwide and emphasizing the importance of wellness considerations at all scales of the built environment from rooms to cities. Both case studies offer fully integrated and comprehensive wellness design approaches creating resilient and life-enhancing wellness through each of the architecture and urban design scales. The book will be of interest to practitioners and students working in urban design, landscape architecture, architecture, planning, and affiliated fields.

"The authors have written a groundbreaking book addressing the emerging trend of designing for wellness, not only in health care settings, but also in places for living, work, learning, play, and worship. This book speaks not only to architecture and urban planning, but also strongly emphasizes the benefit of designed and built environments that enhance the full continuum of wellness supporting the body, mind, and spirit. There is a pragmatic flavor to the book offering a wealth of examples, serving as a useful reference for those who develop, plan, design, and build human places. I strongly recommend this book to students, faculty, health professionals, planning and design professionals, and the public at large."

Ronald L. Skaggs, *FAIA, FACHA, FHFI, LEED AP, Chairman Emeritus, HKS, Inc., Former President, American Institute of Architects, Chancellor AIA College of Fellows, USA*

"*Wellness Architecture and Urban Design* is a clarion call for reimagining our future – a future where design is empathetic, inclusive, and sustainable. It offers an enlightening journey through the principles and practices of biophilic and wellness design, making it an essential read for anyone interested in the future of urban living and environmental stewardship. The book offers a groundbreaking exploration of the profound relationship between our physical spaces and well-being. This work is a rich tapestry, weaving together historical insights, current challenges, and visionary solutions in the realm of design and architecture. It delves deep into the human condition, highlighting how environmental factors and human activities shape our health and happiness. Drawing on years of extensive research and diverse global perspectives, this book is not merely academic; it is a practical guide to transforming our living environments into catalysts for holistic wellness."

Jennifer Walsh, *Founder and Creative Director, AIKR Lab and Institute, USA*

"*Wellness Architecture and Urban Design* is a transformative journey that redefines our understanding of the spaces we inhabit. This book beautifully encapsulates how intentional architecture and placemaking can catalyze wellness on many levels. It's about fostering communities, nurturing the spirit, and inspiring a ripple effect of health and happiness. As Phillip Tabb and Lahra Tatriele share their extensive knowledge, they provide a vision that compels us to rethink our environments and their potential to elevate our lives. Having recently moved from the incessant buzz of New York City to the tranquil hamlet of Mado in Serenbe, my family and I have experienced firsthand the profound impact that connection to nature and thoughtful design can have on well-being. We've become calmer, more balanced, and deeply connected, realizing the stark contrast between our past and present living environments. I am grateful for the insights this book offers and believe them to be an indispensable guide for anyone yearning to create spaces that resonate with our deepest need for connection, wellness, and harmony."

Noa Hecht, *Creative Placemaking Consultant, USA*

"Fivelements Retreat Bali was decades ahead in its quest to incorporate biophilic design principles that nurture the relationships between humans and nature – relationships that heal and sustain life itself. The Fivelements philosophy became the definition of a new eco-luxury experience that positively impacts all seven dimensions of wellness. The founders of Fivelements Retreat understood that true wellness is inseparable from nature, and this shows in every aspect of the resort. From the moment guests enter this awe-inspiring sanctuary, located along Bali's sacred Ayung River, they will experience a holistic approach to wellness, from impeccably designed rooms to exquisite cuisine to unique connections with local healers. I cannot think of a better place to experience the true meaning of wellness design or to understand why it is vital to our industry."

Susie Ellis, *Chair and CEO, The Global Wellness Institute, USA*

Wellness Architecture and Urban Design

Phillip James Tabb and
Lahra Tatriele

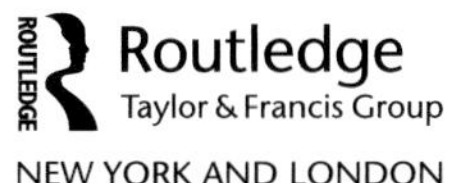

NEW YORK AND LONDON

Designed cover: Photos by Simon Flint (top) and
Serenbe Development (bottom).

First published 2025
by Routledge
605 Third Avenue, New York, NY 10158

and by Routledge
4 Park Square, Milton Park, Abingdon, Oxon, OX14 4RN

Routledge is an imprint of the Taylor & Francis Group, an informa business

Library of Congress Cataloging-in-Publication Data
Names: Tabb, Phillip, author. | Tatriele, Lahra, author.
Title: Wellness architecture and urban design / Phillip James Tabb and Lahra Tatriele.
Description: New York, NY : Routledge, 2025. | Includes bibliographical references and index. |
Identifiers: LCCN 2024014302 (print) | LCCN 2024014303 (ebook) | ISBN 9781032752037 (hardback) | ISBN 9781032752013 (paperback) | ISBN 9781003472902 (ebook)
Subjects: LCSH: City planning—Psychological aspects. | City and town life—Psychological aspects. | Environmental psychology. | Mental health planning. | Mental health policy. | Urban policy.
Classification: LCC HT166 .T32 2025 (print) | LCC HT166 (ebook) | DDC 711/.4—dc23/eng/20240615
LC record available at https://lccn.loc.gov/2024014302
LC ebook record available at https://lccn.loc.gov/2024014303

ISBN: 9781032752037 (hbk)
ISBN: 9781032752013 (pbk)
ISBN: 9781003472902 (ebk)

DOI: 10.4324/9781003472902

Typeset in Univers
by codeMantra

This work is dedicated to future
generations in the pursuit of transformational
wellness for themselves, their families,
their greater communities, and the planet

Contents

Figures

Tables

Foreword

It is increasingly clear that humankind is in the midst of an ever-deepening ecology of crises, both personal and planetary. Largely as the result of our own actions, we are presently experiencing the Sixth Great Species Extinction, as well as the destabilization of all the major ecosystems of land and sea. Megadroughts and spreading deserts, catastrophic floods, uncontrollable wildfires, and other weather-related disasters have now become common around the world. Climate-driven famines and mass migrations are fueling violent conflicts as increasing numbers of people struggle to find food, water, shelter, and the bare necessities of life. Sea levels continue to rise, threatening in this century to flood many of the world's great coastal cities. All of these biophysical crises have already disrupted the fossil-fueled global economy upon which our present way of life depends. The possibilities of societal collapse are no longer the dystopian nightmares of science fiction: they are realities being played out in the daily news.

Unsurprisingly, at a personal level, there is a spreading sense of hopelessness about the future, especially among younger generations. Feelings of powerlessness in the face of these crises afflict rich and poor alike, eroding our personal and collective sense of well-being in the face of what appear to be intractable problems for which there are no viable or even possible solutions. It is within the background of this global context that the authors of this timely book offer us a vision of a way to live together that is capable of addressing all of these issues, if only we choose to design forms of architecture and patterns of settlement that nurture both people and planet. Rather than falling prey to a sense of despair the authors not only provide a vision of the more beautiful world it is in our power to create, but they provide detailed accounts of how communities and groups around the world are already creating ecologically-based communities that reconnect us to each other and the natural world.

Wellness Architecture and Urban Design is not just a book, it is a wholistic new design paradigm for creating resilient and life-enhancing communities of place that is based on two simple but powerful principles: 1) that wellness for humankind cannot be achieved apart from the wellness of the earthworld upon which we depend for life itself, and 2) the foundational idea that the basic unit of sustainability is the mixed use, humanly scaled cooperative community. Given the transdisciplinary scope of this encyclopedic text, the authors have structured the book in a way that leads the reader systematically from definitions of wellness, spiced with inspiring examples of what is already being done around the world, to the final two chapters which provide detailed case studies, one in the United States and the other in Bali, that convincingly demonstrate the global relevance of the Wellness Design paradigm. Each chapter is introduced with an abstract, which gives the reader a concise overview of the scope and focus of the chapter. The main points are helpfully summarized in color-coded tables and exhaustive endnotes which allow the interested reader to follow up with primary sources for each theme covered. This is especially important since the book cuts across so many separate silos of knowledge.

What is unique in the design literature on both wellness and sustainable design is the authors' "Seven Pillars of Wellness" framework, which integrates disciplines which are rarely mentioned in the same breath, but must be integrated in any approach to wellness-based design at any scale of environment. These pillars are: 1) Physical; 2) Mental; 3) Emotional; 4) Spiritual; 5) Social; 6) Financial; and 7) Environmental. Of particular importance is the inclusion of Spiritual Wellness and Financial Wellness, making this transdisciplinary design paradigm the most wholistic and inclusive approach to regenerative, sustainable, and resilient design yet proposed.

The authors also persuasively argue that any truly life-enhancing human ecology must be modular and multi-scalar, ranging from the bioregional and urban planning level to the landscape, architectural, and interior levels of design. Once again, this idea is as obviously necessary as it is routinely neglected in both theory and practice. But this book makes it clear that the challenges that confront us cannot be addressed in any other way. Indeed, any lesser approach based on the present paradigm of separation rather than the proposed paradigm of wholeness and connectivity is likely to only multiply and deepen our problems.

The book closes with two detailed case studies that demonstrate how the Wellness Design paradigm is applicable in the overdeveloped world such as the United States, as it is in less developed places such as Bali, Indonesia, that are challenged with the task to avoid the unsustainable patterns of settlement and ways of life that the United States has perfected. The most fully embodied precedent is the award-winning new community of Serenbe, Georgia, for which author Phillip Tabb is the master planner. This necklace of humanly-scaled hamlets, which are woven into the fabric of the forested landscape of Chattahoochee Hills near Atlanta, Georgia, offers a life-enhancing alternative to suburban and exurban sprawl. Rather than growth by the endless addition of disconnected parts that lengthen distances between life functions in ways that can never be overcome by ever faster and bigger highways, the planning principle of Serenbe is based on the multiplication and the gathering of interconnected wholes within wholes to create an experientially rich community.

The Serenbe community is comprised of six residential hamlets, each of which is built around a different wellness theme: *Selborne*, culinary, visual and performing arts; *Grange*, an organic farm and equestrian activities; *Mado*, multigenerational health and wellness; *Spela,* family and play (under construction); *Education*, schools, international study, and continuing education (planning phase); *Middle Housing*, more affordable housing and a commercial zone connected to the larger existing community (conceptual phase). Seventy percent of the land is and will remain undeveloped. Each hamlet has one face opening onto a narrow serpentine road that connects it to all the hamlets and the world beyond, and the other face opens onto native forests and the many trails that connect to every part of the whole community. A central area at the end of each hamlet provides higher density housing and commercial spaces, providing an identifiable central neighborhood focus. When fully developed, Serenbe will house some 3,000 residents.

The Mado hamlet has been designed as a mixed-use, multigenerational, and ecologically designed biophilic community focused on the practice and cultivation of wellness and the healing arts. The planned *Aging in Place Wellness* campus is adjacent to the *Terra School at Serenbe*, a planned lifelong learning education campus, as well as the community pool to encourage cross-generational interaction. The Medicinal and Edible Landscape and the Mado Food Forest encourage visits by people of all ages throughout Serenbe and beyond, further increasing the likelihood of cross-generational and unplanned encounters among residents and visitors. The many wellness related businesses are mixed throughout the hamlet based on the idea of form-based codes rather than single use functional zoning. In Mado, as is the case throughout Serenbe, a variety of ecologically-based green infrastructure such as vegetated wetland waste systems, bioswales, and bio-habitats, create garden landscapes that integrate function and beauty, demonstrating how we can build with nature, rather than against nature. Every human-made environment, good or bad, is itself a form of environmental education: the all-pervading lesson of Mado, and Serenbe a whole, is that our human ecology and the naturally occurring ecology must be and can be experienced as a single undivided whole in all the areas in which life takes place.

This brief Foreword merely gives a taste of what the reader will find by reading and re-reading this book in depth. Its strength is that it not only provides a comprehensive theory of a new approach to architecture and community design that harmonizes with naturally occurring ecologies of place, but it also provides us with principles, patterns, and precedents at every scale of environment that can inform and inspire the creation of ever new forms of resilient, beautiful, and sustainable communities. Over the course of this century and beyond humankind needs to create thousands of new communities in response to systemic crises that are beyond anything our species has yet encountered. It is estimated that in the lifetime of someone born today there will be as many as a billion and a half climate refugees worldwide by 2100. The United States itself could find several hundred million citizens seeking refuge from rising seas, uncontrollable wildfires, megadroughts and floods, and a cascade of economic and societal breakdowns as existing institutions and systems are overwhelmed. Where will people move to? How will they live?

It is clear that the entire planet will need to build new communities to provide refuge and comfort and to shelter us from the crises that are already on our doorstep. We will not have the capacity for or the luxury of continuing to mindlessly build more and more automobile-dependent, sprawling anti-communities that worsen our carbon footprint and leave us more isolated from the earth and each other. We need to create an economic and cultural revolution that helps us to heal from the traumas of our times, by making it possible for us to meet our basic needs for energy, food, shelter, and cooperative human relationships both locally and sustainably: it is the only way forward for all the peoples of the earth. The forms this will take will be as varied as the cultures and landscapes in which they emerge.

We do not have to wait for systemic failure of our life-support systems to fully emerge: the approach to planning and design described in this book can be applied now at every scale of environment from a backyard to an existing neighborhood, the retrofitting of a dead shopping mall or a life-giving enhancement of an existing school or small town. The ideas in this book are replicable and scalable. I hope this book both informs and inspires the creation of a worldwide network of life-enhancing human settlements in all the varied landscapes and diverse cultures of the earth. Let a thousand flowers bloom! The time to start is now.

Gary J. Coates
ACSA Distinguished Professor
Kansas State University

About the Authors

Phillip James Tabb is Emeritus Professor of Architecture at Texas A&M University and was the Liz and Nelson Mitchell Professor of Residential Design. He served as Head of the Department from 2001–2005 and was Director of the School of Architecture and Construction Management at Washington State University from 1998–2001. He completed a Ph.D. dissertation on *The Solar Village Archetype: A Study of English Village Form Applicable to Energy Integrated Planning Principles for Satellite Settlements in Temperate Climates* in 1990. Among his publications are *Solar Energy Planning* published by McGraw-Hill in 1984, Co-authored *The Greening of Architecture: A Critical History and Survey of Contemporary Sustainable Architecture and Urban Design* published by Ashgate in 2014, Co-edited *Architecture, Culture and Spirituality* also published by Ashgate in 2015. He was author of *Serene Urbanism: A Biophilic Theory and Practice of Sustainable Placemaking* in 2017, *Elemental Architecture: Temperaments of Sustainability* in 2019, *Biophilic Urbanism: Designing Resilient Communities for the Future* in 2021, and *Thin Place Design: Architecture of the Numinous* in 2024, all published by Routledge. Since 2001, Tabb has been the master plan architect for Serenbe Community – an award-winning sustainable biophilic community being realized near Atlanta, Georgia, and his net-zero residence in Serenbe. He is an editor and author of *Wellness Architecture and Design Initiative* for the Global Wellness Institute. He received his Bachelor of Science in Architecture from the University of Cincinnati, Master of Architecture from the University of Colorado, and Ph.D. in the Energy and Environment Programme from the Architectural Association in London. He is a practicing urban designer and licensed architect, and a member of the American Institute of Architects and holds a NCARB Certificate.

Lahra Tatriele is an international wellness executive leading corporate-level growth strategy, business model innovation, concept design and curation, and integrated wellness branding within high growth markets. In 2010, she led the launch of Fivelements Retreat Bali. By 2016, she steered the opening the first urban retreat, Fivelements Hong Kong, in partnership with New World Development, and a city wellness sanctuary, Fivelements Habitat, with Evolution Wellness in the central business district in 2019. Over the course of her leadership, Lahra was responsible for the brand's design and growth strategy resulting in Fivelements as the recipient of over 50 international awards and over 200 editorials spanning health and wellness, culinary innovation, and sustainable design fields. Lahra is also Co-Founder and Principal of Alchemy Concepts and Wellness Communities Italia, working with public and private entities, real estate, and hospitality developers toward embracing an integral wellness strategy as the core foundation for regenerative growth. Previously, she was a co-executive producer of TEDx Ubud on economic empowerment and has received numerous invitations to speak on regenerative wellness and design. Lahra currently serves as Chair of the Wellness Architecture and Design Initiative and is a long-time member of the Mental Wellness Initiative of the Global Wellness Institute (GWI) whose mission is *Empowering Wellness Worldwide*. The GWI's research, programs, and initiatives have been instrumental in the growth of the USD$5.6 trillion wellness economy. Lahra has also had corporate affiliations with the Friends of the Wildlife Foundation in Bali, Indonesia, the Tibet House USA, and the Coral Triangle Conservancy. She received a Bachelor of Science in International Marketing from the Stern School of Business at New York University and completed an executive course in Architectural Imagination from Harvard's Graduate School of Design.

Preface

The human condition is affected by an unprecedented capacity for good and bad consequences for our species caused by the natural and urban environments and the human activity associated with these contexts. Concurrently, the environmental context within which these activities occur is also a benefit or a risk to extremes. Human activity and the natural environment are inextricably linked. And as world population is projected to reach 8.5 billion people in 2030, only six years from now, critical problems are not going away. This increase in the number of people most likely means more ecological degradation, increase in human causes of climate change, increase in conflicts, and higher risks of global-scale heath issues like pandemics. Overcrowding, crime, and food and water shortages are also likely to occur especially in vulnerable locations. To reverse these outcomes to positive wellness benefits is going to require many changes to lifestyle choices and the settled environments within which we live.

Environmental issues include climate change, natural disasters, environmental degradation, deforestation, loss of biodiversity, water scarcity, resource depletion, and appropriate responses to increasing population numbers and migration patterns. With increasing populations, more food and water are needed. This in turn most likely will create increased deforestation in order to create new farmlands, grazing land, and expanded settlements. Another byproduct of population growth is the stress on fresh water. According to UNESCO, between two and three billion people worldwide experience water shortages for at least one month per year.[1] In order to reverse the trend of environmental degradation, planetary wellness principles and strategies are needed to bring our co-existence with nature into balance. Presently there are small pockets or examples where wellness designs have been realized, and there is the need to expand these pockets and proliferate the positive work to even larger scales of influence. There has been a huge surge in the wellness economy from personal care and beauty, nutrition, and spa designs, to wellness tourism and, more recently, in wellness real estate, but more is needed.

The wellness movement is a relatively contemporary concept in part informed by the emergence of the World Health Organization in the late 1940s where health went beyond merely the absence of illness and included states of physical, mental, and social well-being. The work of Halbert Dunn in the 1950s took health to "high-level wellness" which included integrated functions oriented toward maximizing one's potential. John Travis's work in the 1970s promoted self-directed and preventative approaches to well-being rather than focus on "illness-oriented care."[2] The wellness movement was considered to have entered the mainstream in the 1980s and was taken more seriously by the medical academic communities, and included planetary health.

Wellness applied by the design disciplines is also a relatively new practice that was initially born from the planning and design of hospitals, assisted living, nursing homes, and other care-related facilities. In fact, ancient structures were constructed to solicit healing from the gods. Some of the earliest healthcare facilities were built by the Romans as military hospitals. Later, monastic communities became the standard for public hospitals. The "pavilion plan" developed in the middle ages, featured fresh air and natural light. In modern times, hospitals were designed to accommodate greater populations of patients by growing larger and higher with multi-stories. Today, healthcare facilities include addiction treatment centers, birthing centers, blood banks, cancer centers, dental care, optometry care, hospice homes, urgent care facilities, physical therapy centers, and more recently telehealth care support. The shift from curative health to wellness responds to architecture and urban designs with design determinants that implicitly contribute to good health and well-being outcomes.

More recent concepts of wellness design have focused on a variety of scales and with everyday applications. This suggests that wellness should be applied to all urban contexts and building types, from homes to offices, and from schools to shopping centers. Wellness should be infused into all places we inhabit and experience daily. Dr. Edward Valentin puts it as working toward a state of balance collecting "well-moments" over "un-well" moments.[3] Key to promoting greater wellness is the proximity and access to positive wellness-moment environments and experiences. Well moments can be as simple as time spent outdoors, in the sun, near water or breathing fresh air, and they can be experienced as awe or serene moments.

Research into previous literature on health and wellness has helped inform the content of this work. This includes subjects of illness, health, wellness, and physical design disciplines. Also being involved in the planning and design of several of the projects featured in the book gave invaluable insights. This book is based upon previous research into the relationship between wellness and the built environment conducted by a team of volunteer professionals led by initiative chair Lahra Tatriele and editor Phillip Tabb. Seven other international scholars, health, and design practitioners from Hong Kong, Bali, Dubai, Lisbon, London, New York City, and Jackson, Wyoming, also assisted in the preparation of a draft white paper entitled *Wellness Architecture and Design Pathways*. This work was initiated by the Global Wellness Institute initiative on wellness architecture and design intended to raise awareness and provide pathways for the implementation of an interdisciplinary wellness approach delivering positive health, sustainability, and financial outcomes for existing and future environments. It aimed to provide definitions and clarity on what a wellness architecture and design approach is and the benefits and intended outcomes that result. This was in large part accomplished through the use of many examples worldwide as pathways in the planning, architecture, interior, and landscape design sectors.[4]

An important section of the white paper, Chapter 4, focused on the financial and economic benefits of wellness. This included real estate economics, construction, building operations and maintenance, AI, and renewable technologies.[5] Team members for the white paper included Valentina Cereda, Gove Depuy, Anthony DiGuiseppe, Sherry Fong, Stephen Marks, Kailas Moorthy, Veronica Schreibeis Smith, Phillip Tabb and Lahra Tatriele. Initiated in 2022, the preliminary white paper is anticipated to be complete in early 2024. The paper was organized along the seven pillars or dimensions of wellness benefits, a series of planning and design strategies occurring at varying scales, and a focus on financial or economic wellness.[6]

All design fields affect health and wellness in various ways. This includes issues of sustainability, resilience, placemaking, material science, environmental protection, natural disasters, climate change, and biophilia. Sustainability and resilience are important to wellness in terms of both human and environmental health. Building with non-toxic materials improves the indoor environment where we spend most of our time. The reduction of environmental pollution and advancements in hygiene have contributed significantly to the increase in human health and life expectancy. Climate change is linked to a number of health-related risks, including injuries caused by storms or flooding, and the spreading of insect-borne infectious diseases. Biophilic design, for example, supports a host of health and wellness outcomes, including stress reduction, improved heart health and respiratory function, improving incidences of kidney disease, increased social connections, and spiritual renewal.

Figure 0.1 illustrates the contrasts in the relationship between wellness and non-wellness lifestyles and environments. It shows a health and wellness continuum along wellness principles of design.[7] Normal health *or not-sick* occurs at the intersection of these two realms. This neutral state includes medical noninterference and moderate levels of thriving. Lifestyle choices that promote wellness are a balanced life, healthy diet, frequent hydration, regular exercise, access to fresh air, non-smoking, and a healthy social life. High-level wellness is a process of wholistic functioning achieving fuller and longer life potentials.

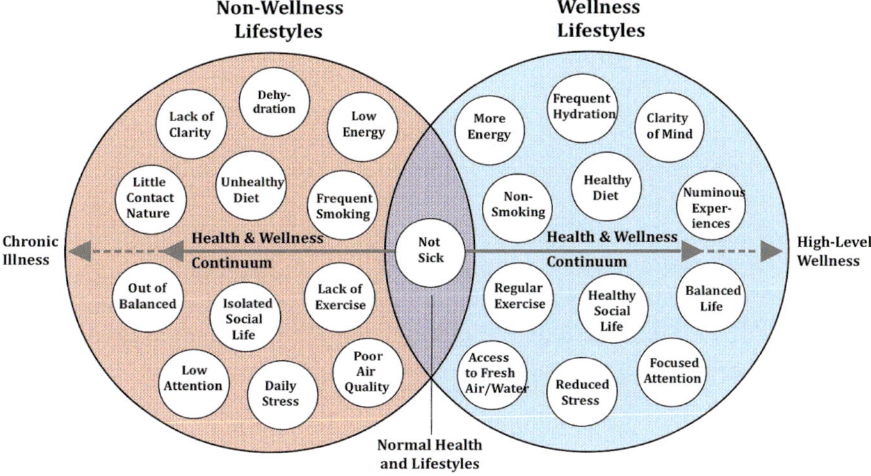

0.1
Lifestyles and Health and Wellness Continuum
(*Source: Phillip Tabb*)

The need for wellness is a top priority for the built environment and places human and environmental health at the center of the design agenda. A more comprehensive and sophisticated wellness lens is at the forefront particularly on personal wellness including better physical health, fitness nutrition, appearance, sleep, and mindfulness. This lens also includes the emotional, social, spiritual, and planetary health in an attempt to address broader scales of influence. The Global Wellness Institute believes that the residential real estate market is the next frontier that will affect the wellness movement. They assert that it is our homes, communities, and the surrounding environments that will directly affect daily wellness behaviors and lifestyles.[8] It is important to see the relationships between health and wellness, their positive benefits, the strategies informing designs for the built environment, and the lifestyle changes that can result with these interactions. While this work focuses on placebound wellness, it does not diminish the importance of between-place wellness, an integral part of modern life. We are in need of strategies that occur on the larger scales and particularly with the movement of goods and people between urban places, from nations to nations, and from continents to continents.

The following chapters address wellness design from a broad and more wholistic point of view to propitiate the integration of positive wellness design and planning measures applied across multiple scales. Also important is the need for accessibility especially through everyday activities which is shown throughout the various scales. It is also important to show that many of the wellness strategies are not costly, but do need foresight. The book is intended to clarify definitions of wellness, explain their connections to the design professions, and elucidate the many benefits that accompany such strategies. The *two case studies* in the last two chapters clearly illustrate the wellness design strategies applicable at the planning and building scales. Focusing on the scale of Mado in Serenbe reveals the importance of wellness considerations with neighborhood planning on the individual and community. And the Fivelements Retreat Bali reveals the inspiring qualities of natural architecture and purposeful well-tourism, and the immersive impacts on individual wellness. Finally, the planning and design strategies are meant to provide guidelines or pathways for interventions in existing urban settings, buildings, interiors, and landscapes and to help guide future growth in new projects toward reimagining a wellness future.

Acknowledgments

Thanks go to Kathryn Schell, Senior Editor, and to Selena Hostetler, Editorial Assistant of Routledge part of the Taylor and Francis Group for their guidance and support throughout the completion of this work. They provided great encouragement, enthusiasm, and valuable feedback throughout the process. Thanks also to Dr. Mona Matthews who engaged in many conversations about wellness design and who edited the entire manuscript. Thanks go to the Global Wellness Institute for initiating the white paper on *Wellness Architecture and Design Pathways*. It was this research effort on wellness architecture and design that offered the impetus to do this book. It provided a refreshing approach to the conventional systems and methodologies and helping project teams to identify and select distinctive design pathways, as well as measure the impact on the wellness for humanity and the environment. Thanks also go to the interdisciplinary team including Valentina Cereda, Gove Depuy, Anthony DiGuiseppe, Sherry Fong, Stephen Marks, Kailas Moorthy, and Veronica Schreibeis Smith for their contributions to the GWI white paper.

For Phillip Tabb, thanks go to Noa Hecht who reviewed the questionnaire for Mado and provided a few of the images and one of the testimonials. Thanks also go to Jennifer Walsh whose enthusiasm about the experience of wellness and nature are unmatched, and for the support of Ronald Skaggs, FAIA who is one of the most influential architects for health worldwide. Special thanks to Gary Coates who wrote the Foreword and provided images of the Vidar Clinic. His insights were invaluable. Thanks also go to the Nygren family, Serenbe Community, and Mado residents for their gracious support of the concept of wellness and for inputs into this work. Thanks go to my family, especially to my sons Michael and David, and to Shea, Kristin Tabb, to my grandsons Emrys, Caius, James, and Jack Tabb, my sister Janice, and brother-in-law Richard Nourse.

For Lahra Tatriele, thanks go to all those who helped create Fivelements Retreat Bali, especially to Chicco Tatriele, my partner and husband in co-creation, Wayan Bawa, our Balinese friend and partner, who inspired local philosophy and tradition as part of this project, and Ketut Arthana for bringing our vision for Fivelements to life and guiding us through an extraordinary Balinese design journey. Thanks also go to our entire Fivelements team, partners, and guests who continue to trust the vision and believe in the power of Love in Action. And a special acknowledgment goes to my three children, Mya, Sasha, and Luca, my parents, Gordon and Beverley Finch, and my dear brother, Leighton, for their unyielding love and support.

NOTES

1. UNESCO, *Imminent Risk of Global Water Crisis, Warns the UN World Water Development Report 2023* (Accessed December 22, 2023), https://www.unesco.org/en/articles/imminent-risk-global-water-crisis-warns-un-world-water-development-report-2023
2. Travis, John, *Illness and Wellness Continuum, 1972* (Accessed June 12, 2023), https://www.houseofhealth.co.nz/wellness-continuum-blog-1-physical-health/
3. Valentin, Edward, Wellness and Its Importance for Our Daily Lives (Accessed November 6, 2023), https://saportareport.com/wellness-and-it-is-importance-for-our-daily-lives/thought-leadership/families-first/
4. Marks, Stephen, Kailas Moorthy, Veronica Schreibeis Smith, Valentina Cereda, Anthony Guiseppe, Sherry Fong, Gove Depuy, Lahra Tatriele, and Phillip Tabb, *Wellness Architecture and Design Pathways*, Global Wellness Institute, 2023.
5. DiGuiseppe, Anthony, and Sherry Fong, "*The Economics of Wellness Architecture and Design*," *Wellness Architecture and Design Pathways* (2024).
6. Global Wellness Institute, *Wellness Architecture & Design Initiative* (Accessed October 1, 2023), https://globalwellnessinstitute.org/initiatives/wellness-architecture-design-initiative/
7. Tabb, Phillip, *Biophilic Urbanism: Designing Resilient Communities for the Future* (New York, NY: Routledge, 2021).
8. Global Wellness Institute, *Wellness Lifestyle Real Estate & Communities* (Accessed October 3, 2023) https://globalwellnessinstitute.org/what-is-wellness/what-is-wellness-lifestyle-real-estate-communities/

1 WELLNESS DEFINITIONS AND OVERVIEW

INTRODUCTION

What does it mean to be well? When asked "How are you?" we most often say "I'm good" or "I'm well." This answer is often vague and in general means that life and especially wealth and health are in a reasonably good place. The response is intended to move beyond any detailed explanation of the myriad of dimensions to how we might really feel – how we physically, mentally or emotionally feel, how are social or spiritual lives are, or how we are doing financially. Yet these are the conditions that do define our experience of wellness. Why we should care is not only important to our individual health, but also our social well-being and the environment within which we all live. Each of these levels is interrelated and affect the quality of a more holistic wellness. So, perhaps it might be posited that wellness gives us a survival advantage; it always has. Meaning that addressing health and wellness-relevant issues of person and place can indeed give benefits or an advantage that in part advances our very survival. Having high levels of wellness can enable us to overcome difficulties, gives us flourishment, help us to self-actualize, be happy, live longer, and experience life satisfaction. This book is intended to address these dimensions as they inform wellness benefits and design strategies on individual, social, and planetary levels. This book does not focus on healthcare architecture or hospitals per se, but rather it presents preventative principles and premeditated design concepts aimed at a larger audience of city and building dwellers, visitors and users of all building types, and hopefully influencing wellness in the activity of everyday life.

HEALTH AND WELLNESS DEFINITIONS

Health and wellness have been terms used interchangeably. Health has been referred to as freedom from disease, pain or defect with normal physical and mental functions. Health is also considered as a state allowing for coping with all the demands of everyday life. And finally, health is a state of balance within the social and physical environments.[1] The term *haelan* derives from Old English meaning to make whole, sound, or well.[2] It is a baseline state of well-being. The World Health Organization defines health as "a state of complete physical, mental, and social well-being and not merely the absence of disease." Well-being, as defined by the Stanford Prevention Research Center (SPRC) is "a holistic synthesis of a person's

DOI: 10.4324/9781003472902-1

biological, psychological, and spiritual experiences, resulting from interplay between individuals and their social, economic, and physical environments that promotes living a fulfilling life." The SPRC's global longitudinal study, Stanford WELL for Life (WELL), uses new methods to understand, measure, and promote multiple dimensions of well-being across countries and cultures. The study's objective is to understand what it means to be well and how we can increase our well-being, shifting the lens of chronic disease prevention to focus on understanding and enhancing well-being. The built environment in which we live our daily lives can positively impact our well-being.[3]

The term *welnes* is derived from the Old English for *wel meaning* abundantly or in good fortune, and *nes* or a word-forming element denoting action. Taken together wellness suggested behaviors that result in happiness, self-actualization, and optimal health. Wellness was considered the opposite of illness. More recently the term by Kenneth Cooper was further advanced as the concept of wellness as a lifestyle.[4] This suggests that human interactions occur with both space and duration of time that frames a wellness experience. Wellness is a process. This includes processes like holistic living, self-healing, preventative care, and active wellness practices. What we eat, how we move, with whom we interact, and our interactions with nature are contributing factors to wellness. The National Wellness Institute defines wellness as an active process through which we become more aware of, and make choices toward, a more successful existence.[5] The buildings and communities within which we live can also contribute to this notion of wellness:

- Health – *refers to the* ***state*** *of complete physical, mental and emotional diseases, and not merely the absence of illness or infirmity. Health includes diagnosis and predisposition of disease and any unexpected injury.*
- Wellness – *refers to a more holistic* ***process*** *of balanced, enhanced, and preventative well-being and is more inclusive adding social, financial, environmental, and wellness to an active self-directed process and change of lifestyle.*

When people focus proactively on prevention and improving their vitality, they adopt attitudes and lifestyles that decrease disease, improve health, and enhance their quality of life, and sense of happiness and well-being. According to the Berkeley Well-being Institute, wellness is proactive, preventive, and driven by self-responsibility. The growth of wellness is the extension of this consumer value and worldview. The Global Wellness Institute defines wellness as "the active pursuit of activities, choices and lifestyles that lead to a state of holistic health" It is an active process of being aware and making choices that lead toward optimal health and well-being outcomes.[6] Closely associated with holistic health, wellness is integrative and multi-dimensional and includes physical, mental, emotional, social, financial, environmental, and spiritual dimensions. Although considered an individual proactive pursuit, wellness is significantly influenced by the physical, social, and cultural environments in which we live, including our built environments. Prioritizing wellness as a central concept in planning and design processes can play a significant role in ensuring built environments not only sustain people living in cities, villages and rural regions but also regenerate and revitalize these built areas, leaving the people and the environment around them better off than before and on a trajectory toward recovery, revival, and increased vitality.[7]

The differences in health and wellness can easily be seen in the architecture that reflects them. Healthcare buildings have long been created to attend to people who are ill, are suffering from disease, or recovering from accidents. Early history sees the caring for the sick in their homes and later in churches. Florence Nightingale was influential following the Crimean War of 1854 recognizing the need for clean hospital wards. This included providing patients with access to natural light, air, landscape, attention to diet, as well as a clean, sanitary environment. An outgrowth was the pavilion configuration, which later shifted to a platform typology, and finally to the layering designs of the larger hospitals of today. In the 1980s, evidence-based research and design, although not a new concept, began to influence the hospital environment.[8] Building types that are associated with health-oriented facilities include hospitals, clinics and medical offices, surgery centers, birthing centers, blood banks, hospices, assisted living, nursing homes, urgent care facilities, and rehabilitation centers.

Wellness architecture, as distinct from healthcare architecture, is relatively new. It focuses on broader, more preventative and nudge-oriented or suggestive planning and design approaches that encourage wellness behaviors and lifestyles. It permeates all building types and planning scales, and attempts to influence healthy lifestyles toward an inclusive integration of all the wellness benefit categories. In a broader sense it also includes responses to natural disasters, resiliency, renewable resources and stewardship of the broader environment generally, and nature's benefits are focused on access for everyone and integration with everyday life activities.

WELLNESS HISTORY

Health has long been a concern for our survival and positive experience of life. Original sources of wellness ideas can be found in deep history, thousands, even millions of years ago. Early primates and humans survived and maintained relative wellness through their abilities to control the terrestrial elements, their food supplies and dietary habits, their strong social connections, and adaptability. From a health perspective, the hunter-gatherer lifestyle of Pleistocene groups is generally considered particularly advantageous.[9] Spanning a wide period of time and based on artifacts and human remains, therapeutic herbs and natural substances were likely used in prehistoric medicine. There also is supernatural evidence found in burial sites and cave paintings. Disease was "*dis-ease*" or lack of ease, and being out of balance and discordant, sometimes attributed to mythological and malevolent spirit sources. And finally, a powerful wellness survival strategy was migration due to dramatic climatic changes and scarcity of food and other resources.

"The concept of wellness is not modern at all, but ancient, deriving from the most basic human drive: to live longer, healthier and better."[10] Indian Ayurveda and Traditional Chinese Medicine some 5000 years ago, sought to bring harmony and balance into daily life. They used physical methods such as Acupuncture, Tai Chi, Qigong, Baduanjin, or Yijinjing, and administered herbal medicines. Ancient Egyptians, also 5000 years ago, practiced bone setting, dentistry, simple surgery, and the use of natural medicines.[11] Ancient Greek medicine 2500 years ago and Ancient Roman medicine, around 2000 years ago, focused on preventing sickness as well as treating disease. Hippocrates is credited as being possibly the first physician. Roman strategies for wellness are most known for the building of vast networks of aqueducts, sewers, and public baths contributing to public health. These traditional systems focused on both curative and preventive methods of disease. They further emphasized one's lifestyle – nutrition, physical activity, quality sleep, moderation, ethical behavior, development of positive thoughts and emotions – and perceived healthcare as holistic with an aim of achieving balance and harmony of body, mind, and spirit.[12]xii These wellness considerations remain important today. Early Christian concepts of health derived as gifts of God focusing on stewardship to self and service to others in "*health, sickness and suffering*."[13] This also included lifestyles choices emphasizing moderation and kindness.

In the Middle Ages most people lived in rural servitude and were subject to contagious diseases, such as the Black Death and leprosy, childbirth deaths, and generally low life expectancy. Early medical practices included herbal remedies, antiseptics, medicinal oils, and midwives. Monastic environments were often centers of health and wellness, and it is from their practices that the term "*hospital*" derived. It was in the Renaissance that modern medicine began, but it was at the turn of the 18th century that marked the modern medical revolution.[14] The earliest evidence for the Western use of the term *wellness* is from 1654, in a diary entry by Sir Archibald Johnston, lawyer and politician. Its meaning is the opposite of "illness" or the "state of being well or in good health." By the 19th century, new intellectual movements, spiritual philosophies, and holistic medical systems had proliferated in the United States and Europe. Alternative healthcare systems emerged, such as naturopathy, homeopathy, osteopathy, and chiropractic, focusing on holistic mind-body-spirit healing and illness prevention. These systems marked the origin of our modern, thriving wellness industry.

The 19th century marked a great advance in public health with advances in scientific knowledge about the sources and means of controlling disease as well as public responsibility for responding to it. Known as the "*great sanitary awakening*," filth was seen as the cause and vehicle of disease transmission.[15] By the mid-20th century, however, evidence-based medicine, and a focus on the treatment of illness gained favor over much of the preventative approaches, resulting in the omission of alternative systems from mainstream medical education. In the 1950s, Halbert L. Dunn's work on *High-Level Wellness*, published in 1961, introduced the idea of "wellness" and the impact of our environment on personal wellness.[16] Dunn's work later inspired American professionals in the 1970s who together are considered the "fathers of the wellness movement," including Dr. John Travis, Don Ardell, and Dr. Bill Hettler, among others. They created their comprehensive models of wellness, developing the first university campus wellness center, and establishing the National Wellness Institute and National Wellness conference in the United States. They defined wellness as more dynamic, going beyond health to reaching a happy, balanced, quality of fulfilled life. Soon after, the WHO released its definition of wellness with a shift toward prevention and health promotion, this marked the official start of the wellness movement.[17]

In 1962, Rachel Carson's "*Silent Spring*" was an awakening of the environmental movement and a critical look at pollution sparking greater concerns about public health. In 1970, Earth Day started as one of the largest grassroots movements in environmental awareness and the Clean Air Act set national air quality and automobile emissions standards both of which closely parallel wellness. Pesticides were banned and the Clean Water Act was passed in 1972. In 1973, the scarcity of OPEC oil and the dependence on fossil fuels spawned the alternative technology industry and leaded gasoline was phased out. Beginning in 1982, toxic building materials were addressed, and many were banned. Many new programs and legislations were set into motion resulting in environmental action. The EPA radon protection program began in 1988. Awareness of climate change occurred as early as the late 1800s by Swedish scientist Svante Arrhenis. Global warming as a function of human behavior began to become a public concern 100 years later, and was a politicized issue in the 1990s.

Over the two decades from 1980–2000, there were more government-sponsored programs in the U.S. focused on health and healthy lifestyles. Through the '90's many of the world's most elite medical institutions, including Harvard, Stanford, Yale, Johns Hopkins, and the Mayo Clinic, began to feature Integrative Medicine departments, including with a focus on evidence-based wellness. The wellness movement soon spread to European nations, and by the end of the 20th century, there was the birth of workplace wellness programs. In the late 1980s companies began to focus on psychological well-being as part of their workplace wellness initiatives, and in 1986, the Occupational Safety and Health Administration began to encourage the implementation of stress-related mental health programs in the workplace. This also was a time of self-discovery, of fitness, spas and self-care, and self-help experts who brought wellness into the mainstream. Another contributing factor to the focus on wellness was the consistent global rise in chronic diseases and obesity which continues to lead to unsustainable healthcare costs. More governments have begun shifting their focus on prevention and wellness to combat the skyrocketing costs of healthcare. By the 21st century, the concepts of wellness, healthy living, and nutrition hit a dramatic tipping point as we began to see them permeate and transform every industry from food and beverages to travel and tourism, and more recently, architecture, design, and real estate development.

In 1973, the evolution of the concept of biophilia began in modern times with Erich Fromm in 1973. Edward O. Wilson in 1980 published his book on biophilia that revealed the health and wellness relationship between humans and nature.[18] Later, in 2008, Stephen Kellert edited a volume on biophilia that further investigated the wellness outcomes of biophilic design and presented 72 attributes to that design.[19] In the early 2000s, Dan Buettner traveled worldwide investigating what he called "blue zones," where the demographics revealed extreme longevity. He discovered that certain lifestyle choices contributed to this phenomenon.[20] Richard Louv's "Last Child in the Woods," underlined the importance of the relationship between children and the outdoors in order to overcome what he called "*nature-deficit disorder*."[21]

In the early 2000s came the rise of eating disorders, the rise of influenza virus, salmonella, SARS and *E. coli* outbreaks, and an increase of morbid obesity. According to Emily Pau, eating disorders, like anorexia, rose 3.5% from 2000–2006 mostly in women and young girls as many desperately strived to copy the ultra-thin figures promoted in the fashion industry and on social media.[22] During this time, solid meals were replaced with liquid alternatives, and portions of servings at restaurants were smaller. In America, the lack of health care insurance and access to prescription drugs for millions were problematic. Yet for the wellness movement, the "*Healthy People 2000*" was a national strategy with its focus on physical activity, fitness programs, improved nutrition, physical education in schools, and personal self-care that began to turn the tide toward wellness. In the decades that followed, a parade of dietary trends emerged, such as the Atkins Diet, Raw Foods Diet, NutriSystem, Keto Diet, and the Juicing Diet. The decades also saw increases in the awareness of food quality as defined as organic, vegetarian, vegan, gluten-free, and non-GMO. In addition to nutrition, closer attention was paid to exercise and fitness.[23]

The early 2000s was also a time of growing awareness of climate change as a result of human activity, growing environmental degradation, and forest loss. According to the Global Forest Watch, 8% of the world's intact forest landscape has been lost since 2000 due to fragmentation, logging, and development.[24] Water and air pollution are also of concern with household air and water pollution on the decline, and outdoor pollution has risen. In addition, according to the United Nations, the number of natural disasters worldwide since 2000 has reached 7,348 taking 1.23 million lives. It is clear that recent history has shown the critical need for wellness strategies for climate mitigation and natural disasters.

In 2023, the GWI released an updated Global Wellness Economy Monitor. According to the GWI report the wellness market was worth $4.9 trillion in 2019 and then shrank during the COVID-19 pandemic. Since 2000 it has grown to $5.9 trillion as a result of the medical world, with governments and consumers placing greater value on prevention and wellness. The report stated that wellness expenditures in 2020 have grown and are now extending to the wellness real estate market ($398 billion), mental wellness ($180.5 billion), public health ($611 billion), prevention and personalized medicine, healthy eating, nutrition and weight loss ($1 trillion), physical activity sector ($976 billion), traditional complementary medicine ($519 billion), personal care and beauty ($1.1 trillion), wellness tourism ($651 billion), spas ($104 billion), thermal and hot springs ($43.3 billion), and workplace wellness ($51 billion).[25]

In 2018, the Global Wellness Institute released *Build Well to Live Well*, the first in-depth research to analyze the $134 billion global wellness real estate and communities sector (previously Wellness Lifestyle Real Estate) exploring how community environments can positively impact personal wellness. The report found that real estate and communities that intentionally put people's health at the center of design, creation and redevelopment are the next frontiers in real estate. The Wellness Architecture & Design Initiative of the Global Wellness Institute hones even further on the built environment, further researching and understanding pathways for the implementation of an interdisciplinary wellness design approach, which delivers health, sustainability, economic, and spiritual outcomes for existing and future designs and environments. Wellness trends in the early 2020s include strategies to overcome loneliness, expansion of wellness tourism worldwide, a focus on workplace wellness, advancing the biotech beauty market, addressing weight and obesity, clean blue spaces, wellness and spiritual implications, neuroscience and

ANCIENT	5000 BC	ANCIENT EGYPTIAN MEDICINE
		ANCIENT CHINESE MEDICINE
		ANCIENT AYURVEDA MEDICAL SYSTEM
	250 BC	ANCIENT GREEK MEDICINE
	50 BC	ANCIENT ROMAN WELLNESS
	100 AD	EARLY CHRISTIAN SPIRITUAL HEALING
	500-1450	MIDDLE AGE MONASTERIES AS HEALING CENTERS
	1654	ARCHIBALD JOHNSON "*WELLNESS*" TERM
	1796	SAMUEL HAHNEMANN HOMEOPATHIC MEDICINE
	1850	THE GREAT SANITARY AWAKENING
	1851	FLORENCE NIGHTINGALE HEALING WARDS
MODERN	1946	CENTERS FOR DISEASE CONTROL & PREVENTION
	1948	WORLD HEALTH ORGANIZATION
	1961	HALBERT DUNN HIGH-LEVEL WELLNESS
	1962	RACHEL CARSON "*SILENT SPRING*"
	1970	CLEAN AIR ACT
	1972	CLEAN WATER ACT
	1972	JOHN TRAVIS WELLNESS CONTINUUM
	1973	AWARENESS OF DEPENDENCE ON FOSSIL FUELS
	1980	EDWARD O. WILSON BIOPHILIC WELLNESS
	1990	KENNETH COOPER WELLNESS LIFESTYLES
	1990	MARGARET SWARBRICK WELLNESS PILLARS
	1991	KAY ROBERTS SERENITY SCALE RESEARCH
	2005	DASHER KELTNER AWE EMOTION RESEARCH
	2006	AL GORE "*AN INCONVENIENT TRUTH*"
	2008	STEPHEN KELLERT BIOPHILIC ATTRIBUTES
	2010	DAN BUETTNER "*BLUE ZONES*"
	2014	GLOBAL WELLNESS INSTITUTE
	2015	MADO FIRST INTEGRATED WELLNESS HAMLET
	2021	WELLNESS COMMUNITIES & REAL ESTATE

WELLNESS TIMELINE
Events Leading to the Development of a Wellness Movement

1.1
Wellness History Timeline
(*Source: Phillip Tabb*)

multisensory integration, models of wellness hospitality, and expanding wellness influences on the cities, infrastructure, and capital improvements.

Planned in 2007 and currently largely complete, the Mado Hamlet, featured in Chapter 7, is located in Serenbe Community outside of Atlanta, Georgia and is one of the first purpose-built residential developments or intentional neighborhoods designed around wellness. When complete Mado will house 575 dwellings with a host of wellness businesses, functions and services. Woven throughout the neighborhood are a fitness center, swimming pool, yoga studios, farm-to-table restaurant, dentist, veterinary clinic, aging in place campus, k-12 school, many health and wellness live-work units, and access to hundreds of acres of forested open space. Wellness retreats, like Fivelements Retreat Bali featured in Chapter 8, and the wellness tourist destination industries are ever-increasing in demand.

Modern conceptions of wellness began in the 20th century and are seen as a holistic and multi-dimensional model of health. While modern medicine and scientific discoveries moved the medical professions ahead, holistic medicine was still common. It was not until J.I. Rodale launched his *Prevention* magazine in the 1950s, when Halbert Dunn put forward his concept of high-level wellness in the early 1960s, and John Travis in the 1970s focused on wellness practice and his development of an illness-wellness continuum, that the wellness movement began to advance particularly in the United States. Now wellness has migrated into planning schemes, infrastructure designs, tourism, destination retreats, building designs, building systems, material selections, furnishings, and real estate to name but a few.

Human activity impacts the land on Earth causing irreversible changes in climate, biospheric integrity, biodiversity, and ecological systems' flows. In response planetary health is an outgrowth of preventative health initiated in the 1970s and 1980s and promotes vitality and sustainability of the Earth's natural systems. To Susan Prescott, et al., planetary health is important and fundamental to maintaining trans-generational vitality at scales of person, place, and planet. Prescott goes on to explain that sustaining vital natural systems, narrative health processes, planetary consciousness, nature-relatedness, and the development of new normative behaviors are now necessary.[26]

WELLNESS CONTINUUM

A wellness continuum describes the increasing and decreasing effects of wellness benefits as developed by John Tavis in 1972.[27] It plots various stages from utter poor health or near death to high-level wellness. Between these extremes is a neutral space of neither illness nor wellness. To Donald Ardell, the continuum spans from *worseness* to *wellness*, which is affected by health hazards, nutritional health, and physical fitness.[28] As can be seen in Figure 1.2, high-level wellness is influenced by purpose in life, life satisfaction and spiritual growth, and wellness lifestyles, while near death and chronic illness are a function of inactivity, poor lifestyles, smoking, high alcohol use, loss of vitality, and social isolation. This continuum is also related to what is referred to as a treatment paradigm (treatment pathology and disease prevention) occurring on the illness side of the diagram and usually involving surgery, therapy, and drugs; while the positive side of the diagram supports a wellness paradigm usually involving healthy lifestyle choices with good nutrition, physical activity, emotional balance, positive social interactions, zest for life, and purposeful spiritual growth.

The wellness continuum reinforces the idea that wellness is not static or one-dimensional, but rather an ongoing process or dynamic progression that can vacillate between illness events and degrees of wellness. The treatment paradigm, reliant upon drugs, herbs, surgery, physical therapy, psychotherapy, acupuncture, blood transfusions, radiation, and palliative care to name a few, can move one to the neutral space. The wellness paradigm moves from the illness and neutral space to greater balance, integration, nutrition, physical activity, and healthier social, financial and spiritual well-being. While the continuum model is a useful visual tool in emplacing the wellness concept, it should be noted that it is a simplification of complex and often contradictory dimensions of health.[29] It is a simple visual tool that allows one to place their wellness on a risk-to-prevention scale.

- Near Death – *an experience of coming close to dying in medical or non-medical setting.*
- Chronic Illness – *conditions requiring ongoing medical attention or limiting activities.*

1.2 Wellness Continuum

(*Source: Phillip Tabb*)

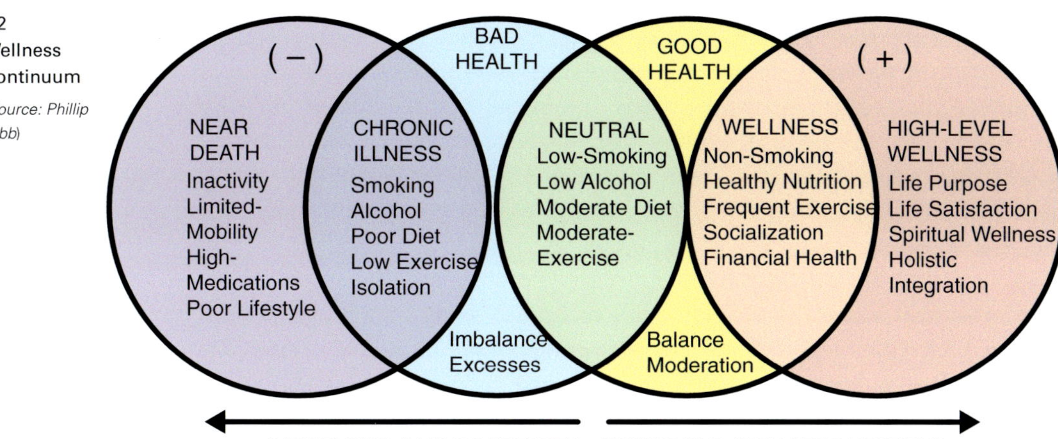

- Neutral Health – *state of medical noninterference and moderate levels of thriving.*
- Wellness – *daily practices attaining holistic and successful health outcomes.*
- High-Level Wellness – *the process of holistic functioning achieving fuller potential.*

WELLNESS BENEFIT PILLARS

A wellness benefit is seen as a tangible health advantage and process promoting health and fitness, and in spiritual terms it suggests *doing* well or *doing good*. Wellness pillars are a broad category of wellness benefits, and are explained in detail in Chapter 2. Physical wellness involves the physical body, its maintenance, exercise, hygiene, quality of sleep, as well as preventing illness or injury. In some instances, it also includes nutritional health and a balanced diet. Cognitive wellness relates to mental processes, clarity, focus, and memory. Emotional wellness covers positive feelings and the ability to understand, communicate and transcend difficult emotions. Social wellness involves the connections and relationships with others whether it is family or community and beyond. Financial wellness is the pillar devoted to living within your means and planning for your future appropriately. Environmental wellness is a function of immediate outdoor spaces, community, and surrounding environment. It involves both our impact on the environment and the environments impact on us. Spiritual wellness relates to living values, a sense of purpose, and meaning in life. Taken together these pillars constitute what may be considered holistic and even high-level wellness. It is further important to understand that the multiple pillars are interrelated and can influence and impact one another.

Created in the early 1990s by Dr. Margaret Swarbrick were what she called "*dimensions of wellness*." Swarbrick's version was used in cases of mental health challenges and included eight dimensions. The model included intellectual rather than mental, and occupational wellness benefits were often excluded from more widely published classifications. The model focused on key daily habits and routines especially within the occupational environment, and encouraged new wellness-oriented behaviors.[30] Financial wellness in contrast focused on the satisfaction with current and future financial situations. Sometimes vocational wellness was considered a pillar that focused on developing life enrichment and contributions to work.

The Global Wellness Institute saw the wellness benefits as multidimensional and included six dimensions. In the GWI white paper on Wellness Architecture and Design Pathways, seven pillars were discussed. GWI sees the wellness benefits as an active pursuit toward an optimum state of health and wellness. Extrapolated from the many publications on the pillars of wellness are the following seven core wellness pillars considered good models of self- and environmental-stewardship discussed in this book:

- Physical wellness – *nutrition, restful sleep, movement and exercise.*
- Mental wellness – *creativity, positive thinking, mental acuity and focused attention.*
- Emotional wellness – *well feelings, supportive sharing, and coping effectiveness.*
- Social wellness – *interactions, relationships, connectedness and sense of community.*
- Financial wellness – *economic benefits, increased value, efficiency and productivity.*
- Environmental wellness – *positive interactions with nature with negatable pollution.*
- Spiritual wellness – *holistic connections, transcendence, and life purpose.*

HIGH-LEVEL WELLNESS

High-level wellness was a concept developed by Halbert Dunn and first published in 1961 that promoted interrelatedness, high level functioning, balance, purposeful direction, and maximizing one's potential. And in 1976, in his book, Donald Ardell advanced high-level wellness as an alternative to doctors, drugs, and disease, and as being highly effective with self-responsibility applied to the varying degrees of high-level wellness.[31] High-level wellness occupies a prominent and desirable position on the wellness continuum where degrees or levels of wellness spanning from chronic illness to normal health to high-level wellness exist. What is important to understand is that wellness is not a static state, but rather a dynamic process that vacillates within all of us, and high-level wellness is achievable through the conscious actions and lifestyle choices we promote in our everyday lives.

Characteristics of high-level wellness include flourishing, attaining purpose and meaning in life, life satisfaction, mastery, optimism, and positive affect. *Human flourishing* is a state of optimal functioning and well-being across our individual lives.[32] According to Haugan and Dezutter, *purpose and meaning* are mediating variables in psychological health, and they contribute to vitality and motivational forces for survival.[33] *Life satisfaction* is associated with lower mortality and risk of hospitalization, and an influence on wellness behaviors.[34] *Mastery* is associated with better physical and mental quality of life.[35] *Positive effects*, including experience of happiness, longer lives, and positive responses to chronic diseases, occur across a wide range of health outcomes.[36] According to Donald Ardell, high-level wellness requires giving care to the physical self, being mentally constructive, channeling stress energy positively, expressing emotions effectively, being creative with others, and connecting to the environment.[37] To Ardell, there are five dimensions to high-level wellness: self-responsibility, nutritional awareness, stress management, physical fitness, and environmental sensitivity.

High-level wellness is broad in its application extending from organizations, buildings and communities, to nations, eco-regions, and humankind as a whole. Here the discussion of high-level wellness must include the health of the Earth's biosphere and natural systems. This includes the wellness-determinants directed toward infectious diseases, harmful lifestyle behaviors, human population growth and migration patterns, and irresponsible use of natural resources. Unfortunately, this includes the prevailing of wars, terrorism, natural disasters, and harmful crimes. Increased population and urban clustering are cause for rising housing costs and the more quickly spread of diseases.[38] Planetary health was defined by the Rockefeller-Lancet Commission of Planetary Health as "*the health of human civilization and the state of the natural systems on which it depends*."[39]

High-level wellness also includes spiritual dimensions and outcomes with concepts of whole health, including physical fitness, good nutrition, flourishing, longevity, positive family and social interactions, and relations to nature. This also is enabled by wellness planning and design measures occurring at all scales of the built environment. High-level wellness involves giving good care to your physical self, using your mind constructively, expressing your emotions effectively, being creatively involved with those around you, and being concerned about your physical, psychological, and spiritual environments. High-level wellness seeks an ever-increasing quality of life integrated with planetary wellness.[40] The term planetary health denotes the interconnections between personal health and place or settings at all scales. Important is the ability to translate high-level wellness determinants to the planning and design fields in order to facilitate supportive environments and settings promoting high-level wellness. Key attributes of high-level wellness are:

- High functioning – *often categorized as anxiety, depression or autism, but in the context of wellness it is the positive process of adaptable health-oriented choices with positive physical, emotional, psychological, and social functioning.*
- Maximizing potential – *an evolving process of actualizing one's goals, direction, calling and capabilities of the whole person occurring day to day. Attracting positive social connections, accumulating the appropriate tools, and living in supportive environment(s).*
- Balance and integration – *the maintenance of completeness and according to Halbert Dunn, the integration of body, mind, spirit, and environment.*[41]

- Positive lifestyle choices – *with healthy nutrition, daily physical activity, frequent experience of nature, financial health, and positive social interactions.*
- Purposefulness – *not only is important to problem solving, but the attainment of higher-level completeness and transformations. Perseverance, vision, resilience, and lived experiences are important to purpose.*

WELLNESS SCALES OF APPLICATION

In order to achieve the greatest impact on wellness design strategies and benefits, there should be broad applications. This is to ensure providing wellness opportunities to all walks of life and pervading lifestyles. Wellness benefits and strategies span a variety of scales from rooms to buildings, and from neighborhoods to cities. It is important to understand that each scale provides certain sets of individual, social, or environmental benefits. Most are either concurrent, complementary, or unique to the scale. For example, access to nature can take the form of an indoor plant, a walled-in garden, a view to the ocean, a walk in the woods, or a vacation to a national park. Even flying across the country in an airplane or viewing the vast night sky can be awe-inspiring. The benefits can occur on pro-individual, pro-social, and pro-environmental levels. It is the purpose here to provide through these scales of application a broad and encompassing set of wellness design strategies.

- Planning and urban design scale – *issues include air and water pollution, inadequate access to green and blue spaces, reduction of arable agricultural land, dependence on the automobile and lack of public transportation, abundance of derelict land, response to city-scale natural disasters, and inadequate and non-renewable infrastructure capacity.*
- Architecture scale – *issues include increased visual and physical indoor-outdoor relationships, increased responses to light and spatial quality, reduced use of toxic building materials, improved design for energy conservation and other renewable resources, improved responses to climate and weather conditions, and natural disasters.*
- Interior scale – *issues include improved interior spatial quality, natural lighting and ventilation, use of non-renewable and toxic material selections, reduced noise pollution, improved thermal comfort, and improved access to nature.*
- Landscape scale – *issues include accessibility and increased open, green and blue spaces, and increased use of climate-resistant species, improvement of stormwater management, reduction of water-intensive landscaping, excessive hardscapes, and mono-culture agriculture.*

While there are varying scales of wellness design, it is important to understand and implement a combinatory and integrated approach where each scaler level is not considered in isolation, but rather as an integrated part of the other scales. And that each pillar of wellness benefits is considered across the scales. For example, how can the wellness benefit of physical fitness be encouraged at the planning scale, within a site and building interior, and with landscape features at each scale?

How can they be combined to give synergy to one another, such as physical fitness, organic farming, and community meals? Mado Hamlet discussed in Chapter 7 is a good example of the integrated effects of the wellness strategies across scales in one place.

WELLNESS DESIGN CHALLENGES

There are increasing signs that both human and planetary health are at risk. Physical inactivity, obesity, poor nutrition, substance abuse, mental health, heart disease, cancer, diabetes, injury and violence, airborne infectious diseases, and lack of access to health care are among the most common human health issues. It is alarming that according to the World Health Organization recently released data that 81% of kids between the ages of 11 and 17 are now inactive.[42] Climate change, natural disasters, air pollution, poor water quality, chemical safety, wildfires, habitat destruction, loss of biodiversity, microbes, and destruction due to war are among the most common environmental health issues. It is clear we need to reimagine the survival advantages for us as well as the planet as a whole. Our very survival may be dependent upon a more well-oriented paradigm.

Our behavior is influenced by the environment within which we live. It is important to understand there is a reciprocal relationship between the two. Therefore, the rooms, buildings communities, and ecological regions within which we live influence our well-being. The challenge is to create designs at these varying scales to help elicit or facilitate the wellness benefits. For the purpose of the work in this book, the scales are limited to urban design, architecture, interior design, and landscape design. It, therefore, is the intent of wellness designs to reduce the negative factors and risks of harm to person and environment, to enhance and increase the opportunities for all the positive benefits, and to support accessible and enduring solutions for all as well as vulnerable populations. It is not only a human-centered design approach, but also an environment-sensitive one as well. This includes plans, physical products, services, procedures, strategies, and policies. In order for wellness design strategies to be most effective, they must simultaneously occur at multiple scales of application, and need to be accessible, inclusive, experienced as often as possible, and made economically feasible.

Another challenge is the implantation of larger-scale wellness and planetary health toward sustainable and biospheric designs. And addressing the questions of existing built urban, suburban, and peri-urban environments, such as, "How can they be transformed into high-level wellness?" According to the United Nations, the urban design scale has the potential to be at the forefront of improving community heath in the coming years. However, most modern city designs, especially in the United States, are based on gridded spatial structure, increasing density, accommodation of the automobile (circulation and parking), and little focus on mass-transportation. The challenges for urban areas are many and include implementing revitalized infrastructure, reducing congestion, increasing public transport systems, and creating more natural open spaces. Suburban designs, on the other hand, are lower in density, employ single-use development and functional zoning, and promote automobile dependency. The challenge is restructuring the monolithic spatial character into an accessible mix of critical land uses, in which many support wellness. For example, these include greater access to parks and recreation, suburban agriculture, schools, commercial shopping, workplaces, and healthcare.

What are the large impactful moves that can really have a profound influence and effect on wellness? In other words, where are the wellness planning and design strategies most likely to be effective? Will they be existing, new, urban, suburban, rural, small or large scale, or developed or undeveloped countries? In existing places, wellness design considerations will initially be directed toward "*interesting interventions*" or "*fixing mistakes*," such as the dominance of the automobile, polluted waterways, disaster-prone areas, inefficient infrastructure, improved mass transit systems, overhauled zoning practices, and piecemeal insertions of wellness buildings. In older cities, the wellness interventions will need to be respectful of the existing fabric, inventory of buildings, and community features. They most likely will be additive and piecemeal.

Another major challenge is to create affordable and accessible designs knowing that many wellness strategies can be costly. According to Jamie Gold, in a building environment where wellness design includes amenities like yoga rooms, air and water purification, state-of-the-art fitness centers and circadian lighting, health and fitness are being built into the housing for those who can afford it. However, other wellness design strategies that are far less costly like well-placed windows with a view to nature, meeting of indoor air quality standards, well-lit community gardens, playgrounds and recreation spaces, the inclusion of more and appealing walking paths, sheltered bike racks, and smoke-free environments.[43]

In new developments, more comprehensive, holistic, and integrated measures can be implemented, such as those illustrated in the strategies section on the urban design scale. According to a 2017 Housing and Urban Development Survey and US Census Data, 21% of households are described as rural, 52% as suburban, and 27% as urban.[44] This suggests more careful and targeted interventions in the larger scaled environments, and more integrated and comprehensive approaches in the lower densities and smaller scales. The challenges are complex, terrain-dependent and require commitment, and design for well-being potentially comes with changes in the physical environment and lifestyle adjustments or changes. In order to overcome this "*wellness-deficit disorder*," the prevailing real estate, land planning, architectural, interior design and landscape practices are in need of revision. To gain a survival advantage, the wellness strategies need to be robust and inclusive. Challenges at scale are listed below:

- Large-scale wellness strategies – *occurring at the eco-regional, city and urban scales where issues of climate, natural disasters, land use, density, mixes of use, transportation, urban greenery, streetscapes, and infrastructure are addressed.*
- Medium-scale wellness strategies – *occurring with the campus, single and multiple buildings, passive survivability, local streets, neighborhoods, schools and universities, and urban landscapes.*

- Small-scale wellness strategies – *occurring with healing gardens, courtyards, interior spaces, furnishings and finishes, and material selections.*
- Easily accessible strategies – *porous and encouraging designs occurring in proximity to nature and social spaces close to where people live, work, go to school, and recreate. The ideal is to have pedestrian access with other modes of transport.*
- Daily wellness strategies – *occurring with frequency as a part of daily routines and integrated with wellness lifestyles.*
- Live-work relationships – *achieving work-life balance and with easier access to work. Commuting is incredibly stressful not to mention sustainably inefficient.*
- Financial wellness strategies – *producing both short- and long-term economic incentives and benefits that help drive and enable the right-retail, the wellness industry and wellness real estate development. Providing affordable strategies.*
- Planetary wellness strategies – *suggesting some lifestyle changes, lower and more renewable and efficient energy and resource consumption, nucleated human-centered sustainable development, greenhouse gas sequestering, population redistribution away from vulnerable locations, and revitalizing natural areas (air, land, water, and ecology).*[45]

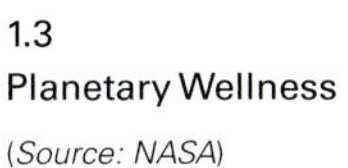

1.3
Planetary Wellness
(Source: NASA)

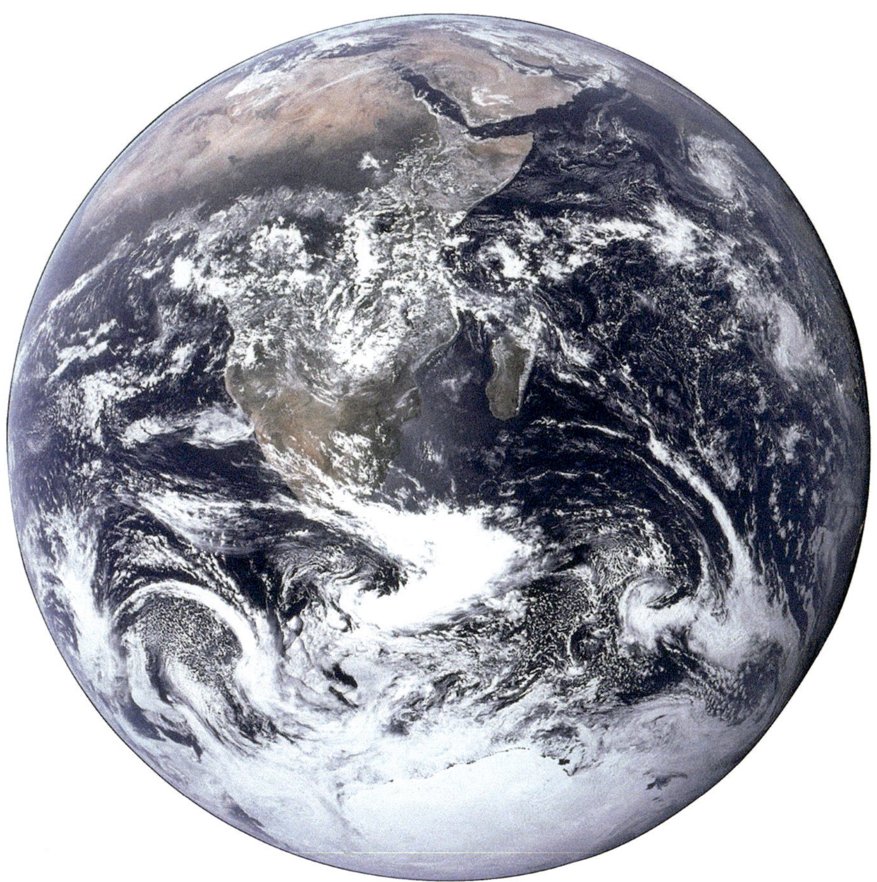

SUMMARY

Wellness as a concept is relatively new, and its applications to the design fields are rare, especially at the urban design and planning scales. However, the history of the wellness movement over the past 50 years is an indication of how important the issue is and the breadth of concerns. The purpose of this book has been to give contemporary definitions to the concept of wellness design, define the dimensions of its reach, and to propitiate physical design strategies that can help elicit the positive benefits. Understanding the range of benefits is important in informing and guiding the wellness strategies in planning and design. It should be noted that wellness benefits and strategies are not curative medical treatments, but rather promote holistic environment and lifestyle choices reinforced through planning and design practices.

According to the National Institute of Health, "approximately 60 percent of premature deaths could be attributed to unhealthy lifestyle factors, including smoking, excessive alcohol consumption, physical inactivity, poor diet, and obesity."[46] This results in the leading causes of death, including heart disease, cancer, stroke, diabetes and dementia. According to the World Health Organization, 23% of all premature deaths can be attributed to environmental factors, including unsafe air, water, sanitation, and hygiene.[47] This underlies the importance of planning and design measures for supporting an integrated model for preventable and positive lifestyle choices and environmental designs. These choices are defined by the seven pillars of wellness.

The following chapters address wellness design from a more holistic point of view with the integration of positive wellness design and planning measures applied across multiple scales and accessible through everyday activities. They are intended to clarify definitions of wellness and elucidate the many benefits. Further, the planning and design strategies are meant to provide guidelines or pathways for interventions in existing urban settings and buildings and to help guide future growth in new projects toward wellness actions in reimagining the future. The work concludes with two detailed case studies at the urban design and architectural scales intended to illustrate the multifaceted methods for achieving wellness design. These case studies are important in that they illustrate in-depth, fully integrated approaches of the wellness strategies on scales from planning to interior design producing a host of wellness benefits.

NOTES

1. Sartorius, Norman, *The Meaning of Health and its Promotion*, (Accessed November 20, 2023), https://www.ncbi.nlm.nih.gov/pmc/articles/PMC2080455/
2. Guidotti, Tee L., *The Literal Meaning of Health* (Accessed July 10, 2012) https://www.tandfonline.com/doi/abs/10.1080/19338244.2011.585096?journalCode=vaeh20#:~:text=The%20English%20word%20"health"%20derives,%2DIndo%2DEuropean%20root%20"*
3. Standford WELL for Life, (Accessed July 21, 2023), https://med.stanford.edu/wellforlife.html.

4. Cooper, Kenneth H., *Overcoming Hypertension: Dr. Kenneth H. Cooper's Preventative Medicine* (New York City, NY: Bantam Books, 1990).
5. National Wellness Institute, National Wellness Institute, *About Wellness*, (Accessed July 10, 2013) http://www.nationalwellness.org/?page=AboutWellness.
6. *Definition of Wellness: Meaning, Dimensions, and Examples*, Berkeley Well-Being Institute, (Accessed July 21, 2023) https://www.berkeleywellbeing.com/wellness-definition.html
7. Global Wellness Institute, *What is Wellness?* (Accessed June 1, 2013) https://globalwellnessinstitute.org/what-is-wellness/
8. Burpee, Heather, *History of Healthcare Architecture*, (Accessed August 15, 2023), http://www.mahlum.com/pdf/HistoryofHealthcareArchBurpee.pdf
9. Alt, Kurt, Ali Al-Ahmad, & Johan Woelber, *Nutrition and Health in Human Evolution-Past to Present*, (Accessed November 20, 2023), https://www.ncbi.nlm.nih.gov/pmc/articles/PMC9460423/
10. Murphy, Douglas, *The History of Wellness*, (Accessed December 5, 2023), https://pacificpsychiatry.com/blog/the-history-of-wellness/
11. National Library of Medicine, *Traditional Ancient Egyptian Medicine: A Review*, (Accessed December 5, 2023), https://www.ncbi.nlm.nih.gov/pmc/articles/PMC8459052/
12. Cohen, Strohecker, A Brief History of Wellness. Wellness Inventory Certification Training, (Accessed July 20, 2023) https://globalwellnessinstitute.org/what-is-wellness/history-of-wellness/
13. Murphy, Douglas, *The History of Wellness*, (Accessed December 5, 2023), https://pacificpsychiatry.com/blog/the-history-of-wellness/
14. Modern Medicine, *The Origin of Modern Medicine*, (Accessed December 5, 2023), https://www.hellovaia.com/explanations/history/public-health-in-uk/modern-medicine/
15. National Library of Medicine, *A History of the Public Health System*, (Accessed December 6, 2023), https://www.ncbi.nlm.nih.gov/books/NBK218224/#:~:text=The%20nineteenth%20century%20marked%20a,of%20nineteenth%2Dcentury%20social%20reforms.
16. Dunn, Halbert, High-Level Wellness for Man and Society. *American Journal of Public Health and the Nation's Health*, 49(6), 786–792.
17. The Surgeon General's Report on Health Promotion and Disease Prevention, (Accessed July 20, 2023) http://profiles.nlm.nih.gov/NN/B/B/G/K/
18. Wilson, Edward O., *Biophilia* (Cambridge, MA: Harvard University Press, 1984).
19. Kellert, Stephen R., Judith H. Heerwagen, & Martin Mador, *Biophilic Design: The Theory, Science, and Practice of Bringing Building to Life* (New York, NY: John Wiley & Sons, Inc., 2008).
20. Buettner, Dan, *The Blue Zones: 9 Lessons Learned from the People Who've Lived the Longest*, 2nd Edition (Washington D.C.: National Geographic, 2012).
21. Louv, Richard, *Last Child in the Woods: Saving Our Children from Nature-Deficit Disorder* (New York, NY: Algonquin Publishers, 2008).
22. Pau, Emily, *Nutrition Through The Decades: 2000s*, (Accessed December 5, 2023), https://www.werise4wellness.com/post/nutrition-through-the-decades-2000s
23. Rowe, Keith, *A Look Back at the Health Trends of the Last 20 Years*, (Accessed December 5, 2023), https://brainmd.com/blog/health-trends-last-20-years/
24. Harris, Nancy, Rachael Peterson, & Susan Minnemeyer, *World Lost 8 Percent of its Remaining Pristine Forests Since 2000*, (Accessed December 5, 2023), https://www.globalforestwatch.org/blog/data-and-research/world-lost-8-percent-of-its-remaining-pristine-forests-since-2000/
25. Global Wellness Institute, *Global Wellness Economy Monitor 2023*, (Accessed December 5, 2023), https://globalwellnessinstitute.org/industry-research/global-wellness-economy-monitor-2023/

26. Prescott, Susan, *Planetary Health: People, Place, Purpose, Planet,* (Accessed November 22, 2023), http://www.drsusanprescott.com/planetary-health.html
27. Travis, John, *Illness and Wellness Continuum, 1972,* (Accessed June 12, 2023) https://www.houseofhealth.co.nz/wellness-continuum-blog-1-physical-health/
28. Ardell, Donald, *High Level Wellness: An Alternative to Doctors and Drugs, and Disease,* (Emmaus, PA: Rodale Press, 1977), pp. 87–91.
29. Wellspring, *Key Concept #1: The Illness-Wellness continuum,* (Accessed November 6, 2023), http://www.thewellspring.com/wellspring/introduction-to-wellness/357/key-concept-1-the-illnesswellness-continuum.cfm.html
30. Swarbrick, Margaret, *Mapping Mental Health: Dr. Swarbrick & The Eight Wellness Dimensions,* (Accessed August 15, 2023), https://alcoholstudies.rutgers.edu/mapping-mental-health-dr-swarbrick-the-eight-wellness-dimensions/
31. Ardell, Donald, *High-Level Wellness: An Alternative to Doctors, Drugs, and Disease* (Emmaus, PA: Rodale Press, Inc., 1976).
32. Logan, Alan, Brian Berman, & Susan Prescott, *Relevance to Personal and Public Health,* (Accessed November 8, 2023), https://www.mdpi.com/1660–4601/20/6/5065#:~:text=Human%20flourishing%2C%20the%20state%20of%20optimal%20functioning%20and,in%20the%20context%20of%20health%20and%20high-level%20wellness.
33. Haugan, Gorill & Jessie Dezutter, *Chapter 8, Meaning-in-Life: A Vital Salutogenic Resource for Health,* (Accessed November 8, 20923), https://www.ncbi.nlm.nih.gov/books/NBK585665/
34. Bi, Kaiwen, Shuquan Chen, Paul Yip, & Pei Sun, *Domains of Life Satisfaction and Perceived Health and Incidence of Chronic Illness and Hospitalization,* (Accessed November 8, 2023), https://bmcpublichealth.biomedcentral.com/articles/10.1186/s12889-022-14119-3#:~:text=As%20a%20promising%20health%20asset%2C%20life%20satisfaction%20has,intake%20restriction%29%20%5B%204%2C%205%2C%206%2C%207%20%5D.
35. O'Kearney, E. L. et al., *Mastery is Associated with Greater Physical and Mental Health-related Quality of Life in Two International Cohorts of People with Multiple Sclerosis,* (Accessed November 8, 2023), https://pubmed.ncbi.nlm.nih.gov/31756608/
36. Pressman, Sarah, Brooke Jenkins, & Judith Moskowitz, *Positive Affect and Health: What Do We Know and Where Next Should We Go,* (Accessed November 8, 2023), https://www.annualreviews.org/doi/10.1146/annurev-psych-010418–102955
37. Ardell, Donald, *High-Level Wellness: An Alternative to Doctors, Drugs, and Disease* (Emmaus, PA: Rodale Press, Inc., 1976), p. 10.
38. Kopec, Dac, *Person-Centered Health Care Design* (New York, NY: Routledge, 2021), pp. 30–31.
39. Haines, Andy, *Addressing Challenges to Human Health in the Anthropocene Epoch – an Overview of the Finding of the Rockefeller-Lancet Commission on Planetary Health,* (Accessed November 6, 2023), https://link.springer.com/content/pdf/10.1186/s40985-016-0029-0.pdf
40. Prescott, Susan, Alan Logan, & David Katz, *Concept of High-Level Wellness in the Planetary Health Paradigm,* (Accessed November 8, 2023), https://www.mdpi.com/1660–4601/16/2/238
41. Halbert Dunn, *High Level Wellness* (Pitman, NJ: Charles B. Slack Publisher, 1977).
42. *Physical Activity for Kids is Out of Control: Policymakers Are Taking Action,* (Accessed August 30, 2023), https://mail.yahoo.com/d/folders/1/messages/AIExDVFm0c9JZO95kgLDCEzt89A
43. Gold, Jamie, *Making Wellness Design Affordable With Builder Incentives,* (Accessed December 6, 2023), https://www.forbes.com/sites/jamiegold/2019/02/08/making-wellness-design-affordable-with-builder-incentives/?sh=424fff2d2bf8

44. *Urban. Suburban. Rural. How Do Households Describe Where They Live?*, (Accessed October 20, 2023), https://www.huduser.gov/portal/pdredge/pdr-edge-frm-asst-sec-080320.html#:~:text=According%20to%20data%20HUD%20and,describe%20their%20neighborhood%20as%20rural.
45. Prescott, Susan, Alan Logan, & David Katz, *Concept of High-Level Wellness in the Planetary Health Paradigm*, (Accessed November 8, 2023), https://www.mdpi.com/1660-4601/16/2/238
46. Li, Yanping, An Pan, Dong Wang, Xiaoran Liu, Klkodian Dhana, Oscar Franco, Stephen Kaptoge, Emanuele Di Angelantonio, Mi Stampfer, Walter Willett, & Frank Hu, *The Impact of Healthy Lifestyle Factors on Life Expectancies in the US Population,* (Accessed January 17, 2024), https://www.ncbi.nlm.nih.gov/pmc/articles/PMC6207481/#:~:text=A%20meta%2Danalysis9%20of,physical%20inactivity%2C%20poor%20diet%2C%20and
47. Zarocostas, John, *Millions of Deaths from Environmental Causes are Preventable, says WHO*, (Accessed January 17, 2024), https://www.ncbi.nlm.nih.gov/pmc/articles/PMC1479630/

2 WELLNESS ARCHITECTURE AND URBAN DESIGN BENEFITS

INTRODUCTION

In what ways can planning and design solutions contribute to human and environmental health and wellness? Health and wellness benefit both human beings and the environments they inhabit including both natural and built places. Human-centered benefits are directed to the dimensions of wellness including our physical bodies, mental health, emotional well-being, social connections, and spiritual growth. As seen in Figures 2.1a and 2.1b, there certainly is a difference between the experience of illness and joy. Financial health is also seen as a wellness benefit, personally and occupationally. The environmental-centered benefits are directed to the natural environment around us and the cities and buildings we occupy, as seen with the industrial air pollution and clean cityscape in Figures 2.1c and 2.1d. The contrast between these two environmental conditions is moving – one is polluted and the other is endowed with clean air. Spiritual wellness is an understanding and acceptance of our connection to the world and our place in it leading to personal peace and purpose. Wellness is an everyday process and is inextricably linked to the place and where we exist.[1] These places include where we live, work, learn, shop, recreate, dine, worship, and otherwise occupy. They are the contexts within which we interact and function, and if these places are healthy places, there is a greater chance of achieving wellness. Lifestyles are based on tangible and intangible factors of individuals and groups, and their actions, living behaviors, conditions, habits and style of living reflect values, attitudes, cultures, and world views. And, for them to become wellness-lifestyles means a balanced, holistic, and purposeful choice.

WELLNESS BEHAVIORS

Wellness manifests broadly across several contexts as pro-individual, pro-social, and pro-environmental behaviors especially as they influence lifestyle choices. Pro-individual behaviors are actions taken to improve personal health, lifestyles, and welfare. Pro-social behaviors are those intended to reduce loneliness, and help other people with actions that are characterized by a concern for other's rights, feelings, and welfare. Pro-environmental behaviors are those which minimizes the negative impact of one's behavior on the built and natural environments. Following are further descriptions of these behaviors:

DOI: 10.4324/9781003472902-2

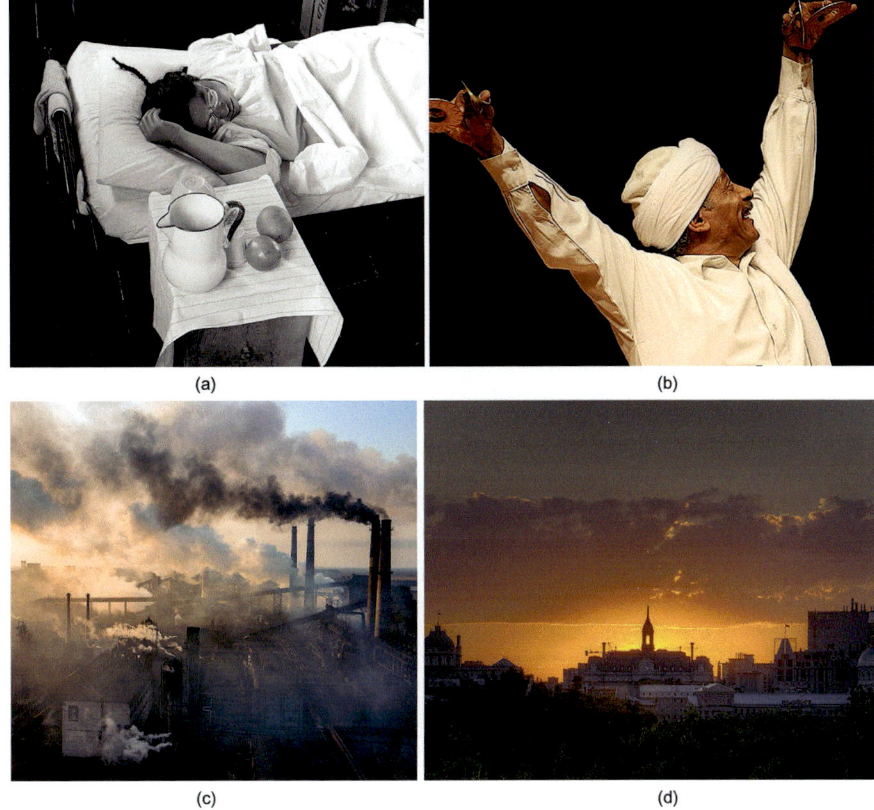

2.1
Wellness Benefits
a) From Illness,
b) To Wellness,
c) From Air Pollution from Industrial Plant, d) To Clean Cityscape

(*Sources: Wikimedia Commons and Shutterstock*)

- Pro-individual behaviors (interpersonal) – *manifest with health-related lifestyles and an increase in well-being and positive health effects physically, emotionally, mentally and spiritually particularly with stress reduction, increased activity, improved nutrition, the perception of having more time, and with a clear purpose in life. Awe-eliciting and serenity-eliciting experiences might offer effective ways of alleviating the feeling of time starvation and temporal density. Wellness experiences can improve mood, increase life satisfaction, and can create clarity of mind and critical thinking. They contribute to the "small self-effect" and self-transcendence and the experience of humility.*[2] *And finally, pro-individual behaviors can lead to positive post-experience accommodation.*
- Pro-social behaviors – *are a broad class of behaviors defined as involving social support, reduced loneliness, and with costs for the self, resulting in benefits for others. They result in a diminishment of perception of the individual self and its concerns. They manifest with positive social relationships that promote interaction, friendship, generosity, empathy, gratitude, sharing, community building, and developing desirable traits. They include socially-responsible behaviors to infectious diseases like COVID-19, and potentials for greater life satisfaction and longevity. Wellness experiences can create a greater sense of connectedness, cooperation, altruism, as well as mutualism.*

- Pro-environmental behaviors – *manifest in positive attitudes about the environment and preservation of nature. They foster biospheric values with awareness of climate change, global forest loss and sustainable living practices, and sensitivity to consumption patterns and their effect on the environment. Wellness experiences also extend to place and the environment leading to environmental awareness, consciousness and action behaviors, thereby potentially reducing the negative environmental and climatic impacts caused by human activities. Pro-environmentalism supports a heightened awareness of environmental problems and the need to modify human lifestyle behaviors.*

CONNECTIONS TO EVERYDAY LIFE

Wellness applied to everyday life means balance, consistency, and care within each of the characteristic areas of one's life, including self, family, work, school, social, recreational, food consumption, and sleep life. It includes major bodily functions such as immune system functions, normal cell growth, digestive, bowel, bladder, neurological, brain, respiratory, circulatory, endocrine, and reproductive functions. Everyday life is the self-evident subjective experience of everyday – how we feel, think, and act on a daily basis. Lifestyle choices are conscious decisions that can lead to a healthier, more productive, and purposeful existence. Imbalance is cause for stress, common among all the wellness pillars, and can lead to permanent damage to one or more of vital organs.[3] It is important that designs for the built environment address this imbalance.

Wellness benefits can occur as momentary "fixes," but in order to maintain longer term effects, the lifestyle activities should be put into practice daily. The strategies that support these practices need to be easily accessible. Like the individuals and families residing in blue zones who experience great longevity, they tend to maintain completeness and wellness from day to day through the fabric of their daily routines. In Dan Buettner's book, *Blue Zones: 9 Lessons for Living Longer*, the key to the people he studied who lived extraordinarily longer lives was the lifestyles they led on a daily basis – heathy diet, exercise, the outdoors, meaningful social interactions, and purposefulness.[4] Everyday wellness is not something applied from the outside like a drug or treatment, but rather it is something nurtured from the inside in terms of lifestyle choices, wellness behaviors, care of the whole self, and stewardship of home, family, friends, community, and surrounding environment that are accessible daily. In this regard, wellness is an inside job and integral to everyday life. It is about living well.

DIMENSIONS OR PILLARS OF WELLNESS BENEFITS

The dimensions or pillars of wellness, developed by Dr. William Hettler in 1976, were originally defined by six approaches comprising a hexagonal model. The number of pillars has varied over the years, but generally are agreed to fall into seven or eight categories. For this work, the seven wellness Planning and Design benefits are based on the physical, mental, emotional, social, financial, environmental, and spiritual categories. They have been identified through decades of evidence-based health and wellness scholarly and scientific research. A justification for this kind of demarcation is the identification of the varying characteristics of wellness that fit one's present condition and lifestyle. Following is a brief listing and summary of the benefit pillars discussed in further detail in this chapter:[5]

1. Physical wellness – *lower stress and blood pressure, improved respiratory function, increased physical activity and energy, lower obesity levels, weight management, increased healing rates, improved circadian cycles, lower addictions, and improved nutrition.*
2. Mental wellness – *improved cognitive ability and appraisal, increased focus and clarity of mind, increased resilience, reduced anxiety and negative thoughts, ability for awareness of present moment (mindfulness), increased attention restoration and soft fascination, and reduced temporal density.*
3. Emotional wellness – *maintaining healthy relationships, improved mood, lower stress levels, experience of positive emotions (awe, serenity, contentment, wonder, and joy), resilience and positive coping, and experience of inner peace.*
4. Social wellness – *creating community, increased social interactions, generosity, mutualism, empathy, compassion, helpfulness, and enhanced collective concerns. Social wellness creates a sense of safety, belonging and security, with increased life expectancy, and the experience of pro-social behaviors.*
5. Financial wellness – *increased efficiency and productivity, increased job performance, reduced absenteeism and presenteeism, positive return on investments, increased market distinction and branding, increased facilities due to economy of scale, and reduced stress over financial matters and security.*
6. Environmental wellness – *producing and experiencing lower air pollution and greenhouse gas emissions, cleaner water, greater access to nature, increased biophilic effect, improved biodiversity and regenerative processes, disaster mitigation, and pro-environmental and biospheric behaviors.*
7. Spiritual wellness – *the addressing of existential questions, increased self-transcendence, experience of wholeness, positive sense of solving problems, invigorated meaning and purpose in life, spiritual arousal, and increased life satisfaction.*

The following sections address each of these wellness benefit pillars with definitions and detailed descriptions. They also include examples and references to seminal works and research. With some of the pillars, there are similar benefits such as stress and anxiety reduction, which have a cognitive, emotional, and potentially a financial benefit. These repetitive benefits are often experiences at all scales of the environment and fall under many if not most of the wellness pillars. There are, however, many benefits unique to each pillar. At the end of this chapter are seven summary tables describing the wellness benefit categories, the listing of benefits to humans and to the environment, and their references. Refer to Figure 2.2 for the seven pillars.

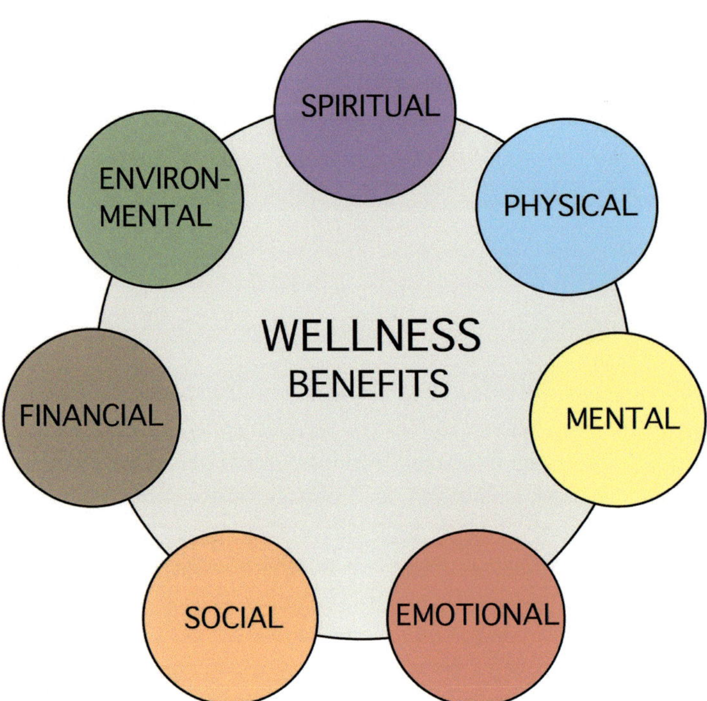

2.2
Wellness Benefit Pillars
(*Source: Phillip Tabb*)

1. **Physical wellness**

Physical health is critical to overall well-being, and can be affected by various factors such as lifestyle, diet, genetics, and level of physical activity. Physical wellness is engaging in daily physical activity, eating fresh and heathy food, managing weight, getting uninterrupted sleep, avoiding injury, initiating preventative care, and preventing illness. Physical activity refers to all movement including during leisure time, exercise, participation in sports, and passive forms such as forest bathing, pedestrian transport to get to and from places, or as part of a person's work. This includes cultivating daily routines of physical activity. And at night sleep efficacy affects physical restoration, wakefulness, focus, and cognitive clarity. Factors affecting sleep include sleep schedule, sleep environment, sound and light, air quality, stress levels, sleep latency, and possible sleep disorders.

Sedentary behavior, poor diet, smoking, spending too much time indoors, and lack of access to nature all can contribute to poor physical health. In the United States, indoor inactivity for adults is exacerbated by consuming media that accounts for more than ten hours a day.[6] The planning and design associated with the environmental context can also affect physical wellness. This includes the quality of air that we breathe, water we drink, amount of sunshine and daylight we receive, the accessibility to natural outdoor spaces for exercise, and even the aesthetic quality of the places we inhabit. Close proximity to disaster-prone locations and those with frequent extreme weather events, toxic landfills, and low-frequency electromagnetic powerlines can negatively affect physical health. In the context of wellness architecture and urban design, the physical benefits occur through site location, design intentions, wellness considerations for planning and design, and in the encouragement of wellness behaviors including increased activity, balanced diet, reduction of illness factors, and increased socialization.

Increased activity, especially on a daily basis, produces powerful wellness effects. According to the Centers for Disease Control and Prevention, the average adult needs 150 hours of moderate-intensity physical activity over five days, which is a little over 30 minutes a day.[7] Exercise enhances stress reduction with improved mental focus and can add variation. The immediate benefits are weight management, reduced health risks, building strength, and improved functioning. Bicycling and walking to work have shown positive connections to heart health, physical activity, weight control, and longevity. Key benefits follow:

- Increased daily physical activity.
- Increased physical performance.
- Strengthens bones and muscles.

Obesity is a major public health issue and is complex, multifactorial, and is shaped by age, social interactions, and the physical environment. It is characterized by abnormal or excessive size and amount of fat cell accumulation. Overweight and obesity produces problems related to heart health, blood pressure, diabetes risk, sleep apnea, musculoskeletal disorders, and some cancers. According to the National Institute of Health, obesity can be reduced by dietary modifications and energy expenditure modifications.[8] Social connectedness and peer group support affect health outcomes, including obesity.[9] A major cause is a sedentary lifestyle and inactivity, which results in an energy imbalance between calories consumed and calories expended. Supportive environments and communities are fundamental in shaping people's choices, with access to healthier foods and regular physical activity, and therefore preventing physical stress, overweight, and obesity.[10] Key benefits follow:

- Increased daily exercise.
- Reduced physical stress.
- Enhanced social networks.

Food is essential, and nutrition is how food affects the health of the body. Improved nutrition is a critical part of wellness. It is the process of consuming, absorbing, and using nutrients from food which is necessary for growth, development, and maintenance of life. Eliminating or reducing energy-dense (fatty) foods can support physical health. Above all, drinking water every day is essential for good health by flushing out toxins, lubricating joints, influencing energy levels, and preventing dehydration. According to an article published by *Nutritional Psychology*, healthy dietary patterns include nutrient-dense food items like fruits, vegetables, whole grains, beans, nuts, lean meat, and low-fat dairy.[11] From a planning and design perspective, this means greater proximity and access to clean water and good nutrition (local farms, gardens, and grocery stores). Key benefits follow:

- Well-balanced diet.
- Access to healthy food and healthy eating patterns.
- Increase drinking water.

A wellness benefit of physical activity is improved heart health. Risk factors to good heart health include high blood pressure, high LDL cholesterol, smoking, obesity, unhealthy diet, and physical inactivity. According to the National Institutes of Health, moderate and vigorous physical activity added to a daily routine affects aerobic activity, strengthens the heart muscle, widens capillaries, lowers blood pressure, lowers triglycerides, and manages blood sugar and insulin levels.[12] The three types of exercise generally accepted to benefit heart health are (1) aerobic exercise, (2) resistance training, and (3) stretching, flexibility, and balance exercises. Exercise done regularly is likely to reduce the chances of suffering of a sudden heart attack or other life-threatening cardiac events. Key benefits follow:

- Reducing cardiac Illness factors.
- Managing blood pressure.
- Reducing HDL cholesterol.

Physical activity can improve respiratory function. Activity increases the need for oxygen which in turn exercises the diaphragm, heart, and lungs. Stopping smoking reduces the risk of heart disease and chronic lung disease including lung cancer. Physical exercise increases lung function by bringing oxygen into the body, providing energy, and removing carbon dioxide, the waste product created when you produce energy. Oxidative stress has also been linked to asthma and COPD, and chronic inflammation in the lungs also leads to these conditions. Over time, vascularization in muscles also improves respiratory function, further improving gaseous exchange and metabolic capacity. The American Lung Association recommends that adults get 15 minutes of moderate physical activity per week.[13] The combination of physical activity and smoking cessation functions in cardiorespiratory fitness. It should be noted that excessive physical activity can lead to maladaptations and difficulties.[14] Key benefits follow:

- Increased oxygen supply.
- Diaphragm strengthening.
- Cardiorespiratory fitness.

The immune system can be balanced with physical activity, healthy diet, maintenance of weight, enough sleep, moderate-to-no alcohol, and not-smoking. The immune system can be protected by social behaviors when exposed to infection risks, such as COVID-19. Physical activity could provide physical, psychological, and emotional benefits and contribute to the prevention and treatment of various diseases, such as cardiovascular disease, diabetes, cancer, hypertension, obesity, depression, and osteoporosis.[15] Spatial distancing, providing sanitation protocols, sheltering in place, quarantining, and sanctuary spaces are among the strategies for the mitigation of spread of communicable diseases. Innate and adaptive immunity can be strengthened with appropriate sleep. Key to the effectiveness of the physical activity depends on the frequency, duration, and intensity, while over exercising can suppress the immune system.[16] Physical activity helps the body react more quickly to viruses, and more efficiently with vaccines. Further physical activity affects nutritional influences and the gradual deterioration of the immune system. Key benefits follow:

- Response to seasonal colds, flu, and COVID-19.
- Mitigating spread of communicable diseases.
- High-quality sleep.

Oxidative stress occurs when there are too many unstable molecules, called "*free radicals*," in the body, and if the system cannot detoxify, then it can lead to cell and tissue damage. Social isolation contributes to oxidative stress. It can be reduced with physical activity, quality sleep, healthy diet, limited alcohol consumption, and no smoking. A moderate and programmed physical exercise has often been reported to be therapeutic both in adulthood and in aging, since it is capable of promoting fitness, and physical activity and intake of antioxidant compounds can protect the body from oxidative stress.[17] Locating buildings and communities close to parks and natural areas can help promote fitness, and away from electrical transmission lines can mitigate ill health related to electromagnetic sensitivity and the increase of allergies, chronic fatigue syndrome, neurological disorders, auto immune system diseases, cancers, and Alzheimer's disease.[18] Key benefits follow:

- Avoiding carcinogens.
- Consuming high antioxidant foods.
- Reducing social isolation.

Walkable trails in nature, jogging along a beach, playgrounds, pedestrian cities, parks, fitness centers, gymnasiums, swimming pools, back yards, using stairs, and even nature-friendly streetscapes are good examples where physical wellness occurs. Yet more nuanced designs can encourage physical activity and wellness, such as courtyards, terraces, balconies, sidewalks, and building stairs. According to Dan Buettner's study of Sardinian centurions, the everyday exposure to the steepness of the street and pathway slopes contributed to long life.[19] Incorporating physical activity and contemplative practices into daily routines can help balance neurochemicals and the hormones that lead to happiness.[20] Figure 2.3 shows jogging exercise along a beach and everyday circulation along steep paths and stairs in Cortona, Italy. Refer to Table 2.1.

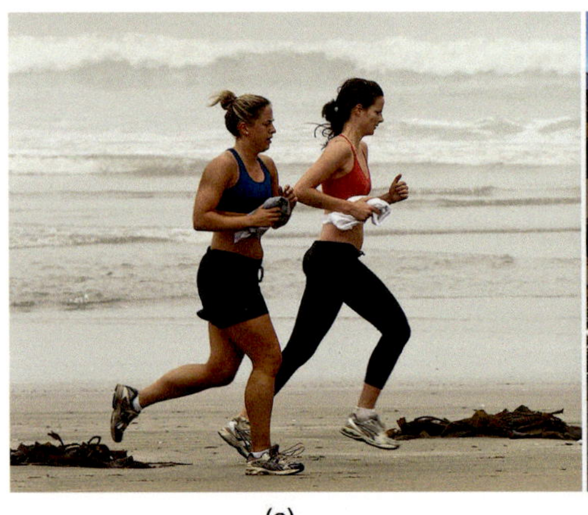

(a)

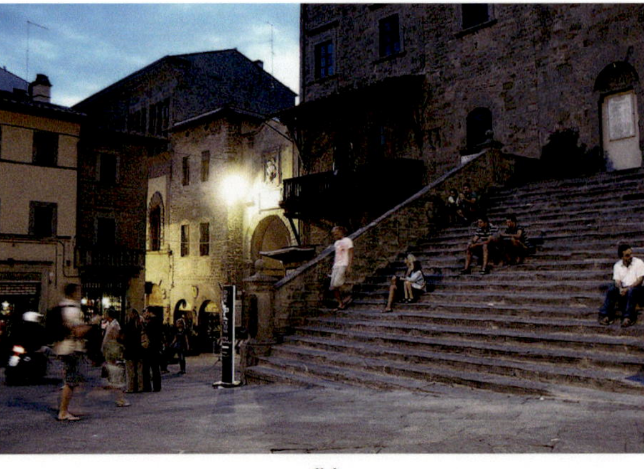

(b)

2.3
Physical Wellness
a) Joggers Along a Beach, b) Cortona, Italy
(*Source: Wikimedia Commons*)

2. Mental/cognitive wellness

Brain health is a broad state of functioning across cognitive, sensory, social-emotional, behavioral, and motor domains.[21] Mental or cognitive wellness is more than mental health as it affects our positive flourishing, resilience, and high-level functioning. It nurtures mental clarity, focuses attention, creativity and productiveness, and supports a positive sense of self. According to the World Health Organization, mental wellness is defined as "a state of well-being in which the individual realizes his or her own abilities, can cope with the normal stresses of life, can work productively and fruitfully, and is able to make a contribution to his or her community."[22] Put simply, it means the ability to think clearly, learn, and remember.

Improved cognitive function can take the form of clarity of thinking. Cognitive function also includes mindfulness and the conscious awareness of the present moment. Another benefit is the ability to activate all the senses and perceive more detail within situations and environments. Clear thinking decreases confusion and external distractions and increases performance for prioritization and more rapid decision making. According to a National Institutes of Health study, improvements in cognitive dysfunction were accompanied by improved workplace productivity.[23] Cognitive health is affected by genetics, age, educational level, and lifestyle factors including physical, emotional, social, and spiritual benefits. Cognitive wellness can also be accompanied by a need for accommodation or the assessment and reframing a mindset or mental schema after either positive or negative experiences. Key benefits follow:

- Enhanced perception.
- Presence of mind and possible need for accommodation.
- Increased production and workplace performance.

The benefits of developing focused attention skills are plenty and can assist in well-being as well as success in other areas. Focused attention and concentration that is selective, discriminating, and sustained over a period of time is a benefit of mental wellness. It affects perception, attention, concentration, and memory. Motivation stimulates attention to detail as well as global features (bigger picture).[24] And sustained attention is the ability to maintain focus and alertness over time resulting in quicker and improved prediction abilities and task completion leading to a sense of success and well-being. Focused attention can be increased with less ambiguity and complexity, and fewer distractions. Focused attention is influenced by personal factors such as level of motivation and activity and emotional state, environmental factors such as reduced and intense distractions, and stimulus factors such as complexity, ambiguity, and novelty of the incitement. Key benefits follow:

- Focused attention.
- Increased motivation.
- Sustained attention.

Cognitive coping mechanisms address and manage stressful events and situations. They put events and situations into perspective and appraisal with understanding root causes and possible resolutions. Avoidance coping occurs by ignoring stressful problems or issues, and results in a host of negative effects. Active coping refers to a coping style that is characterized by solving problems, seeking information, seeking social support, seeking professional help, changing environments, planning activities, and reframing the meanings of problems. According to a *National Library of Medicine* article, factors affecting stress and cognitive function include the intensity of stress, its origin, and its duration.[25] These stresses can be caused by a single event or by continuing worrisome situations. Key benefits to coping with cognitive stress follow:

- Cognitive perspective.
- Understanding causes (origins).
- Resolution pathways.

Although cognitive behavior reflecting trust and cooperative relationships is subject to debate, the link is important as a cognitive wellness benefit.[26] Cognitive trust occurs with the belief in someone else's competence, capabilities, reliability, and dependability. The credibility dimension is a combination of honesty, reliability, and expectancy. Benevolence in trust refers to the well-being of others. Cooperation, in turn, occurs with situations and behaviors that contribute to others' welfare. According to the National Institutes of Health, trust is seen as a chronological mental process involving three elements of expectation (process outcome), interpretation (rational and emotional evaluation), and suspension (moderating interpretative knowledge).[27] Trust occurs across different social groups such as family, friends, or strangers, different issues such as money, work, and relationships, and communication modes such as face-to-face versus digitally. Key benefits follow:

- Rational reasoning.
- Cognitive cooperation.
- Cognitive trust.

High-quality sleep is a positive outcome of healthy cognitive function and tends to facilitate outgoing behaviors and self-confidence. It affects a variety of functions including attention, language, reasoning, decision making, learning, and memory. Sleep plays an important role in consolidation of different types of memory and contributes to insightful, inferential thinking, and helps with empathy and lessens aggression which reinforces positive pro-social behaviors.[28] Lack of sufficient sleep or sleep duration is cause for cognitive decline, and is somewhat linked to one's chronotype – early or late rising. Circadian rhythm regulation plays a crucial role in people's healthy lives affected by factors consisting of cosmic events related to the universe and earth, environmental factors (light, night and day duration, temperature and seasons), and stress levels, sleep habits, and lifestyles.[29] Circadian rhythms are affected by melatonin, cortisol, and other hormone levels. Key benefits to high-quality sleep follow:

- Improved cognitive function.
- Improved circadian rhythms and sleep health.
- Increased energy.

Memory is one of the most important cognitive processes that affects learning, conceptual processes, problem solving, and decision making. It allows people to retrieve, learn, encode, retain, and process knowledge and information. It is essential in developing personality, personal history, and retention of common knowledge. Imagination relies on memory as building blocks. Age-related memory change (forgetfulness) is normal and can be lessened with wellness activities including physical activity, puzzles, social activities, healthy diet, reducing alcohol consumption, and performing services within the community.[30] For people suffering from dementia-related disorders initial visual and spatial cues are important, including those improved by the *serial-position effect* developed by Hermann Ebbinghaus which is accuracy in the recall of the first and last items in a series.[31] Recollection and navigation are improved and reinforced by clear space sequencing, rhythm patterns, and the use of color clusters. Semantic memory is an important accumulation of general knowledge gained throughout a lifetime and is essential to healthy cultural and social interactions. Key benefits follow:

- Memory cognition.
- Serial-position effect.
- Activating the imagination.

John Steele's notion of "*temporal density*," occurs with cognition where any given interval of time is filled and saturated with a myriad of events, processes, information, and thoughts.[32] Time is dense requiring great mental and emotional attention and affords little solitude or the ability to attune to wellness benefits. Too much density is difficult to assimilate and experience the present moment fully. Processing multiple mental problems deludes the ability to focus on single issues. Overthinking and fixating on certain situations, problems, shortcomings, and past mistakes can affect well-being and mental peace.[33] Reducing mental temporal density creates an openness with greater receptivity and the ability to focus on the most important problems. This allows for a clearer mind that is present-centered. Being present activates the mind for greater breadth and creativity, and a fuller experience. Key benefits follow:

- Reducing temporal density.
- Reducing mental noise and stress.
- Increasing present-centeredness.

Cognitive-rich spaces have the potential for experience of embodied information, meaning, and education and symbolic content. Cognitive function includes processes of perception, learning, memory, understanding, reasoning, judgment, intuition, and language skills.[34] Place types like historic cities and sacred sites, museums, libraries, visitor's centers, and schools are infused with both implicit and explicit information. Retail spaces, markets, and grocery stores also are full of content, and there are semantic-rich spaces like religious and ceremonial structures. These spaces of enrichment can cause stimulation of the brain and brain activity, increase resilience and motor learning, encourage active learning, and they can exist at varying scales from cities to rooms. According to Stephen Kellert, intellectual satisfaction and cognitive prowess can be facilitated through designs reflecting nature and nature's abstractions.[35] And, according to Dan Buettner's study of Sardinian centurions, active coping and problem solving helps with mental health, stress resilience, and cognitive longevity.[36] Close family, friends, and community social connections also positively affect cognitive health. Figure 2.4 shows a man concentrating on a pool shot and a boy solving a geometry problem. Refer to Table 2.2 for a summary of cognitive benefits.

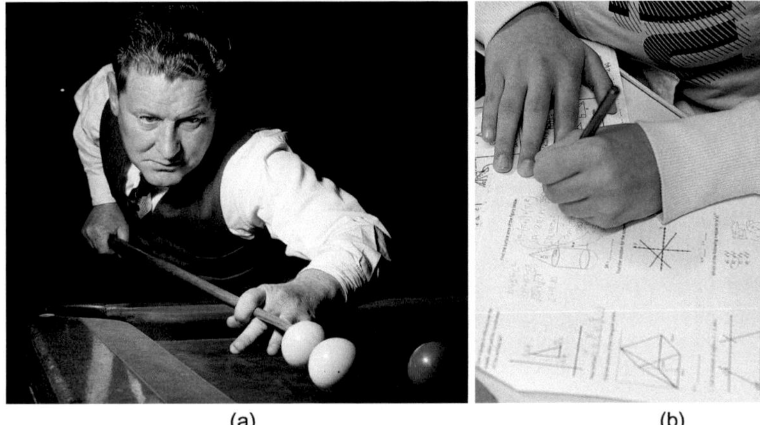

(a) (b)

2.4
Mental Wellness
a) Focused Attention and Concentration,
b) Creative Problem Solving

(Source: Wikimedia Commons)

3. **Emotional wellness**

Emotional wellness is related to how we feel and affects our relationships, our ability to handle stress and overcome negative emotions, the quality of our sleep, our response to grief, productivity, and overall mental health.[37] There are more than 30 emotions of which anger, fear, disgust, sadness, happiness, and surprise are the prime ones. These emotions serve to interpret, guide, protect, inform, and initiate appropriate behavior. Mood disorders are the most disabling and prevalent illness worldwide and range from depression to mania.[38] Emotional wellness addresses negative emotions and promotes the positive ones. Being adaptable and resilient suggests self-awareness and the ability to manage emotions. One of the most important wellness benefits is the experience of positive emotions leading to improved mood and happiness. Moods are feelings that influence thoughts, behaviors, and actions. Moods are less specific and less intense than emotions and can vary greatly from angry, ashamed, depressed, and indifferent to curious, calm, optimistic, and happy. The experience of *good moods* is usually accompanied by reduction of stress and anxiety, good sleep, and pro-social behaviors. Happiness leads to lower heart rates and blood pressure, improved mental health and executive functioning, support of the immune system, and an increase in pro-social behaviors.[39] Key benefits follow:

- Being in touch with emotions.
- Increased good moods.
- Experience of happiness.

Other important wellness emotion benefits are the reduction of stress and anxiety. Stress commonly occurs in three types: *acute* (brief events), *acute episodic* (frequent), and *chronic* (persistent). It typically occurs over a short term and is externally generated with the experience of irritability, fatigue, racing heart, changes in appetite, and difficulty breathing. Anxiety is generally longer-term and internally generated involving persistent uneasy feelings such as restlessness, panic, fear, and dread. Stress and anxiety can result in high blood pressure, apprehension, tension, excessive worry, and loss of sleep. Sleep disorders often accompany stress and anxiety and affect the continuity and quality of sleep. Sleep appears to be essential to our ability to cope with emotional stress in everyday life. According to the Mayo Clinic the following are stress relievers: assert oneself, be active, connect with others, be creative or musical, and laugh more.[40] Key benefits follow:

- Emotional stress reduction.
- Anxiety reduction.
- Reduction of insomnia and sleep disorders.

Adaptability, resilience, and emotional intelligence also lead to emotional wellness. Adaptability refers to the ability to recognize, regulate, and manage emotions and mood swings. This includes the management of impulses and behaviors, and the ability to navigate challenges and difficulties. Emotional resilience is the ability to adapt to stressful situations and environments. Emotional intelligence affects our ability to foster long-term relationships, to succeed in school or work, and to help formulate a sense of purpose. Popularized by Daniel Goleman, emotional intelligence refers to our ability to perceive, observe, evaluate, and even control emotions.[41] The wellness benefit derives from our ability to understand and respond to emotional changes and regulation resulting in improved mental health, job performance, and relationships. Key benefits follow:

- Emotional adaptability.
- Emotional resilience.
- Emotional intelligence.

Serenity and its relationship to emotion theory, health and wellness, and spirituality first appeared in the nursing literature in the mid-1960's when it was identified as an important outcome for terminally ill patients. Serenity is defined as sustained inner peace. The experience of the serenity cluster of emotions (serenity, calmness, contentment, and joy) results in positive wellness benefits. Based on the nursing profession's serenity evidence-based research, a nine-factor serenity scale developed by Kay Roberts and Cheryl Aspy, identified serenity as sustained inner peace, sense of connectedness and perspective, trust, contentment, beneficence, and present centeredness. Both serene and the peaceful qualities of thin places contribute to these emotional experiences.[42] Thin places are locations or settings where a thin veil exists between the secular world within which we live and a wellness environment that possess an energy that is qualitatively different. Thin places functioning in serene ways give us experiences, even if momentary, that are extraordinarily beautiful, incredibly tranquil or contemplative, and insightful, and they contribute to individual, social, and environmental benefits. Three of the more critical attributes of serenity are listed as follows:

- Experience of inner haven.
- Sense of connectedness and belonging.
- Present centeredness.

Like cognitive temporal density, emotional temporal density occurs when any given interval of time is filled and saturated with a myriad of events, processes, moods and emotions. Reducing temporal density contributes to clarity of mind, emotional openness, and the experience of the present. It is being grounded with the ability to be aware and conscious in the present moment and becoming receptive and resonant with the qualities of wellness. According to John Steele, temporal density creates a cognitive and emotional thickness separating us from the present and direct experiences.[43] The emotional responses to temporal density can lead to emotional dysregulation creating outbursts, anxiety, depression, and difficulty in regulating emotions that feel overwhelming. A cluttered and confusing environment can reflect temporal density in contrast to a more peaceful and serene environment. Key benefits follow:

- Reduced temporal density.
- Becoming open and receptive.
- Grounded, serene, and centered.

The biophilia hypothesis posits an innate biological and genetic connection between humans and nature, including an emotional dimension to this connection. Biophilia is the inborn affinity human beings have for nature, other life forms, and life processes.[44] Biophilia's epistemology derives from the two Greek terms *bio* meaning "life," and *philia* meaning "affection or friendly feeling toward." Simply put, it is the emotion of love of life. As a wellness benefit, biophilia connects us to the positive aspects of nature (increased physicality, mental clarity, spiritual renewal, and emotional well-being) as well as fostering biospheric values. Immersion in nature helps improve mood and facilitates positive emotional growth, and in some instances may aid in managing loneliness, irritability, and anger. Beyond the individual and social benefits, connections to nature can promote pro-environmental behaviors. The design attributes include exposure to plants and animals, daylight, the elements, ecological processes and flows, biomorphic forms, color, and spiritual triggers. Key benefits follow:

- Love of life.
- Wellness connections to nature.
- Pro-environmental behaviors.

The ability to transform negative emotional states to positive ones is an indicator of wellness. The emotional benefits include stress reduction, an increase in life satisfaction, developing understanding, and a sense of purpose in life. We seek ways of understanding ourselves and the world around us, therefore, the meaning of life is seen as a positive trait and indicator of well-being.[45] Meaning in life and hope contribute positively to life satisfaction and an increase in emotional well-being especially in difficult times. Life purpose is part of psychological well-being having a sense of meaning and mission as well as direction toward particular goals and aspirations. Life purpose also gives a sense of coherence, especially during times of immense change, and serves to guide self-actualizing processes. Life purpose is linked to pain management, stress reduction, heart health, and longevity. Key benefits follow:

- Life satisfaction.
- Meaning in life.
- Life purpose and longevity.

Wellness planning and design processes intend to provide environments that can help elicit positive emotional benefits for stress reduction, resiliency, acceptance, maintenance, and recovery. Blue spaces and thin places serve to facilitate emotional and spiritual wellness in that they provide safe, quiet, vital, and naturally beautiful spaces. Common characteristics of these kinds

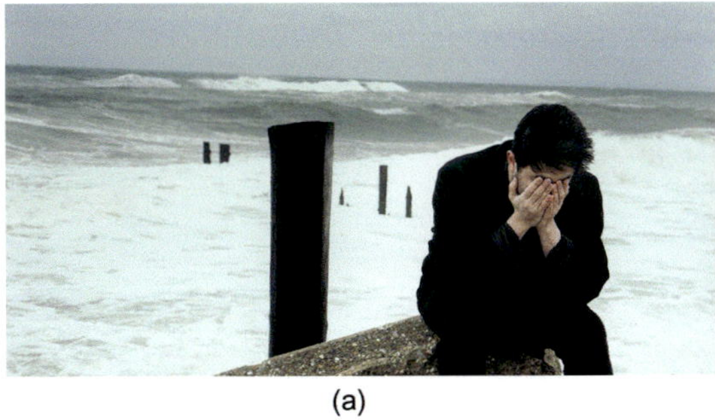

(a)

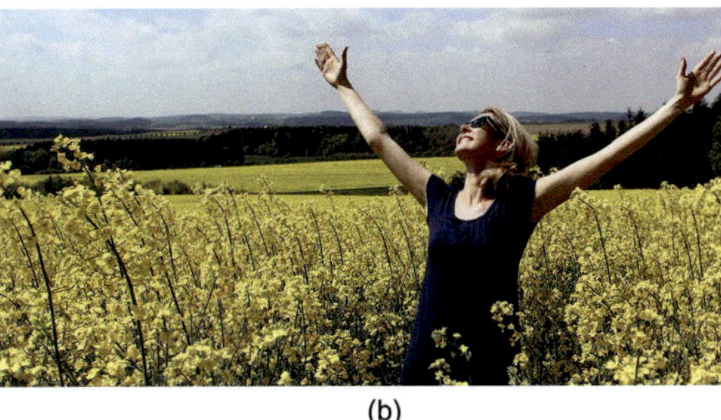

(b)

2.5
Emotional Benefits
a) Processing Grief,
b) Experiencing Happiness

(Source: Wikimedia Commons)

of spaces include identifiable bounding, containment, a sense of place, safe connections to the elements (fire, water, earth, air, and light), and the experience of wonder, fascination, mystery, and awe. The image in Figure 2.5 shows a man experiencing certain emotional distress next to the waves of a beachhead on an overcast day contrasted with a woman enjoying the energy of the sun. Our ability to experience these emotions, center ourselves, and navigate to more positive moods and states is central to emotional wellness benefits. The environmental context is an important contributor to this transformation.

Emotional wellness is important in how one feels and one's abilities to carry out everyday activities and support relationships. According to Dan Buettner's study of Okinawan centurions, reducing anger and quickly letting go of anger contributed to long life.[46] Further positive emotions support interest in physical activities, improved mental states, creativity levels, resiliency, and the ability to handle and even reduce stress. In social contexts, it supports pro-social behaviors, beneficence, and generosity. Emotional well-being is also connected to increased presence and mindfulness.[47] Refer to Table 2.3 for a detailed listing of emotional benefits.

4. Social wellness

Wellness has long been connected to social well-being, which includes the positive relationships we maintain and the quality of interactions with others in both local and global communities.[48] Attachment and belongingness frame the positive effects. Social wellness can have both short-term and long-term influences on mental well-being and physical health, and friendships can function as an emotional support. A higher level of social wellness may be achieved through trust, especially in intimate matters. Several factors contribute to positive social wellness including regular contact, experiencing quality time, engaging in meaningful interactions, joining interest groups, and participating in family, neighborhood, and community events. Social well-being involves sharing, connectedness, being present, listening, and developing and maintaining relationships.

Belonging helps mitigate isolation, loneliness, and low social status and the harm they bring to a person's subjective sense of well-being. Belonging supports human membership and organization and gives a sense of purpose. Belonging increases meaningfulness. It can provide protection and help reduce depression, anxiety, and suicide. The social ties that accompany a sense of belonging are a protective factor helping manage stress and other emotional issues. As a social determinant, it contributes to the continuity of experience toward life satisfaction and longevity. Well-being is closely related to individual and community health, flourishing, and prosperity, and has meaningful participation in a range of daily life activities and occupations.[49] The practice of acceptance, open mindedness, and positive attitudes can increase belonging and support. Key benefits follow:

- Promotes membership, inclusion, support, and value.
- Mitigates depression, anxiety, and suicide.
- Contributes to life purpose, life satisfaction, and longevity.

Positive social relationships foster altruism and beneficence. Altruism connects people and reduces social isolation, and contributes to maintaining a perspective on life. Altruism is good for emotional well-being, and promotes physiological changes in the brain linked with happiness, kindness, and acts of goodness. It also promotes the prevention and removal of harm from others. According to the *Journal of Behavioral Medicine*, altruism results in deeper and more positive social integration, enhanced meaning and purpose as related to well-being, a more active lifestyle that counters cultural pressures toward isolated passivity, and the presence of positive emotions.[50] While beneficence is generally concerned with the caregiver's promotion of well-being toward patients, it also refers to health outcomes and is related to the experience of mercy, kindness, generosity, and charity.[51] Community identification and peer support promote belonging and can help in overcoming loneliness and social isolation. Commuting by automobile, for example, is integral to everyday life providing a transition between private and working life. It can lead to negative impacts on personal and social wellness. Moving to pedestrian, mixed-use communities can reduce commuting miles and times, and can increase opportunities for casual encounters and positive social interaction. Key benefits follow:

- Altruistic behavior.
- Expression of beneficence.
- Increases community participation and reduces isolation.

A marker of social wellness is cooperation as it contributes to openness, trust, and safety. Cooperation involves paying a personal cost (for example, contributing to charity or donating time to a good cause) to gain a collective benefit (a social safety net or giving to a food bank for those in need).[52] It creates communities of human connection and collaboration for the collective greater good. In social contract theory, cooperation contributes to consensus building, group decision making, and work effectiveness. Cooperative behavior encourages the global sharing of knowledge and the ability to tackle shared problems, such as climate change, natural disasters, or economic recessions and depressions. Cooperative behavior was instrumental in reducing the negative effects of the spread of COVID-19 (testing, sequestering, wearing of masks, and social distancing).[53] Key benefits follow:

- Willingness acts to contributing to others' welfare.
- Paying personal costs to gain collective benefit.
- Gaining trust.

Wellness support networks reduce stress, decrease physical health problems, improve emotional well-being, and can lead to longer life. Social connectedness is defined as "the degree to which people have and perceive a desired number, quality, and diversity of relationships that create a sense of belonging, and being cared for, valued and supported."[54] Maintaining an inner circle creates mutual support, and improves mood and self-esteem, especially when it occurs frequently. Network emotional support is an important wellness factor including reductions in high blood pressure, diminished immunity, cardiovascular disease, and cognitive decline.[55] Wellness support is about surrounding yourself with a carefully curated group of people whom you admire and respect and with whom you share common beliefs and values. Social connection, and social media in particular, can raise health and environmental awareness. Key benefits follow:

- Mutual support.
- Curating an inner circle.
- Maintaining over time.

Empathy comes from the Greek word, *empátheia*, which means "passion." Emotional and cognitive empathy is the ability to recognize, imagine, and understand another person's thoughts, feelings, and experiences. Cognitive empathy involves an inclusive ability to accommodate a diversity of viewpoints and having more accurate and complete knowledge and understanding of another's perspective. Emotional empathy is the ability to share, relate, and feel someone else's emotions. Compassionate empathy combines cognitive and emotional empathy promoting pro-social behaviors. Emotional empathy consists of three separate components. First is feeling the same emotion as another. Second refers to one's feeling the same emotion as another. And third is compassion for another person (the most frequent empathy in psychology).[56] Key benefits follow:

- Cognitive empathy.
- Emotional empathy.
- Compassionate empathy.

According to the CDC, "the way we design and build our communities can affect our physical and mental health."[57] Community building encourages socialization, meaningful connections, engagement, and well-being. A healthy community is comprised of membership, influence, integration, and fulfillment of needs and shared emotional connections.[58] There is a shared sense of coherence and identity with common interests. Building community creates physical and social environments that are safe, open and meaningful, and allow for shared experiences and opportunities to learn from one another. Community-building activities should be reported as benefits because they address such root causes of a community's health problems as poverty, environmental hazards, and inadequate housing.[59] Community building in addition to eliciting wellness benefits can function as a survival advantage. Key benefits follow:

- Place sensing and genius loci.
- Shared identity, needs, and emotional connections.
- Communal well-being producing a survival advantage.

Many factors affect a long life including gender, genetics, hygiene, access to health care, diet and nutrition, exercise, lifestyle, and social connections. According to the National Institutes of Health, people who have healthy lifestyle choices and habits can extend life a decade more than those who do not.[60] Longevity is affected by loneliness and social isolation and with a higher risk of disease, disability, and mortality. People with strong social connections live longer. And the environmental quality and daily contact with nature can also extend life. Poor air and water, depletion of natural resources, soil deterioration, low nutritional food, and natural disasters contribute to morbidity. High consumption of alcohol, drugs, and tobacco are some of the lifestyle variables known to have toxic consequences and greatly increase the risk of serious diseases. A seven-year research study found participants with larger social networks were about 45% more likely to live longer.[61] Key benefits follow:

- Reduced loneliness.
- Positive lifestyle choices (diet, exercise, non-smoking, moderate alcohol use, etc.).
- Increase social interactions.

Where social wellness improves communications, relationships, and community building, certain planning and design strategies can contribute to positive social wellness and pro-social behaviors at both the planning and individual building scales. Provision for both indoor and outdoor social spaces from parks and plazas to patios and family rooms can invite gatherings and support social functions. Rituals and celebrations for weddings, funerals, graduations,

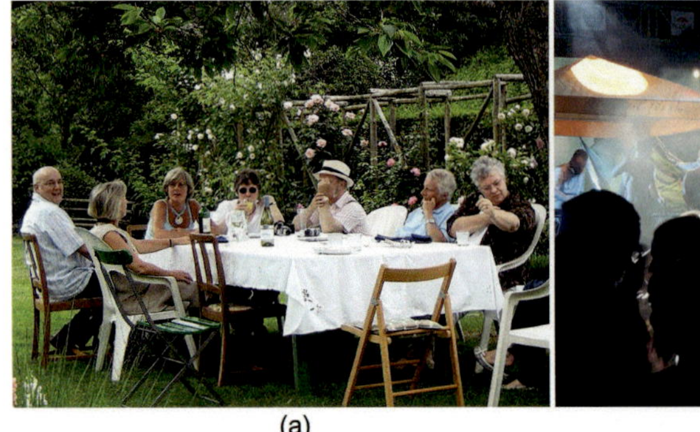

(a)

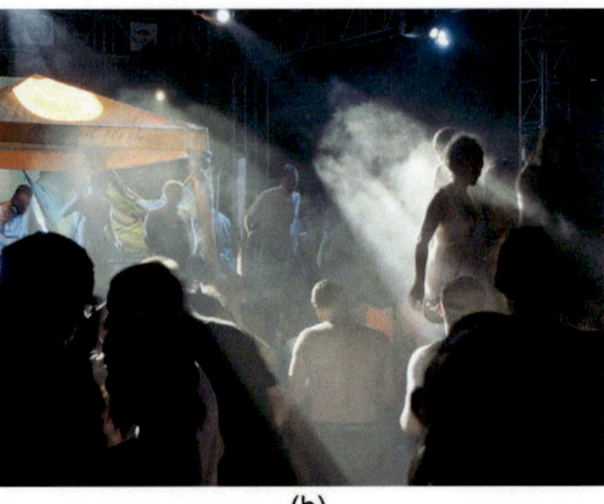

(b)

2.6
Social Wellness
a) Family Outdoor Dining, b) Friends Gathering Party

(Source: Wikimedia Commons)

birthdays, and many religious practices, give a sense of meaning to families and friends. Food is a powerful elicitor in community building and in making place. Forming social support systems contributes to wellness and longevity. Gatherings of friends and family meals are an effective allurement as seen in Figure 2.6. Refer to Table 2.5.

5. Financial wellness

Wellness is a branch of the economy that is increasing the significance of financial benefits to building locations and designs, nutrition reforms, land values, and access to nature and other health-oriented amenities. According to the US Consumer Financial Protection Bureau, financial well-being is having financial security and financial freedom of choice both in the present and future.[62] In turn, financial wellness can reduce *financial toxicity* and financial-related stress. Financial wellness also involves the economic benefits derived from health and wellness designs and functions whether they are individual buildings, retreats, or entire communities. Financial empowerment is considered to possess certain wellness benefits including a sense of security, overall well-being, peace of mind, and stress reduction.

The wellness economy includes many places, destinations, goods, and services including public health prevention and personalized medicine, traditional and complementary medicine, personal care and beauty, health nutrition, mental health, wellness real estate, wellness tourism, and wellness physical activities. According to the Global Wellness Institute, the wellness economy in 2020 was estimated to be $5.6 trillion.[63] People are interested in better health, better fitness, better nutrition, better appearance, better sleep, and better mindfulness. The expanding wellness economy shares growth with food and agriculture, sustainability, planning and design, and biophilia movements. People are seeking deeper cultural experiences and showing interest in going to the source of ancient healing and knowledge. This includes contributing to circular economies of wellness materials, products, and services. Key benefits follow:

- Circular wellness goods and services.
- Wellness tourism.
- Wellness real estate and communities.

Wellness real estate is a fast-growing sector of the wellness economy. The sector includes residential, commercial, leisure, hospitality, fitness centers, and medical properties. According to the Global Wellness Institute, wellness lifestyle and community are defined as homes (buildings) that are proactively designed and built to support holistic health for their occupants and living near one another (community) sharing common interests across many wellness dimensions.[64] Wellness property and design feature intentional wellness elements that are desirable and accessible at all price points. This includes their siting, design, materials, and amenities. Wellness lifestyle real estate is a nascent industry that recognizes, and has the potential to meet, today's immense health challenges. The future of wellness real estate and communities, will generate smarter use of land, nature, resources, technologies, and building systems.[65] Key benefits follow:

- Land and properties that enhance wellness outcomes.
- Integrating wellness mixes of amenities, functions, and services.
- Changing values toward healthy lifestyles.

Return on investment, ROI, is an important benefit of financial wellness. Relative to health and wellness, ROI can include avoided medical costs, reduced absenteeism, improved health outcomes or access to care, increased engagement, or positive experiences. Simply put, investing in wellness planning and design can produce both health and financial benefits. Positive ROI from residential, commercial, leisure, hospitality, medical and rental properties can be achieved by incorporating wellness elements in their siting choices, design, materials, and buildings, as well as their amenities, services, and space programming.[66] Wellness property and design features are becoming more desirable and accessible at all price points. ROI is helped by material durability, reuse, recycling, and, in some instances, local sourcing. People are increasing the value of healthy lifestyles.[67] Key benefits follow:

- Integrating wellness amenities, functions, and services.
- Increasing property values.
- Promoting market uniqueness and brand identity.

Subjective well-being produces less stress, lower turnover, higher levels of satisfaction, and an increase in productivity. The Centers for Disease Control and Prevention, reports that the absenteeism costs to U.S. employers is $225.8 billion annually.[68] Wellness can produce higher energy levels and more efficiency. Loss of productivity can be induced by medical problems and personal financial issues. Low turnover rates can also result in wellness-oriented work environments. Financial well-being means having financial security and financial freedom of choice to enjoy life. Subjective well-being is self-reported and personally experienced, and represents both internal factors, like personality or temperament and outlook, and external factors, such as the quality of social relationships, community, and culture within which one lives.[69] Key benefits follow:

- Improved satisfaction.
- Improved performance.
- Improved cognition and mental focus.

Wellness environments produce less burnout. Reversing the causes of low motivation, lack of direction, illnesses, mental health issues, and stress can reduce absenteeism. Overcoming absenteeism produces financial returns, increases morale and production, and promotes stress reduction in the work environment. Reducing presenteeism through appreciation, collaboration, and encouraging wellness activities. According to the Health Enhancement Research Organization, more than 90% of leaders surveyed said health has a significant or very significant influence on productivity and performance, but that belief must be consistent across all levels of management to truly create a culture of health.[70] While direct measures of productivity are rarely identical across a variety of workplace functions, transaction-based tasks give a good insight into what is possible through design. The reduction of absenteeism and presenteeism, and increase of recruitment and retention add to financial well-being.[71] Key benefits follow:

- Improved production.
- Improved morale and retention.
- Reduced absenteeism, presenteeism.

Distinctive marketing branding is another benefit of financial wellness. Because of the increasing interest and positive benefits of wellness designs, services, and products, it is propitious to promote wellness branding strategies. By having unique, scarce, beneficial, or unusual wellness places, they become more identifiable and therefore economically attractive. Well-branding can be transparent, elicit engagement, and express core values. In a branding survey of roughly 7,500 consumers in six countries, 79% of the respondents said they believe that wellness is important, and 42% consider it a top priority.[72] Health and wellness branding increases positive perceptions related to trust, care, and knowledgeability. Well-branding may aid in capturing greater market share, accelerating new markets, increasing loyalty, and improving the consumer experience. Key benefits follow:

- Health and wellness amenities.
- Integrating wellness functions and services.
- Clustering mixes of use to create access and identities.

Alleviation of debt and financial issues, and the adverse health impacts of unsecured debt can relieve stress, anxiety, sleep loss, headaches, high blood pressure, and depression. On a personal or family level, this includes credit cards, medical debt, student loans, legal financial obligations, high-percentage interest rates, taxes, insurance payments, mortgages, and alimony and child support. Financial wellness creates more security and control, can improve life satisfaction, and prevent hardships. Wellness financial social relationships gain more respect and trust and help reduce financial toxicity and economic hardship. Anxiety about finances can cause sleep deprivation, stress, and panic over everyday activities like getting the mail or opening bills. Altered health behaviors resulting from debt, such as skipping medical care and cutting back on food and utility usage to help pay bills, are one potential mechanism through which unsecured debt may impact health.[73] Separation from family and friends can occur due to a lack of funds or financial support.[74] Regenerative Finance is a focus on practices that help create financial returns focusing on restoring and enhancing economic prosperity, social responsibility, resource sustainability, and environmental well-being. It functions in a circular and holistic way with long-term goals, accountability, and transparency.[75] Key benefits follow:

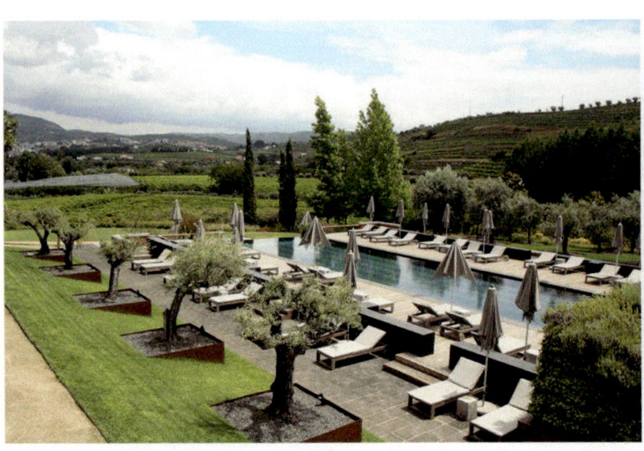

(a)

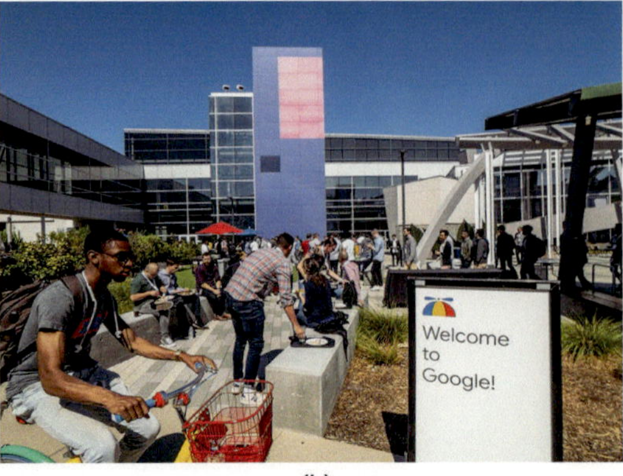

(b)

2.7
Financial Wellness
a) Six Senses Hotel Douro Valley, Portugal, b) Google Mountainview Headquarters
(*Source: Shutterstock*)

- Cognitive and emotional stress reduction.
- Organizing and taking control.
- Social benefits of trust and respect (regenerative finances).

Planning and designing for affordable wellness is challenging, and some strategies that can produce wellness benefits that are not so costly. The Six Senses Hotels, a brand started in the 1990s, is recognized for establishing hospitality environments that are distinctive and diverse in personality using the natural environment, topography, and qualities of the site. The paradise valley of Douro in Portugal exemplifies a well-industry. Refer to Figure 2.7a. The Google workplace environment offers wellness features that include financial benefits. Google workspaces typically encourage "*casual collision*," there are abundant common areas for collaboration, unconventional workspace environments, an atmosphere of innovation, and dog -friendly, with hackable spaces.[76] These strategies contribute to increased creativity, employee satisfaction, productivity, and low turnover rates such as Google Mountainview Headquarters. Refer to Figure 2.b that shows a vibrant outdoor work and social environment at Google. Refer to Table 2.5 listing benefits for financial wellness. Key benefits follow:

- Incorporating "free" wellness elicitors (daylight, fresh air, views).
- Strategies for encouraging physical activity (sidewalks, paths, greenspaces).
- Providing simple social spaces (intimate seating areas, courtyards, balconies).

6. Environmental wellness

Environmental wellness is the positive interactions we have with all forms of the environment and nature as well as with the built environment including our homes, neighborhoods, and cities. It not only refers to wellness to the self but also to the environment and our abilities to preserve, sustain, engage, and give back in positive ways. The co-benefits are directed to both human wellness and planetary health. This includes physical, mental, emotional social, and spiritual human wellness, cleaner air and water, healthier agriculture, reduced risks to natural disasters and extreme weather events, and the spread of diseases. Environmental wellness is a transdisciplinary, interconnected, and inclusive process of the mitigation of the negative impacts of human disruptions to natural systems and the positive benefits derived from the practice of right-livelihood.

The specific environmental benefits include improving connections and opportunities for engagement with nature, utilizing sustainable, renewable, and healthy resources, combating pollution, maintaining a cleaner environment (earth, air, water, energy), reducing greenhouse gasses and increasing carbon sequestering, protecting the biodiversity of the planet so we live richer more vibrant lives, mitigating climate change and natural disasters, improving public health, and creating vital urban spaces. These benefits pervade all scales of human activity from agricultural production of healthy food and the cities we plan in response to planetary population growth to windows on our homes that bring in sunlight and fresh air and to the very fabrics in our clothing. Mitigation and preventative responses to negative climatic conditions, severe weather events, and natural disasters are also important environmental benefits to planetary and human well-being.

Biophilia is the love of nature. Fundamental to the biophilic effect are sets of relationships that occur among nature and its processes, human experiences and lifestyle practices, and the quality of the ever-changing built environment. Correspondingly, nature as the source of these elicitors is reflected in the built environment through its materiality, form, and patterning of daily life. A positive relationship is intended to result in engaging experiences with the support of healthy lifestyles along with associative planetary health.

One of the most important wellness benefits is in improving connections with the natural world and increasing opportunities for daily emersion. Research by Mathew White at the University of Exeter found that people who spent two hours a week in green spaces were more likely to report good health and psychological well-being than those who did not.[77] This reflects the well-documented benefits of biophilia and the love of nature and natural processes, which results in increased physical activity, reduced stress, improved cardiovascular system and respiratory function, and pro-social and pro-environmental behaviors. Access to biomimicry and biomorphic forms can contribute to creative and inspiring design solutions, sustainability, positive health effects, and attention restoration. Environmental concerns contribute to human activities and lifestyle choices that occur on four levels – environmental activism, non-activist public-sphere behaviors, private-sphere behaviors, and organizational behaviors.[78] These activities can contribute to healing, positive mood experiences, and human flourishing. Key benefits follow:

- Increase in physical activity.
- Stress reduction and attention restoration.
- Pro-environmental behaviors.

Both human health and planetary wellness can be enhanced by utilizing sustainable renewable and healthy resources. According to the World Health Organization, energy, especially clean energy, and health are inextricably linked. The public health interests in renewable resources include technical, economic, social, political, and environmental benefits. For energy this includes integrating conservation and safe waste handling practices, and geothermal heating and cooling, solar electricity and hot-water heating, wind energy, biomass, and hydroelectricity. The benefits include reduced global warming emissions, increased security from scarcity, increased economic well-being, decreased terrorism, increased stability, reliability, and resilience, accessibility due to local or regional sources, and finally improved public health.[79] Key benefits follow:

- Conservation practices in everyday life.
- Utilization of natural resources (air, water, solar energy).
- Resource security, stability, and resilience.

Wellness benefits can come from combating pollution toward a cleaner environment (air, water, energy and waste disposal). This includes reduction of greenhouse gas production and increasing carbon sequestering, clean water and sanitation, removal of toxic substances and hazardous wastes, and responses to climate change. Air pollution can lower life expectancy, affect the brain, and reduce the quality of life. Clean water and effective sanitation result in significant declines in disease. Loss of biodiversity can compromise the nutritional value of food. Environmental wellness addresses those physical, chemical, and biological factors that we might not have direct control over but can impact our health anyway.[80] The benefits result in better respiratory function, and relief from allergies and asthma, including improved mood, cognitive health, and longer lives. Pro-environmentalism can raise awareness about the environment and its propensity toward change (often disastrous), encourage interventions to reduce negative environmental impacts caused by human behavior, and encourage the preservation of nature's healthy attributes. Key benefits follow:

- Utilization of clean, non-polluting resources.
- Use of non-toxic materials.
- Pro-individual benefits (physical, mental, emotional).

Mitigating climate change can occur through catastrophic climate and weather events. The overcoming of the psychological distress phenomenon called "*solastalgia*." This includes mitigating natural disasters, such as volcanic events, earthquakes, tornados, hurricanes, forest fires, avalanches, flooding and storm surges, and extreme weather events which can diminish physical safety, health, and wellness. Emotional responses to natural disasters include intense feelings, strained interpersonal relationships, sensitivity to loud noises, repeated memories, and disaster-related stress.[81] Physical responses can include minor injuries, life-threatening injuries, and even death. The negative effects of climate change and natural disasters linger far beyond the event itself, with climate anxiety, loss of habitat, native plants, water, property and buildings, pets, and, in some instances, employment and livelihood. The benefit occurs in the form of mitigation or even elimination of the threats and undesirable events. Key benefits follow:

- Mitigating climate change.
- Response to natural disasters.
- Pro-environmental behaviors.

Protect the biodiversity of the planet's ecosystems including its flora, fauna, microorganisms, soils, and pharmacological products so we live richer more vibrant lives. This includes the protection of the existence and functioning of all forms of life and their relationships to all ecosystems. Benefits support sustained livelihoods, the addition of medical and pharmaceutical advancements, and the preservation of species habitats. Biodiversity loss means loss of nature's chemicals and genes, of the kind that have provided humankind with enormous health benefits, and disruptions affect ecosystem functioning and significance that can result in loss of life-sustaining ecosystem goods and services. Biological diversity of microorganisms, flora, and fauna provides extensive benefits for biological, health, and pharmacological sciences. Ecosystem services affect livelihoods, income, and local migration, and may even cause or exacerbate political conflict.[82] Key benefits follow:

- Direct access to natural resources.
- Pharmaceutical advancements.
- Pro-environmental behaviors.

Health and place are inextricably linked. You cannot have health without place, but you can have a place without health. Thus, the need for wellness benefits includes place creation with responses to access to nature, safe and clean environments, healthy food, the experience of changes of seasons and diurnal fluctuations that can provide signals for particular leisure, recreation, economic activities, and sleep cycles. Aligning with, rather than resisting, the changes can lead to the experience and to the understanding of pro-individual, pro-social, and pro-environmental behaviors. This includes the health benefits of eating more nutritious locally produced seasonal foods. "*Seasonal living*" is a concept that supports greater feelings of interconnectedness with nature and opportunities to amend routines, and is considered an immune system boost. Seasonal living enhances vitality, energetic connections, and renewal. Seasonal body changes also exhibit physical changes, activity levels, and nutritional needs.[83] Key benefits follow:

- Changes in leisure, recreational, economic, and survival activities.
- Nutrition with seasonally produced foods.
- Seasonal living and pro-environmental behaviors.

Wellness benefits can come from the creation of safe and healthy urban spaces and the infrastructure systems that support them. Public spaces are instrumental in creating community and opportunities for socialization, which have positive emotional effects. This includes the addition of amenities, and programmed activities and services. Pedestrianization also contributes to what is called "*sticky urban places*" that support opportunities for meeting, interaction, and enhancing social tolerance. Those things that slow down a pedestrian's pace may be the very things that make a street great – not to mention the reduction of the negative effects of the automobile (safety and pollution). Places like patios, plazas, streetscapes, food carts or trucks combined with attractive seating, street performers, trees and landscape elements, or just lively store windows that draw a crowd, all contribute to making a street more "sticky."[84] Key benefits follow:

- Support of community and sense of place.
- Promoting sticky urban spaces.
- Pro-social behaviors.

The environmental benefits of wellness manifest in positive attitudes about the environment and preservation of nature with biospheric values, awareness of climate change, global forest loss and sustainable living practices, and sensitivity to consumption patterns and their effect on the environment. The numinous sense of connectedness also extends to place and the environment leading to environmental awareness, consciousness, and action behaviors, thereby potentially reducing the negative environmental and climatic impacts caused by human activities. Figure 2.8 illustrates the beauty and environmental benefits of a beautiful beach and sunset in California. It possesses a sense of awe and wonder as well as serene moments. Similarly, the people-friendly pedestrian environment of the Boulder Pearl Street Mall is compellingly sticky and friendly. Pro-environmentalism supports a heightened awareness of environmental problems and the need to change human lifestyle behaviors. The wellness design benefits are intended to positively influence planning, urban design and design strategies for human health and wellness, preserve the natural environment, and incorporate specific approaches to the built environment. Refer to Table 2.6 for a listing of environmental benefits.

2.8 Environmental Benefits a) California Beach, b) Boulder Pedestrian Mall

(Source: Wikimedia Commons)

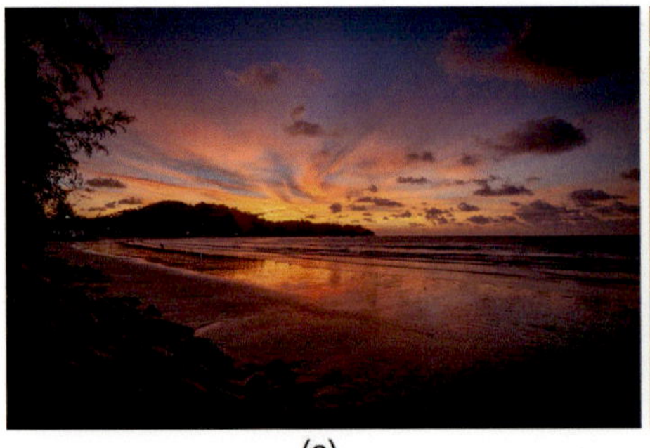

(a)

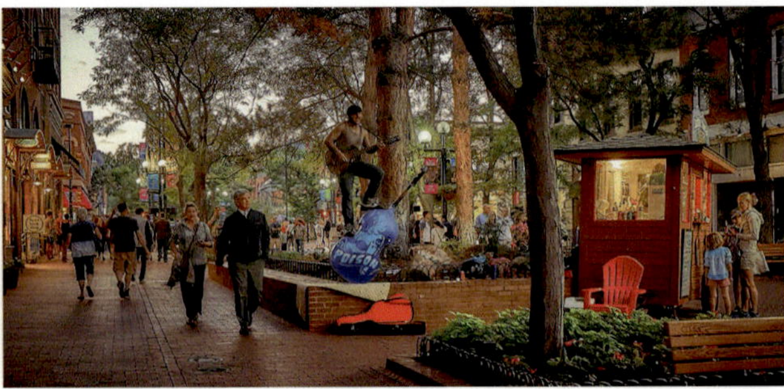

(b)

7. Spiritual wellness

Spiritual well-being ultimately represents our connection to ourselves and the greater world around us. Spiritual dimensions of wellness are about the active pursuit, choices, preventive care, and lifestyles incorporating spiritual experiences leading to processes of holistic well-being. It is the ability to experience and integrate meaning and purpose in life through connection with oneself and others, as well as through other contexts such as nature, the arts, religious practices, literature, or something other and beyond comprehension.[85] A spiritual experience goes beyond the ordinary and can be mystical or euphoric, where there is an awareness of synchronicity, the presence of intuitive thoughts, a sense of ultimate peace and well-being, and a degree of surrender. Spiritual connections to awe experiences include the feeling of being one with others, local place and the larger world, purpose revealing, containing an element of transcendence and a sense of wonder. Spiritual connections to serenity include feelings of calm, inner peace, and slowing of the perception of time.

Many are moving away from traditional religious practice, but yearn for spiritual connections. Research confirms the link between healthy spiritual connections and mental and emotional health. Spiritual experiences contribute to the reduction of stress, increases in positive mental health, in coping strategies, and in individual happiness. Religious and spiritual experiences, like numinous and awe experiences comprise two major experiential qualities, those that are ineffable (indescribable) and those that are noetic (possessing hidden or unexplainable knowledge).[86] Focusing on spirituality in health care means caring for the whole person, not just their disease. Spiritual wellness combines with other benefit pillars to new insights and perspectives, peace of mind, increased kindness and generosity, more social connections with improved relationships, and greater physical health. Spiritual wellness can connect us to cosmic narratives, original causes, spirit of place, source experiences, awe and serene emotions, and purpose in life. Further, it can address existential questions and relieve angst and the experience of a divine presence.

Spiritual renewal can occur in a variety of contexts with differing functions or purposes. Exposure to restorative beautiful natural places and experience of extraordinary architecture can contribute to spiritual renewal. Sometimes referred to as "*thin places*," they can elicit both awe and serene emotions leading to positive benefits. Serene elicitors develop an inner haven, acceptance, belonging, trust, perspective, contentment, centeredness, and beneficence.[87] Awe elicitors are generally vast triggers within thin places that derive from sources that vary greatly sparking wonder, fascination, and inspiration with differing physical, emotional, cognitive, and spiritual responses. These two differing emotional states create both similar and contrasting wellness benefits. Key benefits follow:

- Experience of awe and spiritually stimulating.
- Experience of serenity and spiritually calming.
- The need for accommodation, cross-state retention, and the experience of reflection.

Spiritual experiences change from secular or profane experiences and places to transcendent ones. Secular space is ordinary space that we experience every day, and this includes unremarkable places. Sacred space possesses its characteristics in contributing to charged experiences that include enhanced perception where the senses are heightened, there is a sense of synchronicity and an extrasensory awareness. A spiritual experience goes beyond the ordinary and can be mystical or euphoric, where there is an awareness of the presence of intuitive thoughts, a sense of ultimate peace and well-being, and a degree of surrender. Key to this transcendence is the ability to reduce temporal density and to become more present in experiences of the unknown. Transcendent experiences provide shifts with the small self or individual, with deep inner peace and with prosocial shifts, and support alignments greater than the self.[88] Experiences of cosmic narratives, sensory unity, and interconnectedness are common. Spiritual experiences include the feeling of being one with others, local place and the larger world, purpose revealing, containing an element of transcendence, and a sense of wonder. Key benefits follow:

- Profane and secular experiences.
- Transforming process.
- Experiences of wonder and the unknown.

Awe experiences are vast and elicit ineffable wonder and fascination, and positive emotional valances and transformations. For some time-perception in awe experiences slows down and for others time is expanded. Self-diminishment is the reduction of a salient aspect of self, such as one's own body or its size relative to the awe environment or stimulus. Predicated on the nursing profession's serenity evidence-based research, serenity experiences are peaceful, tranquil, calm, even sedating and free from anxiety, with accommodation emerging in the form of emotional readjustment. Serene environments contribute to creating an inner haven and include elimination of peril and crowdedness, providing proper safe and secure places. Such places include benevolent environmental features, such as gentle and qualitative use of light, balance, and elemental features (fire, water, earth, and air), and importantly, quiet. These experiences challenge our concept of self and the world around us and are the process of adjusting or making sense out of preexisting mental structures and emotional states that were unable to be assimilated during the experience. In a 2018 publication, research showed a six-factor scale of measuring awe emotion.[89] This scale included time, self-loss, connectedness, vastness, physiological (physical sensations), and accommodation. Another scale was initially developed in the 1960s that defined serenity with nine factors as a sustained state of inner peace and spiritual well-being and its universality appeals to a large population of diverse persons.[90] Key benefits follow:

- Awe emotions.
- Serenity emotions.
- Accommodation experiences.

Spiritual experiences can be fostered in places of refuge and sanctuary. Refuge is withdrawal into a safe, sheltered, and protected asylum away from danger. Spaces like these can occur either indoors or outdoors and create opportunities for quiet solitude, peacefulness and relaxation, spiritual renewal, change in moods, reduced stress, and offer isolation from/with communicable diseases like COVID-19. Third places, such as coffee shops, hair salons, and malls, are places where people meet to socialize, express themselves, and support one another. These sanctuary spaces enrich social interaction, a sense of community, and belonging outside of the home and workplace.[91] They foster contentment with safe situations, a high degree of certainty, and a low degree of effort. Key benefits follow:

- Refuge experiences.
- Sanctuary spaces.
- Experiencing the range of wellness benefits.

Spirit of place gives meaning, value, emotion, and mystery to place, and in the context of this chapter, it gives health and wellness benefits. They are most often found in natural environments characterized by features with special geological, topological, hydrological, vegetation, landforms, or those with other visual character. They also occur in places where people live with special cultural, historic, ceremonial, symbolic, architectural, or aesthetic qualities. Spiritual benefits include connections to the spirit of place and the original cause. The beauty and energetic qualities of a special place can amplify, vitalize, charge, and inspire spiritual or transcendent experiences. Often these experiences are characterized by altered perceptions, feelings of connectedness, embodied narratives, and an ancient stirring of the archetypal first place. Sense of place has received considerable attention from social scientists in recent years, and research has indicated that a person's sense of place is influenced by several factors including the built environment, socio-economic status (SES), well-being, and health.[92] Key benefits follow:

- Spirit of place.
- The original cause/feeling.
- Soulful experiences.

Spiritual and existential issues are important factors for well-being and for influencing meaning in life and hope or positive emotions.[93] Spiritual experiences can produce opportunities to help address perplexing and existential issues in an ensemble of feelings in finding meaning while experiencing pain, physical and psychological limitations, and needs frustration. These experiences often spur one to ask questions like "What is the meaning of life?" or "Is there life after death?" There are existential concerns with fear and death, identity and meaning, emptiness and isolation, the unknown, and freedom.[94] Perplexing moments can be filled with difficulty, confusion, and uncertainty, as well as dealing with issues like life changes or climate crisis. According to the National Institutes of Health, we become aware of the existential dimension of health during times of illness.[95] Places of sanctuary, contemplation, caring, and healing qualities can help ease the anxiety and stress accompanying these moments. Key benefits follow:

- Existential issues.
- The unknown.
- Overcoming problems of modernity.

Spiritual healing spaces can contribute to purpose, meaning in life, and life satisfaction. Purpose is a journey that directs our actions and behaviors for life-long goals or simply for daily care. Research demonstrates that meaning is of great importance for mental as well as physical well-being and is crucial for health and quality of life.[96] Research has also found that life satisfaction is strongly correlated with health-related factors like chronic illness, sleep problems, pain, obesity, smoking, anxiety, and decreased physical activity.[97] Subjective well-being receives benefits from relationships, teamwork, and fulfilling work. Meaning in life has been defined as people's subjective judgments that their lives are marked by coherence, purpose, and significance, which emerge from the web of connections, interpretations, aspirations, and evaluations.[98] The progression from birth through death possess moments of celebration and reflection, and the context for life purpose. Key benefits follow:

- Life's meaning and purpose.
- Respecting life's progression and significance.
- Life satisfaction.

Religious and spiritual sites and sacred architecture have consistently had the intention to create a more fluid threshold and transcendent connection between heaven and earth, deity and human, and parish or community to religious institutions and belief systems. Non-theistic believers might see these places and the wellness benefits as opportunities to experience awe, wonder, nature, and the present. Especially charged spaces in many ways are similar to any other building requiring foundations, structure, heating and ventilating systems, and responses to fire regulations. Yet, there is an additional responsibility which is to create space that can become charged, possibly elicit transcendent experiences, and support health and wellness behaviors.

Sacred places, thin places, charged places, transcendent or wellness places often have a certain function or purpose that includes graves, cemeteries, burial grounds, purification and healing sites, sacred plant and animal sites, quarries, astronomical observatories, shrines, temples and effigies, fertility sites, mythic and legendary sites, historic sites, places of spiritual renewal, and healing and wellness. With the experience of such places there often is a "*cross state retention*" or a renewal that is remembered – a kind of spiritual accommodation. Places like the Maggie Centres located throughout the United Kingdom and in Hong Kong, Tokyo, and Barcelona are good examples of the combination of facilities designed for health, wellness, and spiritual growth. They were primarily designed by leading architects to create uplifting buildings

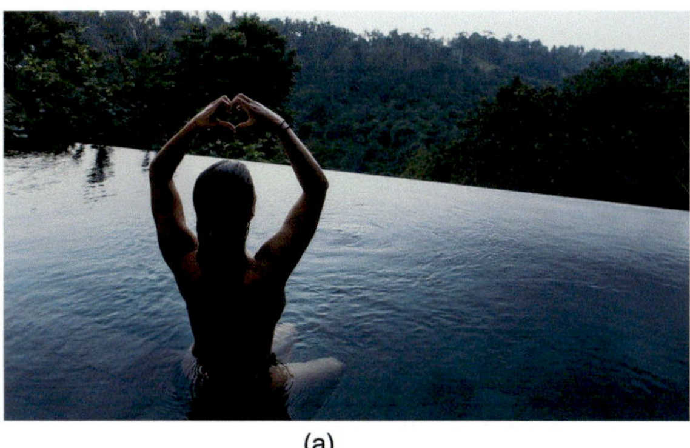

(a)

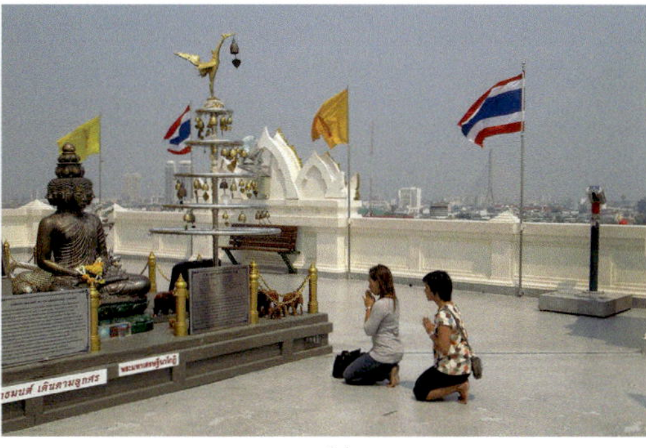

(b)

2.9
Spiritual Wellness
a) Quiet Moment in a Healing Water, b) Prayers at the Temple of the Golden Mount, Thailand

(*Source: Wikimedia Commons*)

to help people with cancer providing support, information, and practical advice. Their focus on good design were intended to help facilitate cancer treatment. Remebering that religious and spiritual benefits comprise two major experiential qualities, those that are ineffable (indescribable) and those that are noetic (possessing hidden or unexplainable knowledge). Refer to Figure 2.9 showing natural and architectural sacred wellness examples. Refer to Table 2.7.

Summary of wellness benefits

Physical wellness reduces the risk of heart diseases, supports positive moods, helps with sleep, and helps control weight. Cognitive wellness increases openness, optimism, curiosity, and participation in trusting relationships. Our emotional wellness helps in overcoming stress, strengthens social connections, builds resilience, and enables us to better cope with loss. With meaningful social connections, we can connect, make healthy choices, and develop better physical, mental, and emotional outcomes. Social places help overcome placelessness. From a financial health point of view, the benefits are understood as one's ability to manage expenses, prepare for and recover from financial shocks, have minimal debt, and provide the ability to build wealth. Although financial wellness underlies all facets of daily living such as securing food and paying for housing, there is inconsistency in the measurement and definition of this critical concept. Environmental wellness reduces pollutants, creates resilience against natural disasters, encourages positive connections to nature, supports physical activity, and supports biophilic patterns. Spiritual wellness gives us connections to a larger community and the world as a whole, greater peace of mind, calmness, and more meaning in life. Filtering through each of these benefit pillars, it becomes clear that certain wellness characteristics are common to each pillar, such as stress reduction, improved cognitive function, improved mood, increased connections to nature, improved life satisfaction, and increased life expectancy. However, a further look into each of the wellness pillars reveals more detailed wellness benefits. There are a host of health and wellness benefits that are a result of lifestyle choices and the environmental contexts within which we live.

The following list of more than 80 wellness benefits are extrapolated from the discussions of each of the previous benefit pillars. They are intended to provide a quick and condensed guide for planning and design purposes. The tables at the end of the chapter, 2.1–2.7, further summarize the wellness benefits relative to the wellness benefit pillars according to pro-individual, pro-social, and pro-environmental factors.

1. **Physical benefits**
   Increase physical activity (boosts energy).
   Physical performance Improvement.
   Bone and muscle strengthening and balance.
   Reduce inactivity and obesity.
   Enhanced social networking (reduces isolation).
   Improved nutrition (access to healthy food).
   Improved respiratory function.
   Improved heart health.
   Strengthened immune system.
   Improves sleep quality (restful and restorative sleep).
   Free radicals' reduction in oxidative stress.
   Mitigating measures of protections from natural disasters.
2. **Cognitive benefits**
   Increase cognitive ability and clarity of thinking.
   Improved memory and concentration.
   Increase focused attention and sustained attention spans.
   Addressing complex problems and situations.
   Reduction of mental stress (worry and tension).
   Increase in creative and logical thinking.
   Increase memory cues according to serial-position effect.
   Improved sleep at night and wakefulness during the day.
   Increase mental energy and less of a sense of fatigue.
   Improved mental performance at work and play.
   Cooperative social cognition and interactions.
   Reduction of cognitive temporal density (too much information, considerations, issues).
3. **Emotional benefits**
   Improve positive emotions and mood.
   Relief from depression and forms of mania.
   Emotional stress and anxiety reduction.
   Emotional resiliency and adaptability.
   Development of emotional intelligence.
   Increase serenity emotions (inner haven connectedness, present centeredness, silence).
   Reduction of emotional temporal density (too many ill feelings, considerations, issues).
   Increase present centeredness and presence.
   Reduction of insomnia and sleep disorders.
   Increase emotional effects of biophilia (love of nature, life forms, and natural processes).

Increase in life satisfaction.
Increase life purpose and meaning.

4. **Social benefits**

Increase in a sense of belonging to reduce a sense of loneliness and isolation.
Creating a sense of place and places that are cared for.
Improvement of cleanliness, maintenance, and aesthetics of the community.
Support engagement and interaction.
Enhanced social networking.
Defines boundaries of private and public to allow refuge and safety.
Increase altruism and beneficence through care of place and community.
Diminish placelessness which leads to vandalism of place and community.
Inspires creativity by creating a variety of experiences.
Increase life expectancy.
Increase emotional and compassionate empathy.
Increase respect for each other and every living creature.

5. **Financial benefits**

Expanding wellness economy, growth, and development.
Improve productivity and work effectiveness.
Increase return on investment.
Increase property value.
Reduced absenteeism, presenteeism, and turnover.
Increase retention and recruitment.
Enhancing and building on market distinction (wellness branding).
Economic well-being and relationship to personal finance.
Supports of the economy of scale.
Clustering of mixes of use creates synergy and accessibility.
Regenerative benefits (enhancing financial prosperity, social, and environmental wellness).
Cognitive and emotional stress and anxiety reduction.
Providing affordable wellness designs.

6. **Environmental benefits**

Improving connection with nature and opportunities for engagement in nature.
Utilizing sustainable, renewable, and healthy resources (energy, water, wind, geothermal, hydroelectric, biomass, rainwater, etc.).
Combating pollution, a cleaner environment (air, water, waste, soils, plant life, energy).
Reducing greenhouse gasses.
Increase carbon sequestering.
Improvement of public health.
Protecting the biodiversity of the planet so we live richer more vibrant lives.
Preserving ecological zones and processes.
Protecting existing forestland and restoring waterways.
Mitigating climate change.
Positive response to seasonal changes.
Mitigating natural disasters.

7. **Spiritual benefits**
   Experiences of beauty.
   Transformative from prosaic to transcendental.
   Connections to the spirit of place and the original cause.
   Increase opportunities for awe experiences.
   Increase opportunities for serenity experiences.
   Reduces mental and emotional stress and anxiety.
   Improves mental health.
   Creation of sanctuary spaces that allow us refuge.
   Can help address perplexing existential issues.
   Encounters with the unknown.
   Cross-state retention or accommodation.
   Gives purpose and meaning to life.
   Can lead to improved life satisfaction.
   Creation of healthy urban spaces (recreational, social, contemplative, spiritual).

Tables 2.1–2.7 serve to summarize the wellness pillars and their specific wellness benefits and serve as planning and design guidelines. The benefits can also serve to create wellness goals and policies. The tables list the key wellness benefits related to descriptions of pro-individual, pro-social, and pro-environmental associated with each of the benefit pillars. Since the planning, architecture, and interior design scales produce human-centered behaviors and practices, the benefits in these tables tend to favor pro-individual and pro-social behaviors, while the landscape scale favors pro-environmental behaviors.

BENEFIT	PRO-INDIVIDUAL BENEFIT	PRO-SOCIAL BENEFIT	PRO-ENVIRONMENTAL
Increased Physical Activity & Performance	After physical activity is improved cognition, reduced short-term anxiety, improved mood, and improved sleep. Physical activity also can help in weight management, reduction of health risks of heart disease and diabetes. Physical activity strengthen bones, joints and muscles.	Certain activities can increase confidence, peer acceptance, leadership skills and empathy. Exercise in groups can boost motivation, create accountability, build teamwork skills, enhance cognitive function, and builds community.	Green activity promotes physical wellness and can shape the quality and length of time of outdoor interactions. In turn our physical work in the environment can be instrumental in preservation, restoration, food production.
Reduced Inactivity and Obesity and Weight Management	Reduced inactivity means increased physical activity. This increases energy, balances caloric intake with burning, and decreases fat around the waist and total body. Combined with healthy dietary practices, the physical benefits are high.	Increase social networks decrease obesity risks. Another social benefit is overcoming the obesity stigma and associated discrimination. Pro-social relations can positively reduce obesity risk.	Removing environmental barriers and obesogenic environments can encourage walking, bicycle riding, accessibility to recreation areas and increase of physical activities. The lack of surveillance can also influence outdoor activity.

Improved Nutrition	This means a well balanced diet with reductions is fatty foods, sodium and sugar. Maintaining healthy eating habits, with produce variety and high fiber, optimize with higher meal frequency, and hydrate.	There are many social benefits surrounding nutrition and food. The more often people dine with others, the happier and more satisfied with their lives they are. Good eating habits are supported by social dining.	Locally grown plant-based foods reduce and sequester greenhouse gasses. Urban agriculture captures rainwater and mitigates the heat island effect.
Improved Heart Health	Heart health can be improved by physical activity, healthy diet, managed weight, reduced stress, and reduced cholesterol, blood pressure, and consumption of alcohol. Stop smoking.	Meaningful family connections, friendships and social interactions contribute to heart health. Healthy heart can translate into healthy lifestyle which can attract others.	Mitigation of natural disasters and extreme weather events can reduce stress and thereby reduce heart disease and stroke. This includes reduced exposure to pollutants and other environmental stressors.
Improved Respiratory Function	Respiratory function can be improved with regular physical activity and reduction of oxidative stress. Healthy lungs can shorten recovery times from infections, allergies, and influenza. They can improve the immune system.	Removing or isolating second hand cigarette smoke. With infectious diseases, wearing masks, employing social distancing and using cleaning protocols can reduce the spread within social contexts.	Air quality both indoor and outdoor ae important to respiratory health. Bacterial, viral and fungal infections can be spread in the environment.
Improved Immune System	Healthy immune systems protect against harmful microbes, pathogens, bacteria, fungi parasites, and certain diseases. Illnesses and wounds heal faster and there is less fatigue. Immune-supporting nutrition can contribute to immune health.	Suggests maintaining antiviral social environments and interactions. Healthy social relationships help strengthen the immune system. Adverse social experiences can cause isolation, threat and may suppress antiviral immunity.	The immune system is an organ that specializes in responding to environmental exposures. Protecting the immune system means maintaining clean, pollution-free environments.
Reduction of Oxidative Stress	Protects body and cells from free radicals thereby reducing the effects of heart disease, cancer and other lifestyle diseases. Healthy systems detoxify reactive products.	Modern lifestyles contribute to oxidative stress induction through consumption of processed foods, exposure to chemicals in the atmosphere, and lack of exercise.	The wellness benefit is removing negative environmental contributors to oxidative stress include radiation ultraviolet light, tobacco smoke, xenobiotics and other pollutants.

Table 2.1
Physical Benefits

BENEFIT	PRO-INDIVIDUAL BENEFIT	PRO-SOCIAL BENEFIT	PRO-ENVIRONMENTAL
Clarity of Thinking	Includes mindfulness and conscious awareness of the present moment. Increases perception of details within situations and the environment. Decreased distractions and increases performance, prioritization and decision making.	Increased performance is a teamwork and work-force benefit. Mental clarity tends to boost life satisfaction, wellbeing and phycological flourishing.	Easier to pay attention to natural stimuli. Nature helps in self-reflection and introspection thereby aiding in a mental "re-set."
Focused Attention & Concentration	Focused attention can be selective and discriminating and occur over time resulting in improved prediction and task completion. Concentration enables faster comprehension and task focusing with improved memory.	Attention can be directed to others fostering empathy skills, inner-group mindfulness, and emotional intelligence. Focused attention can contribute positively to group prosociality.	Focused attention and concentration can be improved with time spent in nature. Nature's fascination and mystery affects attention restoration, mental fatigue and concentration.
Coping Mechanisms to Address Complex Issues	Cognitive coping is using mental activity to manage stressful events or situations. Responses include gaining perspective and situational appraisal, and creating resolution and problem-focused strategies.	Cognitive behavioral coping skills benefit social interactions. It refers to how we process, interpret and respond to different social signals.	Cognitive coping is particularly important during natural disasters and extreme weather events. Conversely, coping can take the form of reappraisal of the negative effects of human activity on the environment.
Trusting and Cooperative Relationships	The cognitive aspect of trust is trusting behavior motivated by good rational reasons. Cooperation results in a process with common purpose and benefit.	Describes situations and behaviors that contribute to others' welfare, and there is belief in someone else's competence, capabilities, reliability and dependability. Trust can improve social and economic interactions.	Concerns about environmental protection, habitat loss, and mitigation of climate change are outcomes of cognitive cooperation.
Experience of High Quality Sleep	Cognitive health can result in improved sleep which in turn affects gaining insights, integrating information, and facilitates memory consolidation.	Tends to facilitate outgoing behaviors and self confidence. Sleep helps with empathy and lessens aggression.	Sleeping outdoors can replenish oxygen levels, boost serotonin (improving mood, digestion and sleep), and relieve stress.

Improved Memory and Remembering	Memory is one of the most important cognitive processes effecting learning, conceptual processes, psycholinguistics, problem solving and decision making.	Language cognition related to memory supports pro-social behaviors. Research indicates a memory advantage for prosocial behaviors.	Helps overcome biospheric amnesia and reinforce the biophilic effect and our love of nature. People readily remember information processed to survival relevance.
Reduction of Mental Temporal Density	Reducing mental temporal density creates an openness with greater receptivity. This allows for a more grounded experience that is present-centered. Being present activates the mind for a fuller experience.	Reducing temporal density allows for more perceptive and connected social interactions. One is a better listener with increased mental acuity.	Temporal density fosters stronger and more meaningful connections to nature. The environment benefits through increased knowledge about the environment, biospheric values, and positive actions behaviors.

Table 2.2
Cognitive Benefits

BENEFIT	PRO-INDIVIDUAL BENEFIT	PRO-SOCIAL BENEFIT	PRO-ENVIRONMENTAL
Positive Emotions and Improves Mood	Improves health and wellness through improved mood and the experience of happiness. Positive moods include calmness, optimism, curiosity, and contentment. They lead to lower heart rates, reduction of stress and anxiety, immune system support, and better sleep cycles.	Social interactions improve moods and self-esteem. Emotional openness supports social interactions, greater trust and empathy, beneficence and cooperation. Positive emotions promote helping behaviors.	Moods are improved by connections to nature, resulting in biospheric values, and positive lifestyle behaviors and changes. Moods are affected by personal environments. Good moods are supported by natural light, outdoor views, order, cleanliness and comfort.
Stress and Anxiety Reduction	Reduction of short term stress can improve breathing, heart rate, sleep cycles, and can improve appetite. Reduction of longer term anxiety can relieve persisting uneasy feelings, restlessness, panic and fear, and lower blood pressure.	Social support can positively affect stress and anxiety with the forms of listening, advice, guidance, empathy, encouragement, assistance, and even financial help. Supportive connections are linked to lower levels of depression and workplace burnout.	Experience of nature can believe stress and anxiety. Both solitude and silence can contribute to positive emotional shifts. Biospheric values can lead to lifestyle shifts that reduce stress o the environment.

Emotional Resiliency and Intelligence	Ability to recognize, adapt and manage emotions can lead to positive wellness benefits. Having the resilience to transform negative emotions to positive ones. The emotional intelligence reflects self-awareness and the ability for self-management.	Emotional intelligence can lead to social awareness, improved communication with others, and reduction of conflict. It improves empathy. Improves social skills. Can contribute to creating a culture of emotional wellness.	Understanding the environmental influences that affect emotional intelligence can lead to greater biopheric values and action behaviors.
Positive Effects of Serenity and Silence	Serenity experiences foster trust, connectedness, life perspective, a sense of belonging and contribute to present centeredness. It signifies an inner haven that is a safe space for healing and wellness.	The social benefits derive from the serenity experience of self-loss, connectedness and sense of other. Serenity is positively related to pro-social behaviors and negatively related to [physical and verbal aggression.	The environmental influences to serenity experiences includes quiet, physical safety, non-toxic materiality, peaceful places and usually places of natural beauty.
Reduction of Temporal Density and Increase Presence	Reducing temporal density creates an openness with greater receptivity. This allows for a more grounded experience that is present-centered. Being present activates all the senses for a fuller experience.	Reducing temporal density allows for more perceptive and connected social interactions. One is a better listener with increased empathy. Peer presence increases pro-social behavior.	Temporal density fosters stronger and more meaningful connections to nature. The environment benefits through increased biospheric values, positive actions behaviors, and love of nature.
Increase Emotional Effects of Biophilia	The love of nature produces positive emotional effects, reduces stress, supports cognitive function, improves the immune system, improves cardiovascular function, and improves mood and psychological health.	Biophilia nourishes social interactions in many forms and outdoor shared experiences, and reinforces a sense of connectedness. Nature-based color elicits calm, natural light boosts mood, and plants reduce stress and promote kinder behavior.	Produces strong biospheric values and pro-environmental behaviors. It expands the sense of self beyond the individual to the environment and world as a whole.
Increase Life Satisfaction and Purpose	More hopeful meaning in life positively affects life satisfaction, which in turn reduces stress caused by painful events, and improves abilities to cope with adversities, uncertainty, and psychological distress.	Higher life satisfaction can increase altruism, generosity, and volunteerism. Shared activities and experiences fostered connectedness, increased safety and reduced crime also contribute to life satisfaction.	The vastness of awe experiences, the peacefulness of serene environments, and the sheer beauty and wonder of nature contribute to life satisfaction and wellbeing.

Table 2.3
Emotional Benefits

BENEFIT	PRO-INDIVIDUAL BENEFIT	PRO-SOCIAL BENEFIT	PRO-ENVIRONMENTAL
Sense of Belonging	Belonging helps overcoming loneliness and supports human organization and a sense of purpose, and provides protection, and helps reduce depression, anxiety and suicide. It contributes to life satisfaction and longevity.	Belonging socially reinforces alliances, friendships and support. Social isolation, loneliness and low social status can harm a person's subjective sense of well-being. Belonging supports meaningful community activities.	People and communities can benefit from positive experiences of nature, and the environment can facilitate social interactions.
Increase Altruism and Beneficence	Altruism is good for emotional wellbeing, and promotes physiological changes in the brain linked with happiness. It promotes kindness and acts of goodness.	Altruism increases social support. It also promotes prevention and removal of harm from others. The intentional voluntary pro-social behavior benefits others.	Pro-environmental behaviors and eco-centric worldviews can be motivated by self-interest, altruism or benevolence.
Increase Cooperation	Social wellness occurs through cooperation as it contributes to openness, trust and safety. Balanced reciprocity gives social support and reduces stress.	In social contract theory, cooperation contributes to consensus building, group decision making, and work effectiveness.	Cooperative behavior encourages global sharing of knowledge and the ability to tackle shared problems, like climate change.
Networking, Social Support and Inner Circle	Wellness support reduces stress, decreases physical health problems, and improves emotional well-being. Maintaining an inner circle creates mutual support, improves mood and self-esteem.	Inner circles have a positive impact and contribute to increasing personal and social growth. An inner circle is a healthy pro-social context with support, caring, motivation, and invigorated self-awareness.	Social connection and social media in particular can raise environmental awareness.
Emotional and Cognitive Empathy	Feeling the same emotion that another person is feeling and seeing things from another person's perspective, understanding why and how they are interpreting and responding to events taking place.	Maintaining deep human connections and empathy allow us to thrive by providing vital social support and encouragement. More accurate knowledge about others increases the quality of empathy.	Higher levels of empathetic connections to nature can improve environmental behaviors and commitments.
Sense of Place and Community Building	Encourages socialization, meaningful connections, engagement, and wellbeing. There is a shared sense of coherence and identity with common interests.	Building community creates physical and social environments that are safe, open and meaningful, and allow for shared experiences and opportunities to learn from one another.	There are many environmental benefits to sustainable behaviors, land revitalization, community gardens and urban agriculture, and the health effects of lower greenhouse gas emissions.

Longevity	Longevity is effective by loneliness and social isolation with higher risk of disease, disability, and mortality. People with strong social connections live longer.	In older age, a diverse friend group can also help protect healthy cognition and is associated with greater longevity.	The environmental quality and daily contact with nature can extend life. Environmental factors effecting longevity include atmospheric pressure, temperature, percentage of sunshine, and humidity.

Table 2.4
Social Benefits

BENEFIT	PRO-INDIVIDUAL BENEFIT	PRO-SOCIAL BENEFIT	PRO-ENVIRONMENTAL
Expanding Wellness Economy	The wellness economy includes public health prevention and personalized medicine, traditional and complementary medicine, personal care and beauty, health nutrition, mental health, wellness real estate, wellness tourism, and wellness physical activities.	Financial wellness includes many social benefits. Circular economy supports wellness economic activities around materials, products and services. Certain wellness sectors of the economy support pro-social benefits, such as, tourism, nutrition, and personal care and beauty.	Earth-friendly business practice benefits the environment. Circular economies produce reductions in energy usage, greenhouse emissions, and the need for the production of new materials. Wellness benefits include increase biodiversity and limits to habitat disruption.
Wellness Real Estate	Wellness real estate is a fast growing sector of the wellness economy. The sector includes residential commercial, leisure, hospitality, fitness centers and medical properties. Wellness property and design features are becoming more desirable and accessible at all price points.	Wellness property and design feature intentional wellness elements that are desirable and accessible at all price points. Wellness lifestyle real estate is in response to holistic health in buildings. Mixed uses, good school districts and amenities improve real estate markets.	Encourages environmental engagement and endangerment. Realization of the cost benefit of environmental measures. Minimizes negative impact on environment. Reducing carbon dioxide emissions through biophilic and sustainable planning.
Return on Investment	Positive ROI including residential commercial, leisure, hospitality, and medical properties. Wellness property and design features are becoming more desirable and accessible at all price points. ROI is helped by material durability, reuse, and recycling.	People are increasing the value of healthy lifestyles. Positive ROI is helped by material durability, reuse, and recycling. Acting pro-socially enhances perceptions of luck and increases financial risk-taking.	Incentives may include tax credits for environmental and sustainable designs. Environmental investments can produce long-term benefits.

Increased Productivity and Performance	Wellness can produce higher energy levels and more efficiency. It produces produces less stress, less burnout, lower turnover, higher levels of satisfaction and an increased productivity.	Wellness has a positive impact on productivity relative to efficiency, belonging, teamwork, and life satisfaction, and positive social work environment positively effects productivity.	Air quality, noise, lighting and temperature control effect production. Green jobs can create new and emerging occupations that arise to address environmental sustainability needs and pro-environmental behaviors.
Reduced Absenteeism	Causes are low motivation, lack of direction, illness, mental health issues, and stress. Overcoming absenteeism produces financial returns, increases morale and production, stress reduction in the work environment.	Absence has a ripple effect that impacts their workload, their team, and management. Reducing presenteeism through appreciation, collaboration, and encouraging wellness activities.	Reduction of negative environmental factors, especially pollution effects absenteeism.
Distinctive Marketing	Distinctive marketing branding is another benefit of financial wellness, by having unique, scarce, beneficial or unusual wellness places, they become more identifiable and therefore economically attractive.	Wellness branding can build trust with customers, increase your market share, and drive sales.	Strong connections to place and nature can foster distinctive marketing.
Financial Well-being	Debt and financial issues can cause stress, sleep loss, headaches, high blood pressure and depression. Financial wellness creates more security and control, can improve life satisfaction and prevent hardships.	Social support can relieve stress. Wellness financial social relationships gain more respect, trust and help exacerbate economic hardship.	Aligning personal finances and green lifestyles can produce positive impacts on the environment. Low hazard environments can contribute to financial well-being.

Table 2.5
Financial Benefits

BENEFIT	PRO-INDIVIDUAL BENEFIT	PRO-SOCIAL BENEFIT	PRO-ENVIRONMENTAL
Access to Nature	Improves health and wellness through increases in physical activity and energy, stress reduction and improved respiratory function, improved mood and emotional wellbeing, and improved nutrition. Outdoors triggers stimulation of the eye retina.	Provides opportunities for social interaction through recreation, organized sports, chance encounters, and direct contact with nature. Experience of happiness, subjective wellbeing, and existential benefits.	Sense of connectedness, biospheric values, and supports heightened awareness of environmental problems and the need to change human lifestyle behaviors. Fosters appreciation and environmental stewardship.

Reduce Pollution	Personal responsibility of conservation of natural resources and waste recycling practices. Elimination of use of red-list materials. Improved personal health in terms of respiratory and cardiovascular function, and air borne allergies.	Incorporation of community-based waste recycling systems. Greater opportunity for socialization with healthy clean environments. Reduced absenteeism. Noise reduction encourages social interactions.	Reduction of use of toxic resources and fossil fuel based resources, industrial practices and consumer products. Reduced pollution helps enable biodiversity and improves community and business image and loyalty. Reduction of night light pollution encourages night walking.
Conservation and Natural Resource Utilization	Developing individual and family conservation practices saving resources and money. Provides clean air, water and energy, and improved health and wellness (physical, mental, emotional and spiritual wellbeing).	There are financial benefits to natural resources utilization. Protection of resources for future generational use. There are economic benefits through job creation for the manufacture and servicing natura systems' technologies.	Development of conservation practices, reduction of commercialism, and increase use of renewable resources like solar, wind, geothermal, biomass, and hydroelectricity provides cleaner air, water and energy, increases biodiversity, and habitat protection.
Response to Climate Change & Natural Disasters	Reducing negative effects of global warming and natural disasters, and creating safe environments during extreme weather events. This includes passive survivability measures.	Provision of community resilience and passive survivability measure for public safety and health. Creation of pro-social behaviors during times of crisis.	Reduced to degradation to the natural environment, sea levels destructive consequences of natural disasters. Mitigation can protect habitats. Preparedness saves lives, protects property and speeds up recovery.
Protecting Biodiversity & Habitat Protection	Provides food and medicinal plant security. Provides opportunities for recreation, relaxation, education, and stress relief. Inspires a sense of wonder and connectedness	There are socio-economic benefits through recreation, tourism, storm resilience, and natural education. Contributes to place identity. Increases natural capital.	Creates healthier soils, water and air and medicinal plants. Conservation protects pharmacopeia and medical knowledge. Wildlife protection benefits the ecosystems win which they live.
Response to Changing Seasons	Eating locally produced seasonal foods have higher nutritional value, have better taste, reduction of the decline in vitamin C, folate and carotenes. Strengthens the immune system.	Can provide signals for particular leisure, recreation, and economic activities. Supports local small businesses and can increase property value.	Reduces carbon emissions using less harmful chemicals and pesticides. Changing seasons effects the type and diversity of food that is propagated in a given location.
Safe Healthy Urban Spaces	Improves mental health, reduces anxiety and stress, and reduces depression. Provides opportunities for pedestrianization, chance encounters, and physical activity. Improves quality of life.	Supports a sense of community and placebound identity. Provides opportunities for passive and active gathering and social interactions. Increase of economic opportunities. Increase of social tolerance with crime reduction.	With greenspaces, increase of greenhouse gas sequestering and enhancing the biophilic effect. Negates the heat island effect. Provides sunshading.

Table 2.6
Environmental Benefits

BENEFIT	PRO-INDIVIDUAL BENEFIT	PRO-SOCIAL BENEFIT	PRO-ENVIRONMENTAL
Spiritual Renewal	Spiritual renewal can occur in a variety of contexts with differing functions or purposes. It is an inner connection to holiness and inclusivity. Benefits include a renewed sense of purpose and inner peace.	Spiritual renewal reinforces shared purpose, the feelings and welfare of other people, and value of community and civic behaviors fostering compassion. Develops stronger connections to others.	Spiritual insights can promote pro-environmental behaviors related to value-belief-norms, which suggest that the environment has value, may be endangered and is worth preserving.
Transcendent Experiences	Transcendent experiences create enhanced perception where the senses are heightened, there is a sense of synchronicity and an extrasensory awareness. These experiences can allow one to transcend beyond the present context.	Transcendent experiences can lead to a recognition of our interconnection and shared humanity. This in turn promotes altruism, empathy, cooperation and generosity. Shared group transcendent experiences can be powerful, like a music event.	Self-transcendent emotions are often triggered by intense absorption of nature and in turn elicits pro-environmental behaviors and biospheric values.
Awe and Serenity Emotions	Awe experiences are vast and elicit ineffable wonder and fascination. Serenity experiences are peaceful, tranquil, even sedating and free from anxiety. Accommodation to both experiences comes in the form of mental and emotional readjustment.	Pro-social outcomes of awe and serenity experiences increase generosity, helpfulness, compassion, and enhanced collective concerns. They also included concerns for the rights, feelings and welfare of other people.	Awe and serenity help in developing biospheric values, sensitivity towards improving environmental conditions and paying attention to negative impacts.
Refuge and Sanctuary	Spiritual experiences can be fostered in places of refuge and sanctuary. Refuge contributes to peace of mind, present-centeredness, and stress reduction. Sanctuary from disasters, storms and disease.	Refugee places offer asylum for groups of people who have been displaced, including sanctuary cities. Immigrant and displaced sanctuary experiences build pro-social connections.	Environmental awareness arises form the need for refuge and sanctuary from disasters, violent storms and communicable diseases. This also includes sanctuary for wildlife.
Spirit of Place and Original Cause	Spiritual benefits include connections to the spirit of place and the original cause. The locational experience is safe, identifiable, vital and up-lifting. It's a connection to our beginnings.	Places endowed with certain energies, historic significances, cultural values, and beauty attract people creating pro-social behaviors. Celebrations and rituals with others can strengthen a sense of place.	Spirit of place refers to the special and energetic qualities of a particular place that contributes to a re-enchantment and appreciation of the larger environment.

Addressing Perplexing and Existential Issues	Spiritual experiences can produce opportunities to help address perplexing and existential issues. Questions like what is the meaning of life? Is there life after death? They are concerned with existence and purpose of life.	Existential issues help people to better understand themselves in relation to others in the world. Perplexing moments can be caused by relationships and connections to community and sharing with others can reduce stress.	Provides some understanding of the complex issues surrounding the world, the environment and existential questions of our collective roles.
Purpose, Meaning and Life Satisfaction	Spiritual healing spaces can contribute to purpose, meaning in life and life satisfaction. Purpose gives motivation and direction. Meaning gives comprehension and understanding of one's life. Life satisfaction is a benefit of wellbeing.	Optimism stemming from life satisfaction can spread to pro-social behaviors, empathy, and increased cooperation and generosity. Subjective wellbeing receives benefits from relationships, teamwork and fulfilling work.	Positive environmental conditions and experiences correlate to happiness and life satisfaction.

Table 2.7
Spiritual Benefits
© Phillip James Tabb, 2023

NOTES

1. Gesler, Wilber M., *Healing Places, (Lanham, MD: Rowman & Littlefield Publishers, 2003*).
2. Piff, Paul, Pia Dietze, Matthew Feinberg, Daniel Stanccato, & Dasher Keltner, *Awe, the Small Self and Prosocial Behavior*, (Accessed November 10, 2023), https://www.apa.org/pubs/journals/releases/psp-pspi0000018.pdf
3. Kopec, Dac, *Person-Centered Health Care Design* (New York, NY: Routledge, 2021), p. 248.
4. Buettner, Dan, *Blue Zones: 9 Lessons for Living Longer From the People Who've Lived the Longest* (National Geographic, 2012).
5. Moorthy, Kailas & Valentina Cereda, "Wellness Benefits, Chapter 2," *Wellness Architecture and Design Pathways*, Global Wellness Institute, 2023.
6. Kopec, Dac, *Person Centered Health Care Design*, (New York, NY: Routledge, 2021), p. 22.
7. Centers for Disease Control and Prevention, (Accessed September 23, 2023), https://www.cdc.gov/physicalactivity/basics/adults/index.htm#:~:text=Each%20week%20adults%20need%20150%20minutes%20of%20moderate-intensity,to%20the%20current%20Physical%20Activity%20Guidelines%20for%20Americans.
8. Niemiro, Gracem, Ayesan Rewane, & Amit Algotar, *Exercise and Fitness Effect on Obesity*, (Accessed September 22, 2023), https://www.ncbi.nlm.nih.gov/books/NBK539893/
9. Pachucki, Mark & Elizabeth Goodman, *Social Relationships and Obesity: Benefits of Incorporating a Lifecourse Perspective*, (Accessed June 6, 2023), https://www.ncbi.nlm.nih.gov/pmc/articles/PMC4512667/
10. World Health Organization, *Obesity and Overweight*, (Accessed November 2023), https://www.who.int/news-room/fact-sheets/detail/obesity-and-overweight
11. *Nutritional Psychology*, (Accessed September 20, 2023), https://www.nutritional-psychology.org/2021-study-shows-a-complex-relationship-between-diet-physical-exercises-and-mental-wellbeing/
12. National Institutes of Health, (Accessed September 22, 2023), https://www.nhlbi.nih.gov/health/heart/physical-activity/benefits#:~:text=When%20done%20regularly%2C%20moderate%2D%20and,levels%20in%20your%20blood%20rise

13. American Lung Association, (Accessed September 22, 2023), https://www.lung.org/lung-health-diseases/wellness/exercise-and-lung-health
14. Physical Activity, Cardiorespiratory Fitness, and Cardiovascular Health: A Clinical Practice Statement of the ASPC Part I: Bioenergetics, Contemporary Physical Activity Recommendations, Benefits, Risks, Extreme Exercise Regimens, Potential Maladaptations, *American Journal of Preventive Cardiology*, (Accessed November 30, 2023), https://www.ncbi.nlm.nih.gov/pmc/articles/PMC9586848/
15. Yang, Jia, Ciang Li, Taiyu He, Fagyuan Ju, Ye Qui & Zuguo Tian, *Impact of Physical Activity on COVID-19*, (Accessed November 24, 2023), https://www.ncbi.nlm.nih.gov/pmc/articles/PMC9657212/
16. Healthline, (Accessed September 23, 2023), https://www.healthline.com/nutrition/does-exercise-boost-immune-system#exercise-and-immunity
17. National Library of Medicine, (Accessed September 23, 2023), https://www.ncbi.nlm.nih.gov/pmc/articles/PMC5908316/#:~:text=An%20acute%20level%20of%20exercise,antioxidant%20defense%20system%20%5B137%5D
18. Eger, Horst, Klaus Hagen, Birgitt Lucas, Peter Vogel, & Helmut Viot, T*he Influence of Being Physically Near to a Cell Phone Transmutation Mast on the Incidence of Cancer*, (Accessed November 20, 2023), https://www.readkong.com/page/the-influence-of-being-physically-near-to-a-cell-phone-6949353
19. Buettner, Dan, *Live to 100: Secrets of the Blue Zones,* (Accessed September 1, 2023), https://www.netflix.com/title/81214929
20. Kopec, Dac, *Person Centered Health Care Design* (New York, NY: Routledge, 2021), p. 25.
21. World Health Organization, *Brain Health*, (Accessed November 17, 2023), https://www.who.int/health-topics/brain-health#tab=tab_1
22. World Health Organization (Accessed June 4, 2023), https://www.who.int/health-topics/brain-health#tab=tab_1
23. National Institutes of Health, *Assessment in Work Productivity and the Relationship with Cognitive Symptoms*, (Accessed September 23, 2023), https://www.ncbi.nlm.nih.gov/pmc/articles/PMC6676443/
24. Calcott, Rebecca, *How Does Motivation Influence Attention? It Depends on the Context*, (Accessed June 5, 2023), https://sanlab.uoregon.edu/2013/10/20/how-does-motivation-influence-attention-it-depends-on-the-context/
25. Sandi, Carmen, *Stress and Cognition*, National Library of Medicine, (Accessed September 23, 2023), https://pubmed.ncbi.nlm.nih.gov/26304203/
26. National Library of Medicine, *Trust and Cooperative Behavior: Evidence from the Realm of Data-Sharing*, (Accessed December 17, 2023), https://www.ncbi.nlm.nih.gov/pmc/articles/PMC6703688/
27. National Institutes of Health, *Trust is for the Strong: How Health Status May Influence Generalized and Personalize Trust*, (Accessed September 23, 2023), https://www.ncbi.nlm.nih.gov/pmc/articles/PMC10486567/
28. National Institutes of Health, *Sleep and Cognition*, (Accessed September 23, 2023), https://www.ncbi.nlm.nih.gov/pmc/articles/PMC5831725/
29. Farhud, Dariush & Zahra Aryan, *Circadian Rhythms, Lifestyles and Health: A Narrative Review*, (Accessed November 17, 2023), https://www.ncbi.nlm.nih.gov/pmc/articles/PMC6123576/
30. National Institutes of Health, *Memory, Forgetfulness, and Aging: What's Normal and What's Not?* (Accessed September 23, 2023), https://www.nia.nih.gov/health/memory-forgetfulness-and-aging-whats-normal-and-whats-not
31. *Serial-position Effect*, (Accessed January 25, 2024), https://en.wikipedia.org/wiki/Serial-position_effect
32. Steele, John, *Geomancy: Consciousness and Sacred Sites* (New York, NY: Trigon Communications, 1985). And, (accessed November 20, 2023), http://threadsofspiderwoman.blogspot.com/2013/09/john-steele-kali-yuga-and-temporal.html

33. Toshi, Nikita, *Overthinking – To What Extent Can It Damage Your Life?* (Accessed January 25, 2024), https://pharmeasy.in/blog/overthinking-to-what-extent-can-it-damage-your-life/
34. Kellert, Stephen R., *Biophilic Design: The Theory Science and Practice of Bringing Buildings to Life* (Hoboken, NJ: Wiley & Sons, 2008), p. 14.
35. *APA Dictionary of Psychology*, (Accessed September 15, 2023), https://dictionary.apa.org/cognitive-functioning
36. Buettner, Dan, (Accessed September 1, 2023), https://www.netflix.com/title/81214929
37. National Institutes of Health, *Emotional Wellness Toolkit*, (Accessed June 1, 2023), https://www.nih.gov/health-information/emotional-wellness-toolkit
38. Kopec, Dac, *Person-Centered Health Care Design* (New York, NY: Routledge, 2021), p. 251.
39. Meade, Elaine, *6 Benefits of Happiness According to the Research*, (Accessed June 4, 2023), https://positivepsychology.com/benefits-of-happiness/#:~:text=Scientific%20studies%20have%20begun%20to,when%20overcoming%20illness%20or%20surgery.
40. Mayo Clinic, *Stress Management*, (Accessed September 24, 2023), https://www.mayoclinic.org/healthy-lifestyle/stress-management/in-depth/stress-relievers/art-20047257
41. Goleman, Daniel, *Emotional Intelligence: Why it Can Matter More than IQ* (Bantam Books, 1996).
42. Roberts, Kay & Cheryl Aspy, *Development of a Serenity Scale*, (Accessed August 20, 2022), https://www.researchgate.net/publication/15347724_Development_of_the_Serenity_Scale
43. Steele, John, *Geomancy: Consciousness and Sacred Sites* (New York, NY: Trigon Communications, 1985).
44. Wilson, Edward O., *Biophilia* (Cambridge, MA: Harvard University Press, 1984).
45. Ryff, C. D. (1989). Happiness is Everything, or is it? Explorations on the Meaning of Psychological Well-being.
46. Buettner, Dan, *Live to 100: Secrets of the Blue Zones*, (Accessed September 1, 2023), https://www.netflix.com/title/81214929
47. Positive Psychology, *What is Social Wellbeing? 12+ Activities for Social Wellness*, (Accessed June 1, 2023), https://positivepsychology.com/social-wellbeing/
48. Altruism, Happiness, and Health: It's Good to be Good, *International Journal of Behavioral Medicine*, (Accessed September 24, 2023), https://greatergood.berkeley.edu/images/uploads/Post-AltruismHappinessHealth.pdf
49. National Institutes of Health, *Sense of Belonging, Meaning Daily Life Participation, and Well-Being: Integrated Investigation*, (Accessed September 24, 2023), https://www.ncbi.nlm.nih.gov/pmc/articles/PMC10002207/
50. Altruism, Happiness, and Health: It's Good to be Good, *International Journal of Behavioral Medicine*, (Accessed September 24, 2023), https://greatergood.berkeley.edu/images/uploads/Post-AltruismHappinessHealth.pdf
51. *Stanford Encyclopedia of Philosophy*, The Principle of Beneficence in Applied Ethics, (Accessed November 10, 2023), https://plato.stanford.edu/entries/principle-beneficence/
52. Holmes, Bob, *Why People Choose to Cooperate, According to Behavioral Science*, (Accessed November 11, 2023), https://www.pbs.org/newshour/science/why-people-choose-to-cooperate-according-to-behavioral-science
53. National Institutes of Health, *Identifying with All Humanity Predicts Cooperative Health Behaviors and Helpful Responding During COVID-19*, (Accessed September 25, 2023), https://pubmed.ncbi.nlm.nih.gov/33690679/
54. CDC, *How Does Social Connectedness Affect Health?* (Accessed November 11, 2023), https://www.cdc.gov/emotional-wellbeing/social-connectedness/affect-health.htm
55. American Psychological Association, *Manage Stress: Strengthen your Support Network*, (Accessed September 25, 2023), https://www.apa.org/topics/stress/manage-social-support
56. Lesley University, *The Psychology of Emotional and Cognitive Empathy*, (Accessed September 25, 2023), https://lesley.edu/article/the-psychology-of-emotional-and-cognitive-empathy

57. CED, *Healthy Community Design*, (Accessed November 10, 2023), https://www.cdc.gov/healthyplaces/docs/Healthy_Community_Design.pdf
58. McMillan, David & David Chavis, *Sense of Community: A Definition and Theory*, (Accessed November 11, 2023), https://aacimotaatiiyankwi.org/2022/05/10/benefits-of-community-building-for-mental-health/
59. Catholic Health Association, *How Community-Building Aligns with Public Health*, (Accessed September 25, 2023), https://www.chausa.org/publications/health-progress/archive/article/september-october-2011/how-community-building-aligns-with-public-health
60. NIH, *Healthy Habits can Lengthen Life*, (Accessed November 11, 2023), https://www.nih.gov/news-events/nih-research-matters/healthy-habits-can-lengthen-life
61. Greater Good Science Center, *How Our Social Lives Impact Our Health*, (Accessed September 25, 2023), https://greatergood.berkeley.edu/article/item/how_your_social_life_might_help_you_life_longer
62. Turner, Terry, *Financial Wellness*, (Accessed June 2, 2023), https://www.annuity.org/personal-finance/financial-wellness/
63. Global Wellness Institute, *What is the Wellness Economy?* (Accessed June 10, 2023), https://globalwellnessinstitute.org/what-is-wellness/what-is-the-wellness-economy/
64. Global Wellness Institute, *Wellness Lifestyle Real Estate & Communities: Definitions and Core Principles*, (Accessed November 11, 2023), https://globalwellnessinstitute.org/what-is-wellness/what-is-wellness-lifestyle-real-estate-communities/
65. Consumer Financial Protection Bureau, *Why Financial Well-being?* (Accessed September 26, 2023). According to the US Consumer Financial Protection Bureau, https://www.consumerfinance.gov/consumer-tools/financial-well-being/about/, financial well-being is having financial security and financial freedom of choice in both the present and future.
66. Bergeron, Paul, *Wellness Real Estate Market Nearly Doubles in Last Few Years*, (Accessed November 11, 2023), https://www.globest.com/2021/09/30/wellness-real-estate-market-nearly-doubles-in-last-few-years/?slreturn=20231011094116
67. DiGuiseppe, Anthony & Sherry Fong, "Financial Wellness, Chapter 4," *Wellness Architecture and Design Pathways*, Global Wellness Institute, 2023.
68. CDC, *5 Proven Strategies for Decreasing Employee Absenteeism*, (Accessed September 25, 2023), https://blog.hubspot.com/marketing/absenteeism
69. Diener, Edward, *Happiness: The Science of Subjective Well-Being*, (Accessed November 11, 2023), https://nobaproject.com/modules/happiness-the-science-of-subjective-well-being#:~:text=Subjective%20well%2Dbeing%20(SWB),with%20other%20types%20of%20measures.
70. Tabor, Barbra, *Scientific Journal Publishes HERO Study on Leadership Views About Workplace Wellness*, (Accessed September 25, 2023), https://hero-health.org/wp-content/uploads/2015/07/NR_HERO_TAHP_FINAL_072315.pdf
71. Ryan, Catie, Bill Browning, & Dakota Walker, *The Economics of Biophilia: Why Designing with Nature in Mind Makes Financial Sense,* (Accessed November 30, 2023), http://www.terrapinbrightgreen.com/wp-content/uploads/2023/09/EOB2-Terrapin-2023-p.pdf
72. Callaghan, Shaun, Martin Losche, Anna Pione, & Warren Teichner, *Feeling Good: The Future of the $1.5 Trillion Wellness Market*, (Accessed September 25, 2023), https://www.mckinsey.com/industries/consumer-packaged-goods/our-insights/feeling-good-the-future-of-the-1–5-trillion-wellness-market
73. American Public Health Association, *The Impacts of Individual and Household Debt on Health and Well-Being*, (Accessed November 11, 2023), https://www.apha.org/Policies-and-Advocacy/Public-Health-Policy-Statements/Policy-Database/2022/01/07/The-Impacts-of-Individual-and-Household-Debt-on-Health-and-Well-Being
74. WebMD, *How to Feel Less Anxious About Money*, (Accessed September 25, 2023), https://www.webmd.com/balance/features/the-debt-stress-connection

75. Singh, Onkar, *What is Regenerative Finance (RdFi)? A Beginner's Guide*, (Accessed November 29, 2023), https://cointelegraph.com/learn/what-is-regenerative-finance-refi
76. Tabb, Phillip, *Biophilic Urbanism: Designing Resilient Communities for the Future*, (New York, NY: Routledge, 2001).
77. Robbins, Jim, *Ecopsychology: How Immersion in Nature Benefits Your Health*, (Accessed November 11, 2023), https://e360.yale.edu/features/ecopsychology-how-immersion-in-nature-benefits-your-health
78. Pereira, Marybeth & Peter Forster, *The Relationship between Connectedness to Nature, Environmental Values, and Pro-environmental Behaviours*, (Accessed September 25, 2023), https://warwick.ac.uk/fac/cross_fac/iatl/reinvention/archive/volume8issue2/pereira/
79. Union of Concerned Scientists, *Benefits of Renewable Energy Use*, (Accessed June 3, 2023), https://www.ucsusa.org/resources/benefits-renewable-energy-use
80. Correll, Robyn, *How Environmental Health Impacts Our Quality of Life and Health*, (Accessed September 25, 2023), https://www.verywellhealth.com/what-is-environmental-health-4158207
81. American Psychological Association, *Recovering Emotionally from Disaster*, (Accessed September 25, 2023), https://www.apa.org/topics/disasters-response/recovering
82. World Health Organization, *Biodiversity and Health*, (Accessed September 25, 2023), https://www.who.int/news-room/fact-sheets/detail/biodiversity-and-health
83. Kelly, Brielle, *Seasonal Living for Better Health*, (Accessed September 25, 2023), https://www.wellbeing.com.au/body/health/seasonal-living-for-better-health.html
84. Toderian, Brent, *Let's Make Sticky Streets for People!* (Accessed September 25, 2023), https://www.planetizen.com/node/69454
85. Predojevic, Anja, *Spiritual Wellbeing*, (Accessed June 1, 2023), https://www.stress.org.uk/spiritual-wellbeing/#:~:text=Spiritual%20wellbeing%20ultimately%20represents%20our%20connection%20to%20ourselves,art%2C%20literature%2C%20nature%20or%20something%20greater%20than%20oneself.
86. VanderWeele, Tyler, *Spirituality Linked with Better Health Outcomes, Patient Care*, (Accessed June 8, 2023), https://www.hsph.harvard.edu/news/press-releases/spirituality-better-health-outcomes-patient-care/
87. Tabb, Phillip James, *Thin Place Design: Architecture of the Numinous*, (New York City, NY: Routledge, 2024).
88. *Transcendence and Wellbeing*, (Accessed September 24, 2023), https://www.mybestself101.org/transcendence-well-being
89. Yaden, Kaufman, Hyde, Chirico, Gaggioli, Zhang, & Keltner, *The Development of the Awe Experience Scale (AWE-S): A Multifactorial Measure for a Complex Emotion*, (Accessed October 4, 2021) https://psycnet.apa.org/record/2018–35661-001
90. Roberts, Kay & Cheryl Aspy, *Development of a Serenity Scale*, (Accessed August 20, 2022), https://www.researchgate.net/publication/15347724_Development_of_the_Serenity_
91. National Institutes of Health, *Closure of 'Third Places'? Exploring Potential Consequences for Collective Health and Wellbeing*, (Accessed September 24, 2023), https://www.ncbi.nlm.nih.gov/pmc/articles/PMC6934089/
92. National Institutes of Health, *Sense of Place and Health in Hamilton, Ontario: A Case Study*, (Accessed September 24, 2023), https://www.ncbi.nlm.nih.gov/pmc/articles/PMC3400750/
93. Beneficial Effects of Spiritual Experiences and Existential Aspects of Life Satisfaction of Breast and Lung Cancer Patients in Poland: A Pilot Study, *Journal of Religious Health*, (Accessed November 24, 2023), https://www.ncbi.nlm.nih.gov/pmc/articles/PMC9569296/#:~:text=Spiritual%20experiences%20can%20have%20a,emotions%20(Galen%2C%202018).
94. Kretschmer, Madeline & Lance Storm, *The Relationship of the Five Existential Concerns with Depression and Existential Thinking*, (Accessed January 24, 2024), https://www.meaning.ca/web/wp-content/uploads/2019/10/216-13-513–4–10–20180704.pdf

95. National Institutes of Health, *Suffering a Healthy Life – On the Existential Dimension of Health*, (Accessed September 24, 2023), https://www.ncbi.nlm.nih.gov/pmc/articles/PMC8830493/
96. Haugen, Gorill & Jessie Dezutter, *Chapter 8, Meaning-in-Life: A Vital Salutogenic Resource for Health*, (Accessed November 20, 2023), https://www.ncbi.nlm.nih.gov/books/NBK585665/#:~:text=Studies%20have%20shown%20a%20significant,with%20illness%2C%20crises%20and%20death
97. Strine, Tara, Daniel Chapman, Lina Balluz, David Moriarty, & Ali Mokdad, *The Associations Between Life Satisfaction and Health-related Quality of Life, Chronic Illness, and Health Behaviors among U.S. Community-dwelling Adults*, (Accessed June 8, 2023), https://pubmed.ncbi.nlm.nih.gov/18080207/
98. National Institutes of Health, *Sense of Belonging, Meaningful Daily Life Participation, and Well-Being: Integrated Investigation*, (Accessed September 24, 2023), https://www.ncbi.nlm.nih.gov/pmc/articles/PMC10002207/

3 WELLNESS URBAN DESIGN STRATEGIES

INTRODUCTION

In response to extreme weather conditions, climate change, natural disasters, air and water pollution, ubiquitous presence of automobiles, lack of access to nature, and many other negative impacts of the existing built environment, there are concerns about the future wellness of contemporary culture. Planning and design strategies can produce benefits that can help overcome these negative effects of certain planning decisions, lifestyle choices and the adverse qualities of the built environment. Health and wellness are inextricably linked to place. While most of our apparent concerns and efforts to improve the built environment were directed toward sustainability, they in fact focused upon correcting what John Ehrenfeld called "*unsustainability*," that is the unsustainable technologies, buildings and design practices, and continued consumer-oriented living styles.[1] This also includes the lifestyle choices we make that affect our health and wellness. Mainstream values and consumption patterns continue to dominate the production, use, and disposal of goods, and are the proximate cause of the damage to the environment. According to Robbie Hammond and Omar Toro-Vacay, the role of the city has been reimagined countless times over the centuries (cities have been trading posts, political and artistic centers, and, more recently, concrete jungles of retail and offices). But the pandemic served as a wake-up call for just how unwell our cities are – sparking a new recognition of the entangled relationship between the health of the cities and the health of city dwellers.[2] It is cities and the regions within which they exist that pose the greatest challenges and the greatest potential solutions that can influence all scales of wellness.

Urban design wellness is broad in its application extending from buildings and communities to cities and eco-regions, influencing the relationship between the built environment, and the health of the Earth's biosphere and natural systems. This includes the wellness-determinants directed toward human population growth and migration patterns, settlement configurations, means of energy production, transport, infrastructure design, large-scale food production and nutrition, and the need for access to nature and responsible use of natural resources.[3] Planetary health was defined by the Rockefeller-Lancet Commission of Planetary Health as "*the health of human civilization and the state of the natural systems on which it depends*."[4]

The tendency to spend the majority of our time indoors, for some as much as 90%, has separated us from direct experiences of nature. This, coupled with poor

DOI: 10.4324/9781003472902-3

indoor air and water quality, has exacerbated the problem. Inactivity, poor diet, and increased stress have even further disconnected us from achieving high levels of wellness. A response for improved health and wellness can occur with improved planning and design solutions that include the incorporation of certain wellness design principles, design patterns, material choices, and intentional connections to nature. Before a project moves into its planning or design phases, robust goals and objectives should be established through a process of defining the project purpose and understanding human health and wellness needs. Since wellness strategies can be applied to all scales of development, it is important to reinforce connections to produce synergetic effects.

The island of Singapore has envisioned itself as a garden city, which in 1965 initially took the form of a tree-planting initiative and a national parks system. Later the vision of a garden city changed from a "*garden in the city*" to a "*city in a garden*," bringing gardens, natural green spaces, and biodiversity to every resident. With this conceptual shift, the Singapore Park Connector Network (PCN) was created and today is an innovative "*green matrix.*" It provides recreational and greenspaces along underused land and existing infrastructure along roads, canals, and railroads. Taken together, the wellness strategies combine to reinforce the concept of Singapore as a city in a garden, a powerful biophilic and well-being strategy. This occurs equally at the building, streets, neighborhood, city, and island regional scales. Refer to Figure 3.1a showing the preponderance of greenspace integrated into the urban fabric.

In Singapore, wellness planning occurs with the intimate knowledge of, and interaction with, the local environment, natural ecological processes, and its inhabitants. It becomes a pathway for self-understanding and a sense of belonging. Wellness strategies are also being implemented, including strengthening the conservation of wetland biodiversity in northwestern Singapore. This includes the protection of habitats, including mangroves, freshwater marshes, and mudflats to maintain strong accessible connections to urban areas. Surveys conducted by the National Parks Board show that residents are not only using the parks and networks for recreation, physical activity and commuting, but also for social gatherings. In addition, preserving the enormous parkland contributes to a positive climate reduction of carbon dioxide and the production of oxygen. Wellness industries have also

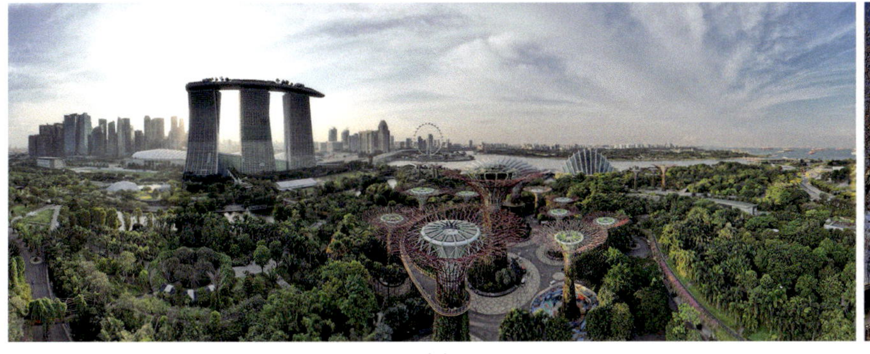

(a)

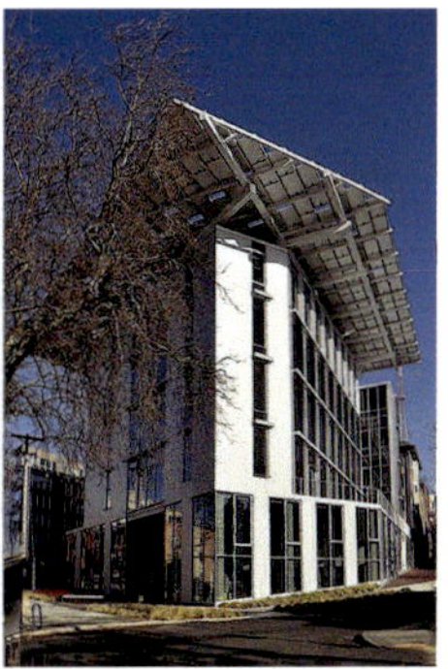

(b)

3.1
Wellness Strategies
a) Singapore Aerial Photograph,
b) Bullitt Center

(Sources: Shutterstock and Wikimedia Commons)

flourished in Singapore within the real estate, recreational, workplace, health care and beauty, traditional and preventative medicine, nutrition, and wellness tourism sectors.[5]

Another example of urban-scale wellness strategies is the Bullitt Center in Seattle, WA, USA. Located on an urban street corner, the Bullitt Center was largely considered to be the most sustainable commercial building in the world at its completion. Propelled by a mission to "drive change" in the marketplace faster and further occurs by showing what's possible today. This significant project began as an intention from its founder, David Hayes, to show what was possible in modern buildings with entirely "off-the-shelf" products so the result would be easily repeatable.

> *To really change the market, the economics of the project had to support it. Today's reality is that economic policy promotes environmental decay. Between negative externalities, discount rates that dictate impermanence, and codes and incentives that favor the status quo, the market frequently demands products and services that leave society worse off.*[6]

By setting a significant goal and adhering to purpose, Hayes and his team were able to achieve the goals of the Living Building Challenge, one of the most stringent certification schemes available to date. Some of the individual wellness elements that led to this success include pedestrian-, bicycle-, and public transport-friendly elements, centrally placed stairways for an active lifestyle, equitable daylighting, operable windows, and a pocket park. Refer to Figure 3.1b showing the Bullitt Center.

The opportunities that emerge from setting a clear and focused purpose early in the planning and design processes, and prioritizing this purpose during all steps of the life of a project are largely overlooked in many city comprehensive planning processes, real estate developments, and architectural projects. Treating each step as an effective strategy for the industry as a whole, rather than an interesting anecdote from a niche market sector, can provide significant value for developers in the long run.[7] The planning and urban design scales offer endless opportunities to influence well-being through wellness lifestyle patterns.

WELLNESS BENEFITS

Wellness is a multi-dimensional set of pursuits, activities, choices, and lifestyles that lead to a state of holistic health, and at the planning and urban design scale, they set the dynamic context for health outcomes. The wellness planning and design benefits are based on the physical, mental, emotional, social, financial, environmental, and spiritual categories. They have been identified through decades of evidence-based health and wellness scholarly and scientific research. Places like the Pontevedra city center in Spain; Prairie Crossing, Illinois; Shearwater in St. Augustine, Florida; Serenbe Community in Georgia; and White Gum Valley in Western Australia show that wellness can be achieved at varying urban scales.[8]

Following is a brief recap of benefits summarized from Chapter 2 to help in relating health outcomes applicable to planning strategies:

- Physical wellness – *lowering stress and blood pressure, improved respiratory function, increased physical activity and energy, lower obesity levels, weight management, increased healing rates, improved circadian cycles, lower addictions, and improved nutrition.*
- Mental wellness – *improving cognitive ability and appraisal, increased focus and clarity of mind, increased resilience, reduced anxiety and negative thoughts, ability for awareness of the present moment (mindfulness), increased attention restoration and soft fascination, and reduced temporal density.*
- Emotional wellness – *maintaining healthy relationships, improved mood, lower stress levels, the experience of positive emotions (awe, serenity, contentment, wonder, and joy), resilience and positive coping, and experience of inner peace.*
- Social wellness – *creating community, increased social interactions, generosity, mutualism, empathy, compassion, helpfulness, and enhanced collective concern. Social wellness creates a sense of safety, belonging and security, with increased life expectancy, and the experience of pro-social behaviors.*
- Financial wellness – *increasing efficiency and productivity, increased job performance, reduced absenteeism and presenteeism, positive return on investments, increased facilities due to economy of scale, and reduced stress over financial matters and security.*
- Environmental wellness – *producing and experiencing lower air pollution and greenhouse gas emissions, cleaner water, greater access to nature, an increase of biophilic effects, improved biodiversity and regenerative processes, disaster mitigation, and pro-environmental and biospheric behaviors.*
- Spiritual wellness – *addressing of existential questions, increased self-transcendence, experience of wholeness, positive sense of solving problems, invigorated meaning and purpose in life, spiritual arousal, and increase of life satisfaction.*

WELLNESS STRATEGIES

Wellness strategies are a mutually supporting set of design approaches that serve as prime actionable elicitors of wellness benefits promoting individual physical health, positive emotional responses, mental clarity, pro-social behaviors, environmental reparation, and spiritual renewal, as defined in Chapter 2. The wellness design strategies are intended to positively influence human health and wellness outcomes, preserve the natural environment, and incorporate specific approaches to the built environment. The strategies are generally planning schemes, physical concepts, design patterns, attributes, and elements associated with the particular scales of application. Across each scale they occur within primary, secondary, and tertiary design responses from larger overarching patterns like renewable infrastructure systems and preservation of large natural areas, to medium responses like wind towers and fountains, and smaller details like shutters, fans, and even a house plant.

These wellness strategies share an important correspondence with sustainability, resiliency, biophilia, and sacred place design as they seek similar positive outcomes for our health and well-being. Most of these strategies are established on science-based outcomes within the public health, health sciences, and environmental psychology fields. Four scales have been selected which are the planning scale, architectural scale, interior scale, and landscape scale. The strategies described in this chapter are neither meant to be exhaustive nor to be the only ways to achieve the intended benefits. They are presented here more as a broader dive into the practical application of a discipline that is still in development and can be seen as in its infancy. The strategies have been shown to produce positive outcomes verified by scholarly and evidence-based research. Each strategy includes a basic description of the planning or design pattern, several examples that show how the strategy has been effectively applied in previous works, and then a list of the most pertinent wellness outcomes to be expected from applying the strategy. Strategies at the planning scale, in part, include and are defined by the following:

- Concepts – *planning schemes and strategies organized around zoning regulations, a masterplan or central idea with explicit goals oriented to health and wellness.*
- Patterns – *models after timeless and repeatable object-oriented planning approaches that are integrative, inclusive, and influence behavior.*
- Attributes – *an inherent and determinant quality describing the characteristics of development details supporting urban wellness.*
- Elements – *urban design scale plans comprised of wellness-oriented zoning revisions, building components, and design elements of parks, streetscapes, infrastructure schemes, water features, and carbon-sequestering materials.*
- Elicitors – *planning and design approaches that function to promote or trigger urban-scale wellness benefits and outcomes.*
- Physicality – *pro-wellness planning and zoning schemes, physical development designs, public spaces, streetscapes, and urban agriculture related to tangible physical and real designs.*

SCALES OF APPLICATION

Wellness planning and design outcomes are intended to include varying scales of application from city planning to intimate gardens. This is intended to provide the largest over-reach for wellness planning and design pathways. Within each scale, there are six to ten examples of useful strategies appropriate to that scale. Strategies applied at a larger scale will often support and influence wellness outcomes with progressively more systemic orders (such as more efficient infrastructure, renewable utilities, waste recycling and water management systems, and urban farming) while solutions applied at smaller scales involve building and landscape design elements (such as protected entries, overhangs, window coverings, non-toxic materials selection, and climate resistant landscaping) and are often more technological (such as installing HEPA air filters in an HVAC system to ensure interior air quality or the use of renewable technologies).

The more wellness-supportive choices made at each of the scales, such as choosing a project location and context safe from natural disasters to implementing biophilic design principles and renewable technologies, the greater the opportunities for wellness outcomes. The health and wellness benefits of the spiritual can also be applied to each of these scales, creating extraordinary places from protection of sacred rivers and historic sites to healing gardens and holy wells. It should be noted that while wellness strategies are most effective when applied to all scales, care should be given where certain strategies may impinge upon or conflict with another (such as the need for densification versus the requirements for solar access). It is the purpose here to provide, through these scales of application, a broad and encompassing set of wellness design strategies.[9]

- Urban design scale – *includes city planning, town planning, neighborhoods, mixed-use development, water management systems, urban parks, pastureland, agriculture, and infrastructure design.*
- Architecture scale – *includes building sites, buildings, climatic form responses, envelope design, fenestration schemes, building elements, material choices, building systems, and indoor-outdoor relationships.*
- Interior scale – *includes interior spatial quality, circulation patterns, furnishings, color, natural lighting and ventilation, and material selections.*
- Landscape scale – *includes connections to nature, parks, urban tiny forests, gardens, edible landscapes, vegetation, ground cover, water features, urban agriculture, and land art installations.*

It should be noted that there are scales both larger and smaller than these four including eco-regions, continents, and the Earth as a whole as well as the micro-worlds of fabrics, pigments, and the atomic level of matter. However, to inform planning and design these four scales have been selected. Each of the wellness strategies found within the four scales follow descriptions that articulate the wellness strategies that possess the wellness benefits toward the wellness outcomes. The STRATEGIES – BENEFITS – OUTCOMES relationship occurs when a strategy is a planning or design measure that provides the benefit of physical, emotional, mental, social, spiritual, financial, or environmental wellness, and the outcomes of specific positive health and wellness responses such as reduced stress, improved respiratory system, mental clarity, improved mood, spiritual renewal, improved productivity, and greenhouse gas sequestering. At the end of this chapter is a summary table describing the design intentions, wellness strategies, and their references.

At the urban design scale, the planning and design strategies address spatial organization and urban functional issues that affect the quality of well-being, human safety, and environmental protection. The urban design scale strategies address mitigating natural disasters and, more specifically, climate change. The introduction of renewable energy resources and infrastructure, carbon sequestering, and reforestation are also important biophilic strategies. Land use diversity and appropriate and useful mixes of use, density, integrated zoning, and urban growth by multiplication rather than by mere addition, are effective wellness approaches. Further strategies include modes of transportation, mobility and pedestrianization, reducing or eliminating the negative impacts of automobiles, creating livable communities and neighborhoods, the introduction of more parks and greenspaces, and finally creation of accessible urban agriculture.

URBAN DESIGN SCALE STRATEGIES

Health and wellness strategies at the planning scale involve considerations for cities, towns, and neighborhoods especially as they are affected by climate, natural hazards, water shortages, and social inequity. The strategies address planning considerations of climate change and location, density, mixes of use, responses to rain and storm-water, infrastructure efficiencies, low night light pollution, and mobility and pedestrianization with access to varying modes of transportation. This scale also considers agriculture and locally produced food. According to Fran Baum, "*The challenge for the twenty-first century is crafting an ecological public health in a way that acknowledges humans as part of the ecosystem, not separate from it and not central to it.*"[10] This suggests more integrative approaches to planning and human activities, especially in the context of health and wellness. Health and wellness benefits from strategies at the planning scale range from improved comfort and respiratory function to stress reduction and improved mental health. They benefit in particular ways as previously discussed in Chapter 2 with physical, psychological, mental, social, spiritual, economic, and environmental outcomes. The planning scale strategies in this section include ecologically responsive form, efficient and renewable infrastructure design, mixed-use zoning and provision of incubators, amenities, and social gathering places, access to public transportation with emphasis on pedestrianization, and community allotments and urban agriculture.

1. **Mitigating natural disasters and climate change**
   Natural disasters affect human habitation and survival, and are caused by the convergence of damaging phenomena and vulnerable human settlements. Natural disasters, such as the Indian Ocean tsunami (2004), Hurricane Katrina (2005), the Kashmir earthquake (2005), cyclone Nargis (2008), the Haiti earthquake (2010), the Tohoku earthquake and tsunami (2011), superstorm Sandy (2012), the Mount Everest avalanche (2014), Hurricanes Harvey, Irma, and Maria (2017), the Hawaii volcanic eruption (2018), the Australian wildfires (2019), and the global COVID-19 pandemic all contributed to a greater awareness of the reoccurring dangers of our relationship and proximity to threatening events. Mitigation strategies for natural disasters at the planning and urban design scale include rethinking locations of future population growth, especially near vulnerable areas near known hazards. Mitigation also means planning for passive survivability and maintaining critical life-support systems (power, water, food, and medical supplies). Planning involves the implementation of resilient communities with the ability to avoid and recover from disasters. Disasters may create different types of losses, many of which may be difficult to quantify, but include loss of property and well-being.

   Climate change and environmental degradation are also the consequences of our contemporary condition, a situation the public has recently recognized.

Human activity in cities and urban areas are the major causes of climate change, and they also hold the greatest opportunity to mitigate it. In 2023 in the United States, climate change affected both increases in summer temperatures especially in the southwest and increases in precipitation in the northeast. Global cooling in winter accompanies global warming and increasing low temperatures, and the number of storms and weather anomalies. Mitigation strategies for climate change at the planning and urban design scale include reducing and stabilizing greenhouse gas emissions in the atmosphere, and promoting renewable resources. This means reducing the burning of fossil fuels in the power, building, and transportation sectors. It also suggests CO_2 sequestering through surface material selection and urban landscaping. According to NASA, this also means adapting to life in a changing climate and reducing risk from the harmful effects of sea-level rise, extreme weather events, and food shortages.[11] Our adverse impact on the environment is not confined to climate change but also extends to other natural systems, giving rise to a complex dynamic of environmental destabilization that has already reached critical levels.[12] Climate change and environmental degradation are also the consequences of our contemporary condition; therefore, the location of new developments and maintenance of existing cities should carefully be considered especially in terms of climate and local ecological processes. Fortunately, most people live in temperate climate zones where there is less need for exaggerated climatic planning interventions. Other climate zones that experience greater extremes can have potential health and wellness risks most often due to droughts, tropical storms, and extreme temperature swings. Climate-related hazards include temperature change, precipitation intensity, windstorms, sea-level rise, and increasing severe weather events.

Examples of climate-oriented planning are focused on extreme polar and desert climates, as seen in Figures 3.2a/b/d, in contrast to the architecture and urban design in the mild Mediterranean climate of Santorini, Greece, Figure 3.2c.

Tromso, Norway is a built example of an extreme Arctic city planned in response to its cold climate characteristics and is a gateway to the north, Figure 3.2a. Summers are short, cool, and mostly cloudy and winters are long, freezing, snowy, windy, and overcast. Tromso is experiencing some effects of climate change with the melting of nearby glaciers, decreasing polar ice, and slightly increasing temperatures. Tromso has a population of over 77,000 inhabitants in which a large proportion of the population lives within the compact city center. Wellness benefits include close contact with beautiful nature including the midnight sun and Northern Lights. The majority of the city exists on the island of Tromsoy adjacent to Tromsoysundet strait. Its form is linear, somewhat compact, low and southeast facing, and protected by local hills to the northwest. The cold climate is a cause for more introverted living, which affects outdoor physical activity and social interactions. However, wellness occurs with its stunning nature, colorful buildings, solar access to south windows, healthcare system, national health insurance, the increase of biotech and health tech industries, high standard of living, and increased life expectancy.

The elemental and ambient environmental forces became potential form-givers as illustrated in Ralph Erskine's boreal climate image of "*Arctic City*" or in the design of his Villa Strom in Stockholm (1961) where its compact form, response to the low winter's sun, and wind-excluding devices responded to the severe sub-Arctic climate. Erskine's interest in climatic design led to his work on the Hedesunda Housing Cluster in Sweden, Figure 3.2b. Erskine's housing project in Hedesunda, built in 1989, employs a dramatic wind protection form concept. The houses have highly insulated shed roofs deflecting the wind over the cluster, while at the same time having the inner vertical façades opened up to views of the river Dalalven and south for passive solar energy gain. The north-side sloping roofs extend high on the interior side directing the cold winds up and away from the buildings and inner courtyard. For a project located in such a cold and inhospitable place, the design shares a response to the climatic conditions of the place while creating a warm sense of community in the inner form of the buildings.[13]

Located on the north end of the island of Santorini, the village of Oia is known for its quiet life, picturesque beauty, and fantastic sunsets. The crater-side buildings are terraced and cascade down the steep slope; on the outer perimeter, the land gently slopes to the Aegean Sea. At the top of the caldera is a pedestrian main street that connects to shopping and restaurants and enjoys sunset views. The overall landscape bears the aftermath of a volcanic eruption. Climatic planning responses are present in the village of Oia and are integrated to create a truly elemental urban environment. This is accomplished through the south-orientation of most dwellings and the high mass construction. Energy costs are high; it is windy and winter temperatures are chilly and humid. Small portable stoves are used for burning bush branches found on the island. Cooling is accomplished through the flywheel effect of the earthen caves and mass construction, and with the use of pergolas and canopies. Light-colored pavements and structures are employed to mitigate overheating from the intense sun. Primarily pedestrian in nature, in many ways it is difficult to articulate where buildings end and the urban fabric begins, Figure 3.2c.[14]

Design responses to arid climates are also important. The image in Figure 3.2d shows the compact city of Zarqa, Jordan. The name Zarqa means "the blue (city)" and once was a small Arab fortress, but now it is the third largest city in Jordan. The summers are long, hot, and arid while the winters are typically cold and mostly clear. The region receives very little rainfall with an annual average of 7.2 inches which is considered arid and comparable to the state of Nevada. The climatic design determinants for Zarqa include the relative density of built form, narrow streets, high mass construction, light-colored buildings, small fenestrations, window screens or shades, flat roofs, rooftop water storage, some rooftop terraces, and interspersion of tree shading.

The planning strategies include the creation of climate-responsive urban forms, the use of renewable infrastructure, movement systems, land use and density mixes, planning for solar gain or shading, and responses to natural disasters. The specific benefit pillars include physical, emotional, social, spiritual,

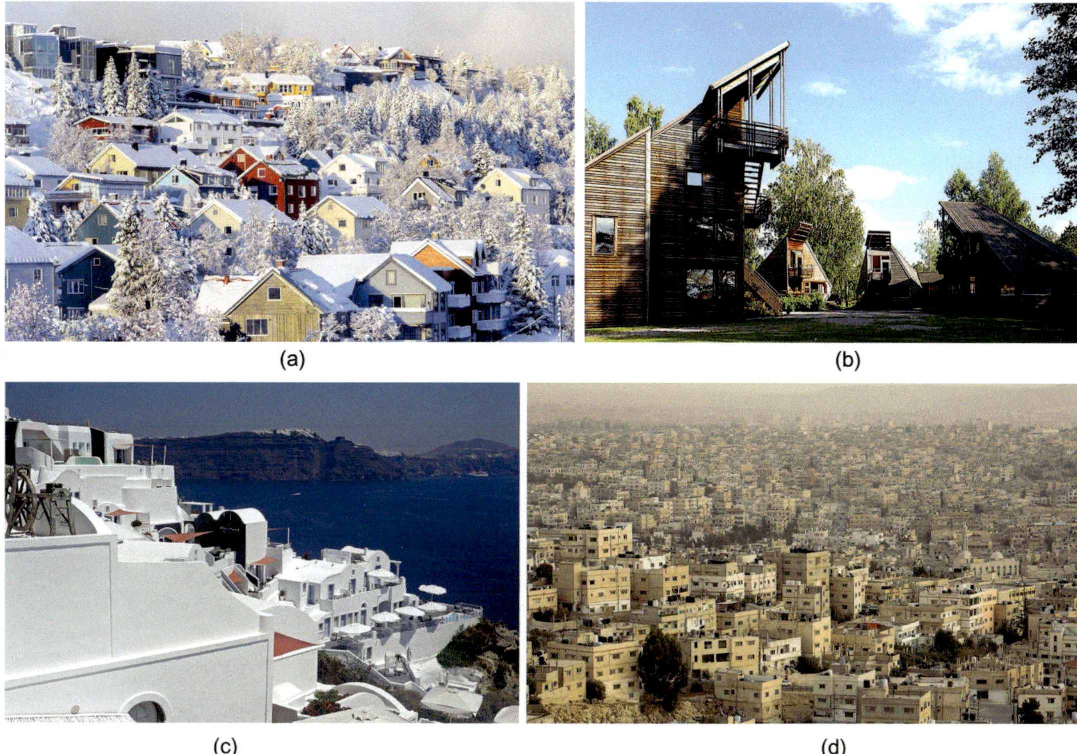

(a) (b) (c) (d)

3.2
Ecological Communities
a) Tromso, Norway,
b) Hedesunda Housing Cluster,
c) Santorini, Greece,
d) Zarqa, Jordan

(*Sources: Shutterstock and Wikimedia Commons)*

and environmental benefits. More specifically, strategies include natural disaster mitigation, maintaining infrastructure during disaster events, lower energy consumption, inclusion of nature within urban form, encouragement of social interactions, potentially lower operating and energy costs, cultural and spiritual connection to place, and pro-social and pro-environmental behaviors.

2. Renewable infrastructure

In the field of geography, infrastructure usually refers to the underlying structure of physical assets and services essential for society to function. This includes the basic spatial structure of buildings and the network of transport (roads, bridges, and subways), as well as electricity, gas, water, and sanitation connections. Green infrastructure encompasses water management including flooding, runoff, filtration, and capturing. The concept of renewable infrastructure is relatively new and is intended to provide for the basic human needs, and use renewable resources to drive the services, including solar and wind energy, geothermal heating and cooling, hydroelectricity, biomass, rainwater collection, storage and filtration, vegetated wetlands for waste treatment, and food production. The challenge is converting existing urban environments, that have been based upon fossil fuel technologies, into renewable infrastructures.

New York City's remarkable High Line Park (2009 and 2011) was designed in three sections by the landscape architecture firm, James Corner Field Operations with architects Diller Scofidio + Renfro. Theirs was a competition-winning proposal created as an aerial greenway elevated above the ground for one mile along Manhattan's West Side transforming the 1.45 mile (2.33 kilometer) section of the former New York Central Railroad spur running through the Chelsea Neighborhood, Figure 3.3a. Originally it was a massive public-private infrastructure project done in the 1930s called "West Side Improvement" that elevated dangerous freight trains 30 feet (9.1 meters) off the street level thereby avoiding conflict with pedestrians and cars on the ground below. The design was described as part promenade, part town square, and part botanical garden – an urban and nature integration or "*agri-tecture*."[15]

ReGen is a term for "regeneration," where the outputs of one system are inputs for another. In biology, it is the process of renewal, restoration, and new growth. ReGen is an integrated and resilient development, and an experimental model neighborhood of regenerative homes conceived in 2016 by James Ehrlich from Denmark. The village of homes, based upon ongoing resiliency research, is designed as energy positive with mixed renewable energy and storage systems, water harvesting and waste recycling, and high-yield organic food growing. Related specifically to wellness design, ReGen provides clean energy, water, and food production. The village design combines a network of farms, blue spaces, pedestrian connections, and regenerative infrastructure with mixes of use and social gathering places. Their concept of a *food hub* addresses the wellness benefits of nutrition, socialization, and emotional well-being. The benefits include encouragement of physical activity, stress reduction, positive social interactions, carbon sequestering, and healthy nutritious food.

ReGen village is located in Oosterwold, Netherlands on a 50-acre (25-hectare) site. The design by EFFEKT Architects enhances resilience against flooding, optimizes biodiversity, employs an integrated renewable infrastructure with water storage facilities and waste-to-resource systems, electricity production, and integrates local farming and food production. The nucleated planning nests around public spaces, vertical food production, and community programs with individual interconnected dwelling-greenhouses.[16] Taken together they form an off-grid neighborhood focused on sustainability, infrastructure, and well-being. Refer to Figures 3.3c/d for an aerial view of the Helsinge Haveby conceptual design and an infrastructure plan.

The renewable infrastructure strategies most likely will be incremental interventions to existing environments but can be incorporated within new planning developments. Specific strategies include the use of renewable energy, collection of rainwater, passive solar heating, photovoltaic solar farms, vegetated waste collection and purification, biomass systems, and geothermal heating and cooling, which are all interconnected into a renewable infrastructural system. Green infrastructure reduces and treats stormwater at its source, and mitigates flood risk by slowing and reducing stormwater discharge. The benefits include improved response to variable external climatic conditions, improved comfort, utilization of free natural resources and CO_2 sequestering, and the creation of resource independence. Specific benefits include stress reduction, lower financial costs and energy consumption, clean air and water, improved public health, and passive survivability solutions in response to natural disasters and severe weather conditions.

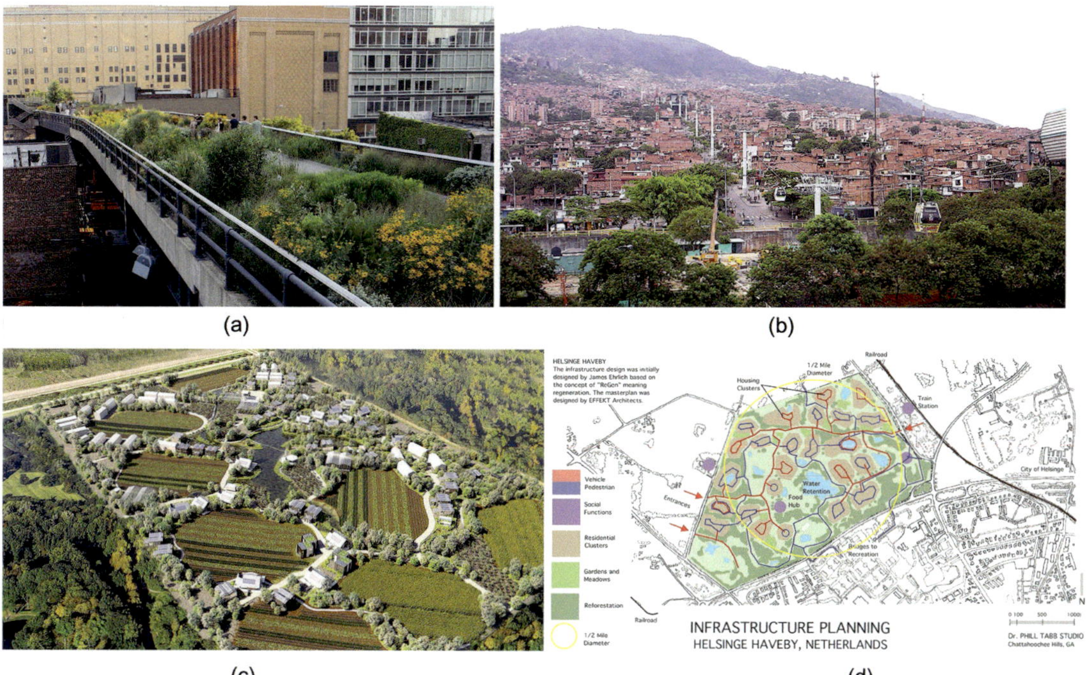

3.3 Renewable Infrastructure a) New York High Line Park, b) Medellin Gondola System, c) Helsinge Haveby Village, Netherlands, d) Helsinge Haveby Infrastructure Plan

(Sources: Wikimedia Commons, Wikipedia, and Phillip Tabb)

3. Land use diversity

Land use diversity, similar to biodiversity, is critical for urban vitality. This can be accomplished through the integration of residential with commercial, civic and recreational uses, and with the inclusion of nature. The benefits derive from the synergies, links, and accessibilities that are generated within an urban setting due to the integration of different goods, services, functions, and activities. In terms of wellness, mixed-use development promotes sustainability, safety, and wellness facilities. Land use diversity includes inclusionary zoning that seeks to promote affordability with employment and housing opportunities for workforce residents.

Seaside, Florida is a small resort community located in the Florida panhandle and is considered one of the first examples of the New Urbanism movement in the United States. Designed by Duany Platter-Zyberk, the planned design features a traditional town grid spatial structure, pedestrian walkways and alleyways, differing building types, and mixes of use. Houses are positioned close to the sidewalks and streets with no private front lawns, though they do have front porches. Most houses have rooftop terraces, decks, or rooms with views to the Gulf of Mexico. The mixes of use include several restaurants, a grocery store, an ice-cream shop, clothing stores, gift shops, a school, a chapel, swimming pools, recreation area, and a post office. This diversity of land use mixes contributes to gathering points, places of interaction, and a sense of community. The activities also contribute to pedestrianization with a diminished need for automobile use to get around.

Seaside is not strictly a residential community meaning that most residents are not permanent residents, rather they visit to experience the gulf and beaches as a second home or vacation destination resort. As such, there exist many health and wellness strategies that generate many benefits. These include pedestrian ease of movement through community walkability seaside activities, control of automobile traffic except on the main county road A-30, and stress reduction with the provision of many quiet places integrated into the physical plan and along the beach. Promotion of pro-social behaviors occurs through the many dining, shopping, and casual encounter opportunities for gathering, and pro-environmental behaviors due to the experience of the abundant sunshine, the elements, and particularly the Gulf of Mexico.

Another example of land use diversity is the village of Titchfield located on the south coast of England in the county of Hampshire. The urbanized portions of Titchfield occurred within a one-kilometer diameter circle and, according to the 1981 census, housed 2,517 people in 891 dwellings. For this population, there was a high degree of mixed use with 67 non-residential land uses, businesses and services, including two schools, four greengrocers, a grocery store, a chemist, medical surgery, a post office, a bookstore, a butcher, baker, hair salon, hardware store, two hotels, a parish church, gasoline station, and four pubs.[17] A photograph taken in 1840 showed the commercial businesses and trades that existed in the central square. They remain today almost intact and in the same locations. It is interesting to see the essential businesses and services necessary for basic everyday functioning clustered together with easy pedestrian access. The wellness strategies include the combination of its walkable density and inclusion of mixes of uses that are accessible, serve critical life-support functions, and the central village square and community green support social interactions. The river Meon and the landscape fingers provide close contact with nature.

Strategies for land use diversity include a move away from single-use zoning to integrated zoning that includes residential, commercial, cultural, institutional, open space, and residual uses including wellness-oriented goods, services, and businesses. This includes planning for closer connections of homes and residential areas to schools, grocery stores, health care facilities, and parks and recreation. This also means planning for public transportation networks, and pedestrian and bicycle movement connections. At the panning scale, sprawl development, redlining, and single-use zoning, as well as automobile-dominant spatial structures are considered detrimental to sustainability objectives and to human health and wellness.

The *15-minute city* which is a mixed-use planning concept that places critical daily necessities and services within a 15-minute walk, bike ride, or public transit ride from any point in the city.[18] Activities like work, shopping, groceries, education, healthcare, and leisure are accessible to all residents. This brings to the forefront the need for clear boundary articulations and the replication of goods and services on smaller scales. The replication of mixes of use could be alleviated to some degree by merchandise delivery services or by theming differing non-residential uses and distributing them over multiple neighborhoods or settlements. Multiplication is not a new concept as villages across the world were initially sustainable in this way when automobiles were not used.

In England for example, 10,000 villages were established in the Anglo-Saxon period (410–1066 AD) and were essentially self-sustaining. However, today, the 15-minute walk to goods and services is desirable in urban, suburban, and peri-urban contexts where people want walkable communities. The diagram in Figure 3.5c illustrates the multiplication of a series of 15-minute settlements as based on the work of Studio PDP. This could be a good model for future growth and densification in lower-to-moderate density locations.

The benefits of land use diversity and spatial mix include places for social interactions, uses accommodating critical needs, products, and services, use of natural resources and accommodating needs locally, with public spaces that respond to a range of users (children through older adults), reduced travel distances, and reduced reliance on the automobile to connect residential districts to critical life-support functions. It encourages synergies and accessibilities bringing together origins and destinations both in terms of concentrated as well as dispersed mixes. Research has shown that a higher mix of land uses or a balance of residential and retail uses generates more walking activity. They include the development of placemaking and community, improved response to variable external climatic conditions, improved connections, stress reduction, increased positive moods, financial benefits, and promotion of pro-social behaviors.

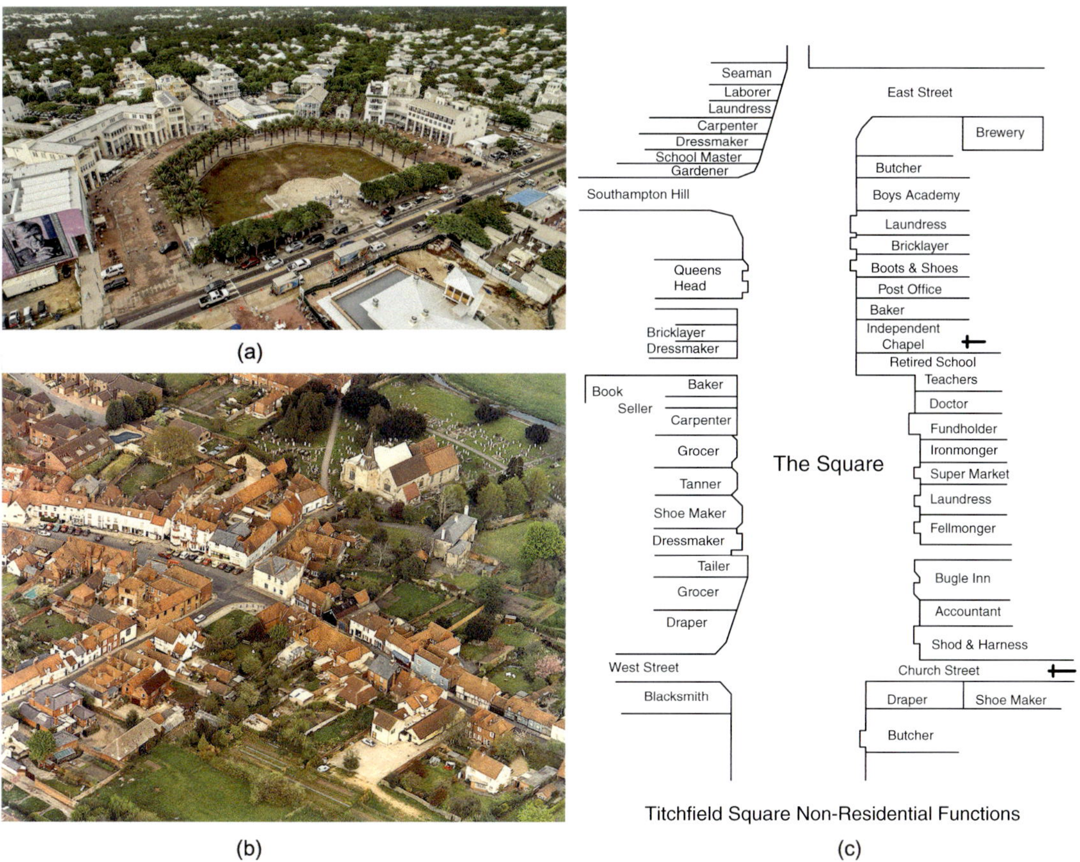

3.4
Land Use Diversity
a) Seaside, Florida,
b) Titchfield Village, UK in 1985,
c) Titchfield, UK in 1840

(Sources: Shutterstock and Phillip Tabb)

4. Growth by multiplication

Until the 1800s, the world's population was less than one billion people; in 1930 it doubled, and 30 years later it reached three billion. By the millennium it reached six billion, and by 2015 the world's population measured more than seven billion people. In that same year over a billion people migrated both within their own countries or abroad. The world population is projected to increase by more than one billion people within the next 15 years, reaching 8.6 billion in 2030, and projected to increase further to 9.8 billion by 2050 and 11.2 billion by 2100. Such growth will have an enormous impact on natural resources and increased consumption.[19]

"*Limits to Growth*" was a pioneering report modeling the interactions and consequences between natural and human-made systems.[20] It was another poignant warning that the growing world population was reaching the limits of its carrying capacity of finite planetary resource supplies. The pattern of exponential growth was analyzed using five variables: world population, industrialization, pollution, food production, and resource depletion.

An important dimension of growth is the actual method and form of the growth. According to architect Leon Krier, growth by addition expanded beyond the human scale.[21] This pattern usually begins at a center and expands outward in concentric circles, either by urban extension, unplanned sprawl, or by infill or conversion of nonurban to urban uses within the urban area. Isolated growth is characterized by development existing outside of the primary urban area. In the industrialized world, this process has been enabled by the automobile, which provides access to employment, education, shopping, and cultural activities.

However, another growth pattern occurs where community size reaches rational human limits, and then grows by a system of multiplication. This pattern suggests an optimum size based on nucleation and pedestrian access to goods and services. When this size is reached, it shifts to another location where the nucleation process begins again. Growth by gross addition might better be achieved through the intelligent multiplication of populations in sync with the carrying capacities of our local ecological regions. This, too, is referred to as "*systemic constellating urbanism*."[22]

One of the determining factors for the size of a settlement (campus, neighborhood, hamlet, small city) is the travel distance for walking and cycling between an urban or neighborhood center and the farthest outlying dwellings. According to the National Household Travel Survey, the average distance in the United States for a walking trip was 0.7 miles and a travel time of less than 15 minutes. The average bicycling distance is 2.3 miles and approximately 19 minutes.[23] For pedestrians at 15 minute and bicycles between 20- and 30-minute trips, the boundary limit can be determined for nucleated neighborhoods. The wellness effects of this pattern of urban form and the resulting pedestrianization are many. Refer to the diagram of Figure 3.5c that indicates a constellation of small, nucleated hamlets connected by a main road, bike paths, and pedestrian pathways. They become a network of wholes within wholes. Settlement land area can be increased in size while maintaining pedestrianization. This occurs with the introduction of public transport systems with access

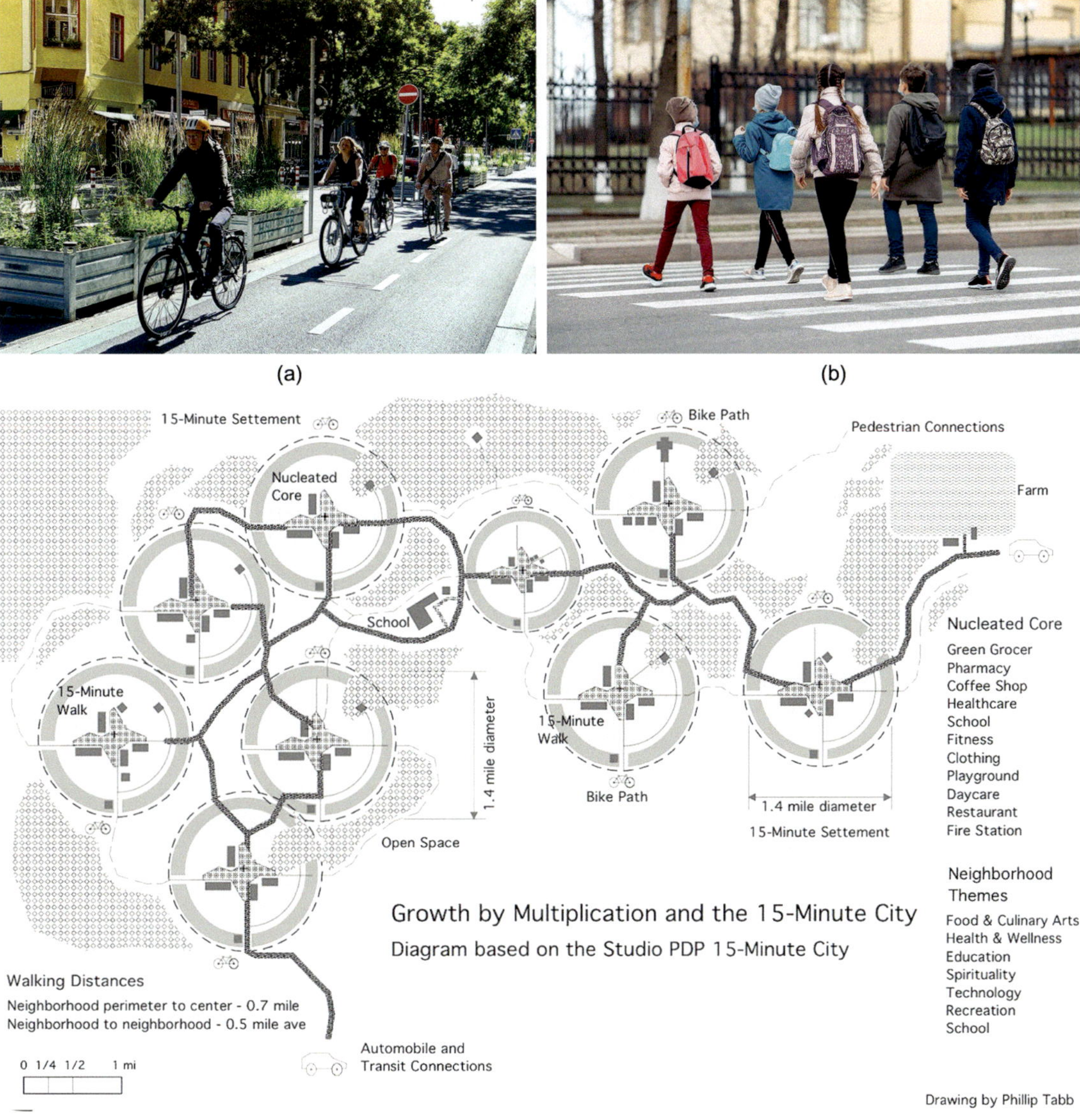

3.5 Growth by Multiplication a) Biking in the Neighborhood, b) Walking to School, c) Growth by Multiplication and the 15-Minute Cities Diagram

(Sources: Shutterstock, Phillip Tabb)

to all residential districts. Transit-oriented development is not a new idea, and there are compact, walkable, pedestrian-oriented, mixed-use communities centered around high-quality public transit systems.

A polynucleated scheme can occur with urban neighborhoods, suburban clusters, or with peri-urban perimeter settlements. Since this describes horizontal territory, the density can vary. Nucleated settlements and neighborhoods can accommodate both dispersed as well as concentrated mixes of non-residential uses. Principle benefits are the inclusion of mixes of use, especially if they represent critical, wellness, and sustainable life-support functions, closeness to agricultural land, increased pedestrianization, increased social interaction, creation of an identifiable sense of place, and increased access to nature and openspace. The wellness benefits include increased physical, emotional, and cognitive health, and support of pro-social and pro-environmental behaviors. If there is a variety of non-residential land uses spread throughout a network of nucleated settlements, then health services co-exist.

Figure 3.5c is a diagram of multiple neighborhoods designed to the 15-minute walking distance. While it is not a real design, it does indicate a theoretical concept of repeating walkable neighborhoods with nucleated centers, non-residential mixed-use themes, and a network of bike and pedestrian paths. Gilston villages near Harlow, UK is a good example of neighborhoods that are multiplied. It is planned for a buildout of 2,300 homes by Grimshaw Architects. This network of villages is part of a larger UK plan to relieve overcrowding around London and provides for some 200,000 new homes across the country. The villages and neighborhoods will incorporate a mix of uses including retail, commercial, institutional, educational, parklands, and employment opportunities as well as affordable housing. There will be extended bus services and extensive bicycle and pedestrian networks. The villages are surrounded by agricultural land, and portions will be designated for biodiversity and wildlife habitats.

5. **Mobility and pedestrianization**

Mobility is an important, if not critical, human need and within the urban environment, it takes on many different modes from walking, biking and golfcarts to automobiles, high-speed trains, and airplanes. From a health and wellness point of view, those modes that support greater physical activity are healthier. Automobile traffic is both a curse and a blessing as it creates danger and stress while also creating convenient and quick connections. Creating people-centered city planning, superblocks, pedestrian walkways and zones, low-traffic neighborhoods, the 15-minute city, and car-free urban spaces are increasing in numbers across the world.[24] The benefits are many with reduced air pollution and greenhouse gas production, lower stress, increased access to nature, improved streetscape aesthetics, and greater safety and opportunities for social interaction. The 15-minute city concept is a strategy in which mixed-use zoning and pedestrian mobility are planned in such a way as to provide critical daily necessities and services within a 15-minute walk or 20-minute bike ride. That is access to shops, schools, doctors, the gym, parks, restaurants, and other cultural activities. This strategy aims to reduce automobile dependency, promote healthy and sustainable living, and increase quality of life.

Pontevedra is a city located in the northwest of the Iberian Peninsula in Spain and has a long history of maritime trade. By the end of the 1990s, Pontevedra was dominated by automobile traffic and congestion, especially within the historic city center not designed for it, and was considered dirty and dangerous. Pontevedra is known for its aggressive urban planning strategy of pedestrianization of its historic city center and creating an automobile-free environment. The plan incrementally limited the use of automobiles and service vehicles and reduced speed limits. One can cross the entire city in 25 minutes. The purpose was to make the city more accessible, especially to the most vulnerable, senior citizens, children, and those who were handicapped. The city estimates that automobile use has dropped 77% and CO_2 emissions have decreased by 66%. Now people walk. Family-centered services have moved from outside to within the city center. Schools, maternity and pediatric services, libraries, cultural activities, and children's boot camps have either remained or have been relocated into the city center.[25] Wellness benefits include increased physical activity, less noise and stress, abundant social meeting places, increased birthrates, and greater access to nature.

The Millennium Footbridge in London is another example of a pedestrianization wellness strategy. Opened in 2000, it functions to connect Bankside with the City of London 1,066 feet (325 meters) across the river Thames linking on axis with St. Paul's Cathedral on the north side and the Tate Modern and Globe Theater to the south. No vehicles are allowed to use it; therefore, it is less dangerous and polluting. Approximately 2,000 people are on the footbridge at any given time. The wellness benefits are its accessibility to important places on both sides of the Thames, the reduction of greenhouse gasses, the ensuing physical activity, and access to the outdoors. The most obvious wellness strategy is the accessibility and connections created by the function of the bridge crossing the river Thames, and other strategies are also present including openness to fresh air, views of the river, a place to meet, and chewing gum art. Refer to Figure 3.6b.

A pedestrian strategy in the US is Nevada City Cohousing. This is a multi-generational rural community in the Sierra Foothills near Nevada City, California. Located on 11 acres (4.45 ha) of land, it accommodates openspace, gardens, walking trails, residences, and commercial buildings. Cohousing is a form of community where there is private ownership of homes while sharing certain community aspects of life. Common to the shared activities are communal meals, greenhouses, laundry, guest facilities, shared equipment, mailroom, and childcare. Typically, cohousing projects are pedestrian-oriented, and automobiles are peripheral with the exception of emergency vehicle access. There are no garages and circulation throughout the community occurs with landscapes and paths. The streetscape is a living space and is friendly and encourages interaction with nature and among the residents. The wellness strategies include strategic connections with nature and one another promoting pro-individual, pro-social, and pro-environmental behaviors. The wellness benefits include positive associations with physical and mental health, and quality of life, life satisfaction, and well-being. There is a sense of community, a decrease in isolation especially for seniors, and increases in social support, safety, and economic security. This example suggests that not only cohousing communities, but also those that are pedestrian in character with close ties to nature can produce the positive effects. Refer to Figure 3.6c.

In the United States there are approximately 1.2 million miles of urban roads and streets. The proportion between rural and urban roads varies from

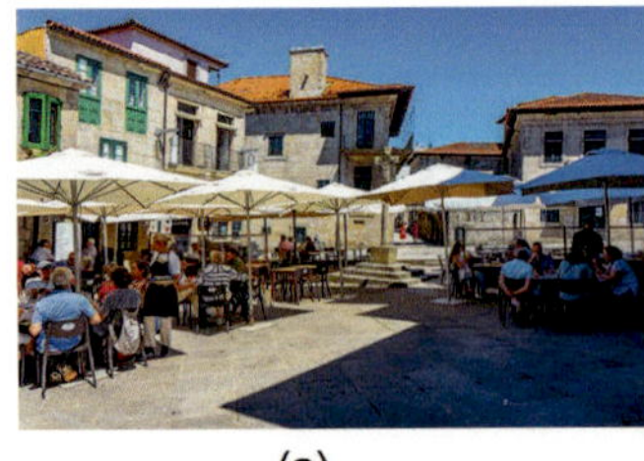
(a)

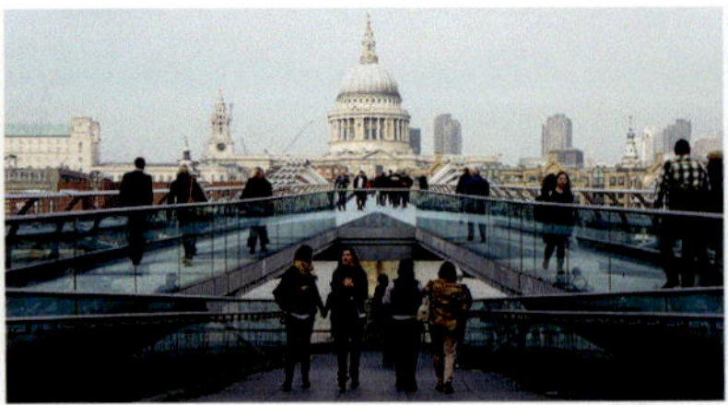
(b)

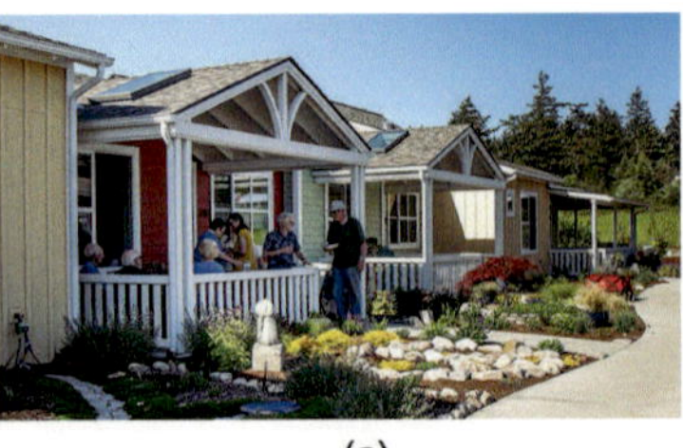
(c)

3.6
Pedestrianization
a) Pontevedra City Center, Spain,
b) London Millennium Footbridge,
c) Nevada City, California Cohousing

(Sources: Alamy, Wikimedia Commons, and Charles R. Durrett)

state to state. Pedestrianization is a reassessment of the function of the commute and the character of streets that connect residential properties. This presents a huge opportunity for pedestrian places. If no longer dominated by automobile access, the streets can become environments that are safe, friendly, more natural, and full of life and vitality. They become social spaces and opportunities for casual encounters and connections to nature. Refer to Figure 3.6c for a pedestrian street image for the Cohousing Development in Nevada City, California. Streetscapes that are human in scale, with wide sidewalks, that are treelined with places to sit, include on-street parking, and have slower automobile speed limits are safer with far fewer serious accidents and higher rates of survival from lifelong debilitating illnesses.[26]

Commuting to work by automobile can produce negative health effects, including elevated stress, increased blood pressure, increased exposure to air pollution, and possible accidents.[27] Average US commute time is nearly an hour (52.2 minutes) per day. Due to reduced exercise, there is an increase in weight along with sleep disorders. Long commutes can cause poor prolonged posture and musculoskeletal problems resulting in compressed veins and arteries in the legs as well as vertebrate compression. Commuting can lead to unhappiness, bad moods, lower life satisfaction, and have adverse effects on socialization.[28] According to *Psychology Today*, research has shown that long commutes have caused depression and can replace healthy time with family and friends.[29] With nearly 90% of daily trips in the US taking place in personal vehicles, it is no wonder that pedestrianization and compact mixed-use communities are a welcome alternative.

The pedestrianization concept of "*free-range parenting*," while controversial is gaining momentum. The concept is not a new one, in fact for generations even centuries, children were allowed to play freely often without parental supervision. In our modern society however, the issue is one of safety versus growth and freedom. The answer lies within the contexts where support and safety exist, and free-range parenting might be encouraged. For pedestrian-oriented neighborhoods that are populated by people, neighbors, and other children, free-range parenting can occur with safety nets. Not every parent will agree, but for those who do, there can be advantages. Benefits include promoting self-confidence and self-sufficiency, engaging with nature and active play, and improving social and communication skills. The negative consequences are usually cited as increased risk of harm without constant supervision, a lack of supportive community environments, and the possibility of neglect ensuing government interventions.[30]

The benefits of pedestrianization include a reduction of automobile use, possible decreases in congestion, crashes, injuries, pollution and noise, and increases in physical activity, lower blood pressure, increased respiratory function, improved cardiovascular and pulmonary fitness, increased positive mood, increased safety, boosts in immune function, while supporting cultural and spiritual connection to place, and promoting pro-social behaviors and pro-(urban) environmental behaviors.

6. Livable communities

Cities are now considered healthier than suburban living in terms of human well-being, with socializing, reduced obesity, engagement with more exercise, a more balanced lifestyle, happiness, and livable urban neighborhoods as the prime elicitors. They provide opportunities for aging in place, promotion of physical activity, have greater accessibility, and have closer access to employment. Livable communities can occur in either cities or suburbs, and have goods, activities, and services that support daily living and are accessible by walking or biking. A wellness community is a group of people living near one another sharing common goals, interests, and experiences in proactively pursuing a holistic lifestyle across its many dimensions.

In 1958 Evarts Loomis, considered the father of holistic medicine, purchased land southeast of Los Angeles and opened the first holistic live-in retreat called Meadowlark which functioned for 33 years. The guests could participate in art and music therapy, classes on yoga and meditation, acupuncture treatments, bodywork, biofeedback training, and therapeutic fasts, all of which led to a deeper understanding of illness and healing.[31]

Another example is the city of Boulder, Colorado that has often been seen as an attractive college town nestled up against the foothills of the Rocky Mountains. With a well-defined city center and university district, the city is further defined by fairly distinct neighborhoods. It is also known for its intellectual diversity and cultural amenities. In 1971, Boulder residents voted for a population growth cap thereby limiting growth by addition, but rather by multiplication and densification from within. Boulder is a walkable community with a greenbelt surrounding the city and trails and bike paths throughout the city. The Mapleton Hill Neighborhood is one of the oldest, established in the 1880s, and has been designated a Historic District. There is a strong sense of community within the neighborhood with its variety of historic styles and types of architecture, picturesque streets and neighborhood school, and close access to mountain trails and the downtown. There are 500 dwellings, one of the oldest elementary schools, hospital facilities, the first public library, and 200 silver maple trees and mature landscaping. Wellness occurs with a strong sense of community, sense of place, access to nature, quiet friendly streets, and access to surrounding amenities. Mapleton Hill is known for its tree-lined Mapleton Boulevard that passes through the neighborhood and into the foothills beyond, Figures 3.7a/b.

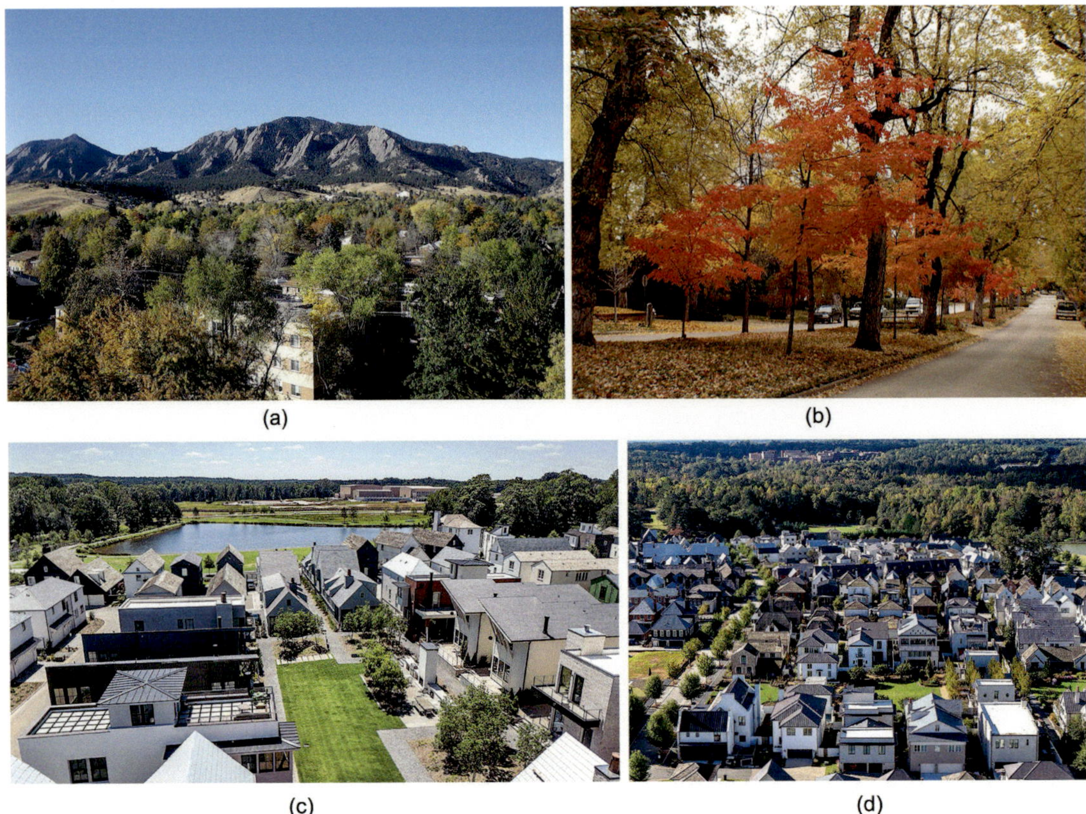

(a) (b) (c) (d)

3.7
Livable Neighborhoods
a) Mapleton Hill Neighborhood, Boulder, Colorado, b) Mapleton Avenue, c) Trilith Openspace, d) Trilith Overview
(Sources: Wikimedia Commons, Lew Oliver, and David Cannon Photography)

Trilith is a new neighborhood and mixed-use development launched in 2016 and being realized outside of Fayetteville, Georgia southeast of Atlanta. When complete, it will be comprised of 1,400 homes and nearly 400,000 square feet of commercial space near the Marvel Studios. There are 600 single-family dwellings, 100 townhomes, and apartments. Residential plot sizes are relatively small ranging between 1,800 and 3,200 square feet. The smaller dwelling types fit a growing market of smaller households. Some 70% of homes are apartments. More than half of the residences face onto a green street or park. The final buildout is estimated at 5,000 residents. The architectural language is inspired by European vernacular village designs. Garages are in the rear of dwellings and de-emphasized. Planned by planner Lew Oliver, Trilith won the 2021 Congress for the New Urbanism Award in the Neighborhood District category, Figure 3.7d.

The masterplan is divided into three areas with residential, commercial, and recreational land uses. There are 235 acres of land dedicated to preservation, with parks and greenspaces comprising 51% of the development. Trilith Village includes coffee shops, restaurants, a multiplex, fitness facilities, retail shops, and community gathering spaces. Nearby are healthcare facilities and the Forest School. It is the combination of density, scale, pedestrianization, and access to the commercial and recreational functions that render it a livable community. Due to its exurban location and forested land surrounding it, Trilith has a strong sense of identity. Close by are the Trilith Studios which grew out of the UK-based

Pinewood Studio. Now the Studio is being branded as not only an entertainment venue, but also as a community ecosystem composed of live-work opportunities.

Both older and newer livable neighborhoods share common characteristics which include scale, diversity of land use mixes, and varying dwelling sizes and types. As seen in Figures 3.7a/b, The Mapleton Hill Neighborhood in Boulder, Colorado is a century old with varying styles and ages of buildings and a strong integration of nature. Figures 3.7c/d are photographs of the newly constructed Trilith Community in southeast Atlanta, Georgia. Each of these communities has a strong identity and sense of place, and is walkable, has a mix of uses, and has close access to nature. Mapleton is established and Trilith is new, but both have a human scale that contributes to wellness.

The strategies include passive survivability that focuses on planning and designing adaptations for adverse weather events and natural disasters, including power outages, extreme temperatures, drought, viral transmissions, and terrorism threats. Critical life-support systems are kept intact and maintained throughout the debilitating event. These add to the livability of a community. Other strategies include the incorporation of land use mixes appropriate to the scale of a small community, the creation of identifiable boundaries and coherent networks of pathways and pedestrian sidewalks, the provision of outdoor public pedestrian spaces, the inclusion of nature within, and more friendly and safer streets. The specific benefits of such strategies include increased activity, lower blood pressure, increased respiratory function, cardiovascular and pulmonary fitness and positive mood, increased safety, boosts to immune function, enhanced cultural and community sense of place, and promotion of pro-social behaviors.

7. Parks, greenspaces, and streetscapes

Around 2009, most of the developed world was urban, making parks and greenspaces greatly appreciated within the urban environment. They provide access to nature, blue spaces, recreation, and urban agriculture as well as other biophilic benefits. The three primary biophilic principles derive from the interactions of the nature-human-built environments, and often are influenced by urban parks and openspaces. As in any triad, one part interacts with the other two creating multiple relationships. The positive outcomes of nature affect humans in beneficial ways, and it is from nature that the built environment materializes. Human interactions are influenced by both experiences of nature and the built environment. According to Kaplan and Kaplan, landscapes today that resemble savannas or are parklike are preferred.[32]

Greenspaces are undeveloped landscapes, wild places, protected natural areas, openspace reserves, wetlands, and water and greenways moving through the urban fabric. Building landscaping, greenroofs, gardens, tree-lined streetscapes, and urban agriculture are also considered greenspaces. While not strictly "green," plazas, squares, courtyards, and promenades contribute to health effects through social interaction. The wellness benefits of parks, greenspaces, and biophilic environments are well documented. According to the Urban Institute, parks and greenspaces intrinsically support healthy and productive lifestyles, contribute to resilient and cohesive communities, and produce positive health outcomes, such as a reduced risk of cardiovascular disease, diabetes, cancer, and heart disease with averted health expenditures. In addition, they can help reduce stress levels and improve mood. Benefits occur with mental, emotional, social, and environmental wellness with physical health impacted the most.[33] The inclusion of parks and greenspaces has economic benefits including increased property values, tax revenues, increased tourism and branding potential, improved environmental health, and improved aesthetics.

Probably one of the most well-known parks is Central Park in the center of Manhattan, New York City, Figure 3.8a. Designed in 1858 to address the recreational needs of the rapidly growing city, its purpose was to give urban dwellers an experience of the countryside, access to nature, bridal paths, a meandering stream and lakes, skating rinks, a zoo, and a variety of landscapes. Designed by Fredrick Law Olmsted and Calvert Vaux, the park has more than 18,000 trees that today provide a habitat for wildlife, cooling the heat-island effect, and is aiding in carbon sequestering. The park encourages walking in fresh air and an escape from the confines of internally conditioned air. The park is sometimes referred to as the "lungs" of the city. During COVID-19, the park provided a newfound place of refuge.

James Oglethorpe established Savannah, Georgia in 1733, which has long been an excellent example of early American planning. Originally it was planned with four squares named after each ward, and by 1851 there were 20-established squares. It is for these 24 nature-filled squares located evenly throughout the original town fabric that Savannah is most recognized. Each of the squares measure approximately 200 feet (61 meters) from east to west, but they vary from north to south from approximately 100 to 300 feet (30–91 meters). Buildings located along the east-west sides of the squares typically house civic functions, while north-south blocks are residential (*tythings*), Figure 3.8b. The key wellness strategy is to incorporate and/or preserve parks and greenspaces at the beginning of the planning process allowing for adequate inclusion and meaningful integration.

The Forsyth Park designed by Fredrick Law Olmsted is located in the center of Savannah and was one of 20 proposed squares in the 1840s. Figure 3.8c shows Forsyth Park which is Savannah's oldest and largest park with 30 acres (12 ha) of land. Its amenities include tennis and basketball courts, grassy fields, scenic wheelchair-friendly paths, an amphitheater, a fragrant garden for the blind, and a quaint café. Lush greenery and Spanish moss-draped live oaks surround the perimeter of the fountain, as well as many park benches, so travelers and locals can sit back, relax, and take in the fountain's majestic charm. The dispersion of the parks within the urban fabric of the older city allows for easy access to their physical, social, and environmental benefits.

In 2010, the automobile-dominated street of Lancaster Boulevard, California was transformed into a vibrant pedestrian streetscape, and is becoming a central hub, shopping district, and community focus in the heart of its downtown, Figure 3.8d. Designed by David Sargent and Elizabeth Moule, it

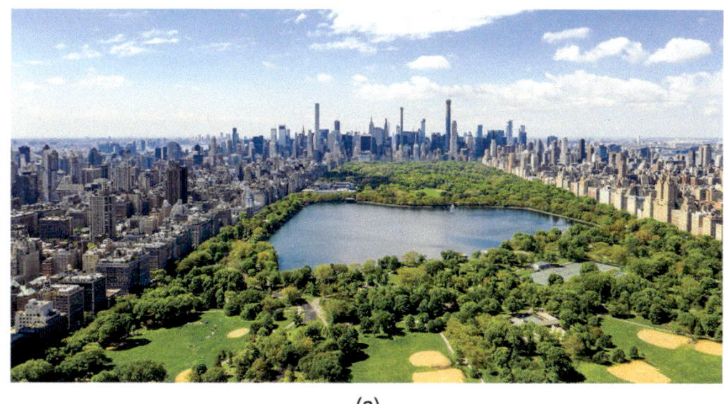

(a)

East Bay Avenue

Reynolds Square

Johnson Square

Ellis Square

East Broughton Avenue

(b)

(c)

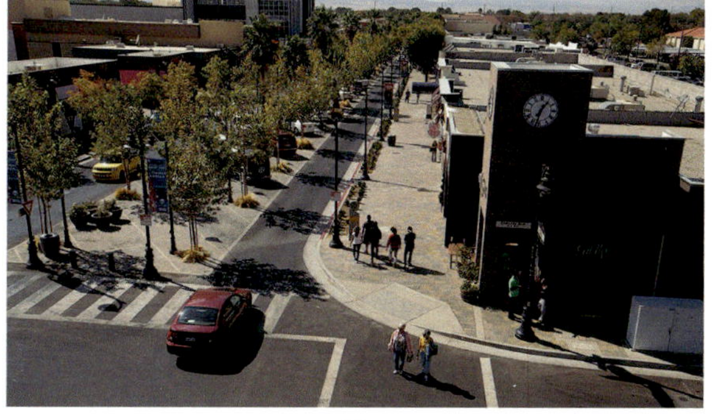

(d)

3.8
Parks and Openspaces
a) Central Park, Manhattan,
b) Savannah, Georgia Park Plans,
c) Forsyth Park, Savannah, Georgia,
d) Lancaster, California Streetscape

(Sources: Shutterstock, Phillip Tabb, and Wikimedia Commons)

comprised a three-quarters of a mile (1.2 kilometer) segment. Streetscape strategies include creating or reinforcing a sense of place, spurring social and economic opportunities, providing shading, carbon sequestering, street vendors, new pedestrian lighting, bike lanes, wayfinding signage, gateway markers, verges, and paved sidewalks. They can be "sticky," in that they are streets posing a challenge to get through, not because of barriers or blockages, but because of so many enticing opportunities to participate in public life. Streetscapes are safe, accessible, sticky, and beautiful providing a wealth of health, wellness, and biophilic benefits.

8. Urban agriculture

Urban farming is a local food system of growing plants and raising livestock in and around cities, as opposed to traditional rural areas. Today, 800 million people around the world rely on urban agriculture for access to fresh, healthy foods. Urban agriculture comprises 15 to 20% of the global food supply. Urban agriculture, which is considered a complement to rural agriculture, includes different scales from commercial agricultural facilities to household-level production and is widely practiced by society in areas of rapid urbanization, cities, suburbs, and towns. Urban agriculture is versatile, allowing for different crops to be grown. This provides urban communities with direct access and control over nutritious and locally-produced food, which creates jobs and boosts the local economy. Urban farming is also good for the environment and positively impacts household food security.[34]

Urban agriculture occurs in several ways including agriculture along streets and in derelict sites, urban land secured for agricultural allotments, growing on building rooftops, and vertical farming. They include farmers markets, rural cooperatives, aquaculture, hydroponics, beekeeping, urban fisheries and forests, animal husbandry, as well as indoor growing practices. Urban farms typically tend to utilize intensive production techniques on smaller land bases, including vertical growing and rooftops. Principal food products are fresh vegetables, herbs, fruit, and meat and poultry. In the United States the average urban and peri-urban farm site size is nine acres.[35] Regenerative urban agriculture is based upon principles of using natural resources (sun, water, soil, biodiversity, and human social interactions).[36]

Most grocery stores have food that travels as much as 1,500 miles to reach the shelves. The concept of a 100-mile diet proposes the idea of ending global purchasing in favor of eating locally by only obtaining food produced within a 100-mile radius of your home. People engaging with the 100-mile diet are considered "*locavores*." The strategy is simple, either growing or purchasing locally grown food including produce, fresh meat, and dairy products. Principal benefits include a lower carbon footprint, less wasteful, fresher food with higher nutritional value, and support for the local economy. This concept also suggests starting home or community gardens. It can reduce "food-miles" or the distance between food sources and home destinations. According to the U.S. Department of Agriculture, 88% of Americans use the automobile to get to the grocery store at an average distance of 2.2 miles. Dispersing urban agriculture can reduce these numbers.[37]

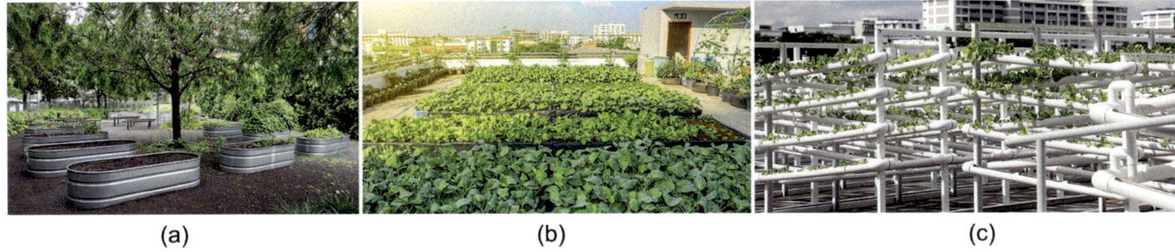

(a) (b) (c)

3.9
Urban Agriculture
a) Urban Allotments in Long Island, NY,
b) Rooftop Farming,
c) Vertical Farming in Singapore
(Sources: Wikimedia Commons and Shutterstock)

Vertical farms are not new as the Hanging Gardens of Babylon were the first known vertical farms. In Armenia, a hydroponic tower was constructed in 1951. More recently, vertical farms were expanded upon by Dickson Despommier. Vertical farming allows for the conservation of land resulting in higher crop yield per square foot of land, reduced water usage, can produce food year-around, can be dispersed and located in denser urban areas and nearer to residential districts for easier access, and easier controls against pests.[38] Some disadvantages include high initial costs, the need for specialized equipment, technologies, and processes, and can be energy intensive. Refer to Figure 3.9c for a rooftop vertical farm.

The strategies include appropriate site locations and urban agriculture zones with easy access to residential districts in city centers and suburbs, encouraging community engagement, and integration and distribution of urban agriculture from farms to parks to gardens. Urban agriculture can absorb and help reduce rainfall runoff. The specific benefits include improved response to variable external climatic conditions, improved nutrition and food security, expanded educational opportunities for children, promotion of biodiversity, CO_2 sequestering, improved indoor-outdoor access, stress reduction, a focus and sense of community, and financial benefits to lower supply chain energy consumption. Indoor urban agriculture need not be as sensitive to seasonal changes. They can support pro-social and pro-environmental behaviors.

9. Rural-urban transect

A transect is a transverse section through a landscape originally used for analyzing natural landscapes and ecological zones for biodiversity, and for surveying waterline perimeters and water bodies. They were used in the 19th century by Sir Patrick Geddes for valley sections to identify the most favorable places for human habitation. Applied to urban planning, the rural-to-urban transect serves to spatially organize urban density along a continuum from low to high density, and to transition green and open spaces along the transect with greater amounts at the perimeter and more public spaces at the center. It is an ordering device designed to create a smooth and fluid transition of a buildup of the built urban form. It can function in small hamlets, neighborhoods, villages, small towns. and even cities although at the larger scales it may be an over-simplified approach, may lose identity due to scale, and may become too "single zoned." In the 1980s the transect was utilized by New Urban planners, such as Leon Krier and Duany Plater-Zyberk. Their work created zones of varying density from rural areas to low-density zones to increasing density of built form and larger mixed-use building types at the neighborhood or settlement center.[39] What renders the transect a wellness strategy is its accommodation of cross-rural agricultural land with vibrant cross-urban cultural activities and opportunities for cross-pollination. The transect incorporates areas of high environmental, agricultural, or scenic quality, a variety of residential (varying housing types) and commercial spaces (higher densities, pedestrianization, retail, mixed use, workplaces, and civic uses) into a distinct yet fluid sequence of spaces. It allows for choice and equity with varying choices of where to live along the transect.

The natural transect in Figure 3.10a shows the transition downhill from the conifer forest to grasslands, and finally to deciduous trees along the streambed and the river water. Density increases as the rural road enters and approaches the village center.[40] The point at which a hamlet is entered is called the "*threshold of dispersion*." Buildings are placed closer to the road and closer to one another. Conversely, the landscape does the reverse with buffers between the road and dwellings at the perimeter. Then they progress to the center with mature trees along paths and walled-in gardens with connections to the village center occurring in the rear. The transect with greenspaces, bus stops, and the central village square are considered "*third places*," a concept addressed by Robert Putnam that are social spaces separate from home and work offering crucial civic engagements and community building.[41] These third places provide opportunities for re-engaging lost social capital. Pictured in Figure 3.10b is an aerial view of a rural-urban transect in Lasowice Village, Poland showing the lower density at the edge and a build-up at the center. The greater density of built forms and indoor-outdoor spaces contribute to a sense of community. What makes these villages so compelling is the fluid transition, the role of architecture in defining space along the transect, and the inclusion of landscape elements from rural land to village centers.

The rural-to-urban transect is an intentional spatial strategy with specific elements of design. First is the changing relationship between the progression of a predominant natural, agricultural or landscape environment to the increasing density of built form. The material character of the transect along streets can vary from rural to urban outdoor rooms. The transect provides three contexts: the rural, transitional, and the urban. Each of these contexts require specific strategies and offer differing sets of benefits with some occurring through each context. The specific wellness benefits from this strategy are access to nature and agriculture, exposure to biophilic attributes, access to social and cultural spaces, experience of sticky streets along the transect, and urban wayfinding. The transect accommodates differing street types and parking solutions that in turn affect pedestrianization and public safety. In communities supporting passive and active solar energy collection, the transect can help inform varying levels of solar access as a function of the density of built form and area requirements of solar collection. At the rural end of the transect, a high degree of solar access can be achieved for all buildings while at the urban end, shorter setbacks and verges, higher buildings, and increased shading can be problematic generally limiting access only to top floors and

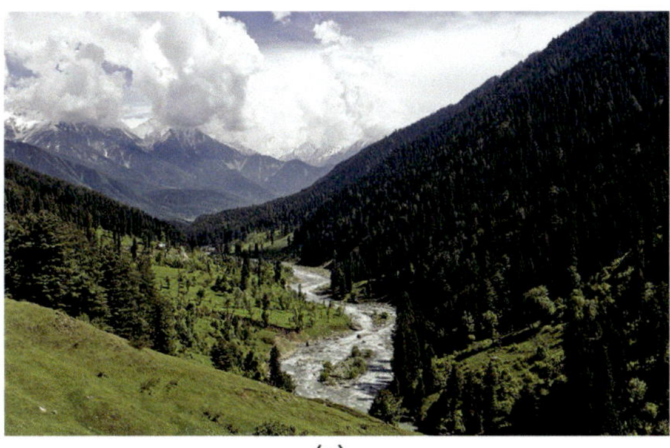

(a)

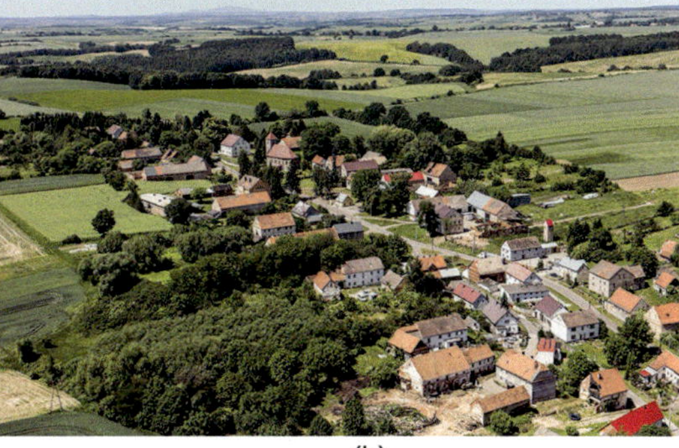

(b)

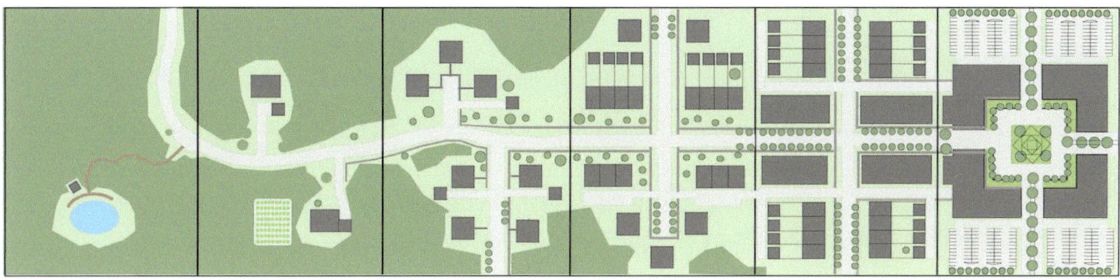

RURAL TO URBAN TRANSECT
Adapted from Thorburn 1971, Krier, 1980 and Duany and Falk, 2020
T1 NATURAL ZONE
Rural land with minimal human intervention.
T2 RURAL ZONE
Lowest density estate housing with landscape buffer.
T3 SUB-URBAN ZONE
Lower density, detached housing with garages.
T4 GENERAL URBAN ZONE
Medium density, attached, and single-family housing.
T5 URBAN CENTER ZONE
Higher density, attached housing, and mixes of use.
T6 URBAN CORE ZONE
Highest density, mixes of use, and central green.
(c)

3.10
Rural-Urban Transect
a) Natural Transect,
b) Lasowice Village, Poland Transect
c) Rural-to-Urban Transect

(Sources: Wikimedia Commons, Shutterstock, and Phillip Tabb)

rooftops. The transect provides biophilic and sustainable benefits as well as synergistically connecting nature to people. It solicits pro-individual, pro-social, and pro-environmental behaviors at the urban scale. Refer to figure 3.10c which is a rural-to-urban transect diagram adapted from Andrew Thorburn, Leon Krier, and Andras Duany and Brian Falk.

Planning and urban design scale summary

The planning scale offers opportunities for specific design strategies to incorporate health and wellness benefits that range from positive responses to ecological and hydrological cycles, climate change mitigation, reduction of greenhouse gas emissions, and encouragement of physical activity through greater pedestrian connections and networks. This scale offers the opportunity to create a more seamless connection between urban (climatic forms, renewable infrastructure, mixes of use, and the positive effects of densification) and nature (parks, green streetscapes, and urban agriculture). This scale also sets the scene and physical context within which the other scales are emplaced (architecture, interiors, and landscapes). Due to the larger impact of the planning scale, wellness design strategies and opportunities can quite easily be addressed with both existing and new construction. The outcomes at this scale contribute to pro-individual benefits through intimate and everyday wellness strategies, contribute to pro-social benefits through fostering community and family and friend gatherings in public settings, and contribute to pro-environmental benefits through protection from negative climatic effects and positive interactions with urban nature. It must be noted here that implementation of these wellness design strategies does not guarantee positive health outcomes but can provide greater opportunities for them to occur. Table 3.1 was originally developed by Gove Depuy and Phillip Tabb.[42]

PLANNING SCALE STRATEGIES

1. Mitigating natural disasters and climate change.
2. Renewable infrastructure.
3. Land Use diversity.
4. Growth by multiplication.
5. Mobility and pedestrianization.
6. Livable communities.
7. Parks, greenspaces, and streetscapes.
8. Urban agriculture.
9. Rural-urban transect.

STRATEGY	DESIGN INTENTIONS	WELLNESS STRATEGIES	WELLNESS OUTCOMES	REFERENCES
Mitigating Natural Disasters and Climate Change	Plan for climate oriented landuse, and networks and settlement form responses to weather and local ecological flows. Mitigate natural disasters. Give identity and sense of place.	Location, orientation, siting, weather mitigation strategies, settlement geometry, density, networks and form responses, land use, densification, reforestation and land reformation, reduction of hard surfaces, and provisions for nature.	Physical harm reduction due to disaster mitigation and climate responses to extreme weather conditions, CO2 sequestering, increase biodiversity, and increase to healthy natural areas, and fostering pro-environmental behaviors.	https://www.niehs.nih.gov/research/programs/climatechange/health_impacts/mental_health/index.cfm https://www.nasa.gov/feature/esnt/2021/reducing-emissions-to-mitigate-climate-change-could-yield-dramatic-health-benefits-by-2030
Renewable Infrastructure	Plan for efficient network responses to utility services, energy, water and waste management, and become a visible nature-benefit. Plan for efficient transportation.	Systems for energy, water, waste disposal, police and fire protection, and telecommunications. Designs for efficiency for greater accessing and utilizing renewable sources.	Stress reduction, improved biodiversity, improved efficiency, provision of critical life-support utilities during power outages and natural disasters. Providing opportunities for access to natural processes.	https://adelphipsych.sg/surprising-effects-of-power-outages-on-mental-health/ https://www.apa.org/monitor/2020/04/nurtured-nature

Growth by Multiplication	Plan for reducing dependence on the automobile, decrease carbon emissions, increase opportunities to experience nature and meet with community members.	Accommodate growth by optimizing size according to cycling and walking distances. Insure landuse mixes with critical non-residential uses. Nucleate settlements and create an interconnected network.	Improved access to nature, increased pedestrianization and social interactions, and increased sense of community. Encourages stress reduction, increased physical activity and pro-social and pro-environmental behaviors.	Donella Meadows, Dennis Meadows, and Jorgen Randers, Limits to Growth (Chelsea, VT: Chelsea Green Publishing, 1972).
Land Use Diversity	Response to wide range of human needs including life support functions, a rich mix of uses, activities, and building types, and reduction of sprawl and single-use development.	Incorporation critical land use mixes supporting heathy and sustainable lifestyles, creating easier access to goods, services and amenities, clustering and densifying to create easy access.	Reduction of automobile travel, improved air quality, increase social interaction and community, increase access to nature, improved mood, increase physical activity, and stress reduction, and supporting pro-social behaviors.	https://www.nature.com/scitable/knowledge/library/the-characteristics-causes-and-consequences-of-sprawling-103014747/ https://www.mdpi.com/2071-1050/13/23/13460
Mobility and Pedestrian-ization	Providing multiple modes of travel, efficient connections, transit-oriented catalysts, with concentration on biking and pedestrianization.	Provision of multiple modes of transport, reduced emphasis on automobile travel and parking, increase bike and pedestrian connections. Increase access to nature.	Improved cardiovascular health, reduced obesity, improved mood and cognitive health, increase activity, increase community interactions, and supporting pro-social behaviors.	https://www.researchgate.net/publication/303891478_Benefits_of_pedestrianization_and_warrants_to_pedestrianize_an_area
Livable Communities & Agrihoods	Creating safe places that foster community, chance encounters, and walkability, mixes of use and human scale, and support of mixes wellness lifestyles.	Providing coherence, high opportunities and appropriate scale, boundaries and sense of place, providing a diversity of building types, integrating nature within, and densifying for pedestrianization.	Sense of community and pro-social behaviors, improved mood, lower blood pressure, reduced stress and anxiety, reduced noise pollution, increase pedestrianization, activity and access to nature.	https://www.urban.org/sites/default/files/publication/32821/412648-Benefits-of-Living-in-High-Opportunity-Neighborhoods.PDF https://www.ncbi.nlm.nih.gov/books/NBK568862/

Parks, Greenspaces and Biophilia	Providing adequate access to openspace for recreation and social interactions. To encourage going outdoors and increasing physical activity. Increase carbon sequestering.	Provide greenspaces around perimeter of settlements and within a network inside. Provide greenspaces along streets to encourage walking and shading.	Increased access to nature, increase physical activity and opportunities for social interactions. Encouragement of pro-social and pro-environmental behaviors. Stress reduction.	https://www.urban.org/sites/default/files/2022-03/the-health-benefits-of-parks-and-their-economic-impacts_0.pdf
Urban Agriculture	Provision of urban farms, allotments, community gardens, tiny forests, food forests, and remediable landscapes that are easily accessible.	Providing land with easy access and vertical farming, planned for food security and reduced food miles, planned for community involvement and education, and planned for seasonal and extended growth.	Increase nutritional value of food, plant-based diet, reduced energy consumption for transport, improved air quality and CO2 sequestering, and increased access to nature, reduced stress around food.	https://foodsecurity.org/uahealthfactsheet/ https://www.fs.usda.gov/Internet/FSE_DOCUMENTS/fseprd865482.pdf
Rural-Urban Transect	Creating integrated links between rural land and urban centers through intentional transitional zoning, building types, and streetscapes.	Varying building front and side-yard setbacks, density of bult form, relationship to curbs, parking, street plantings, urban plazas, and surface materials.	Increase access to nature and physical activity, support of outdoor social functions, increase pro-social and pro-environmental behaviors.	Thorburn, Andrew, "Planning Villages," Estates Gazette Limited, London, UK, 1971. https://oroeditions.com/product/transect-urbanism

Table 3.1
Planning and Urban Design Scale Strategies

NOTES

1. John R. Ehrenfeld, *Sustainability by Design* (New Haven, CT: Yale University Press, 2008).
2. Capolongo, Stefano, Andrea Rebecchi, & Andrea Brambilla, *E-collection – Urban Design and Health*, (Accessed November 17, 2023), https://academic.oup.com/eurpub/pages/urban_design_and_health
3. Hammond, Robbie & Omar Toro-Vacay, *Wellness and Cities: Urban Infrastructure Just Might Save Cities*, (Accessed November 23, 2023), https://www.globalwellnesssummit.com/wellness-cities-urban-infrastructure-just-might-save-cities/
4. Rockefeller Foundation-Lancet Commission on Planetary Health, *Safeguarding Human Health in the Anthropocene Epoch*: https://www.thelancet.com/journals/lancet/article/PIIS0140-6736(15)60901-1/fulltext
5. Global Wellness Institute, *Wellness in Singapore*, (Accessed November 8, 2023), https://globalwellnessinstitute.org/geography-of-wellness/wellness-in-singapore/
6. Hayes, Denis, *Better, Faster, More*, (Accessed December 10, 2023), https://bullittcenter.org/vision/message-from-denis-hayes/

7. Baum, Fran & Matthew Fisher, *Critical Public Health*, (Accessed June 28, 2023), https://www.tandfonline.com/doi/abs/10.1080/09581596.2010.503266
8. Tabb, Phillip, Biophilic Urbanism: Designing Resilient Communities for the Future (New York, NY: Routledge, 2021), p. 9.
9. DePuy, Gove and Phillip Tabb, "Chapter 3 Wellness Strategies," *Wellness Architecture and Design Pathways*, Global Wellness Institute, 2023.
10. Baum, Fran & Matthew Fisher, *Critical Public Health*, (Accessed June 28, 2023), https://www.tandfonline.com/doi/abs/10.1080/09581596.2010.503266
11. NASA, (Accessed November 2, 2023), https://climate.nasa.gov/effects/
12. EPA, *Impacts of Climate Change*, (Accessed November 2, 2023), https://www.epa.gov/climatechange-science/impacts-climate-change
13. Tabb, Phillip, Elemental Architecture: Temperaments of Sustainability (London, UK: Routledge, 2019).
14. Ibid.
15. Tabb, Phillip, Biophilic Urbanism: Designing Resilient Communities for the Future (New York, NY: Routledge, 2021).
16. Ibid.
17. Tabb, Phillip, Solar Village Archetype: A Study of English Village Form Applicable to Energy Integrated Planning Principles for Satellite Settlements in Temperate Climates, Doctoral dissertation, Architectural Association School of Architecture, London, UK, 1990.
18. Schauenberg, Tim, (Accessed October 12, 2023), https://www.dw.com/en/15-minute-cities-what-are-they-and-how-do-they-work/a-64907776
19. United Nations, *World Population Projected to Reach 9.8 Billion in 2050, and 11.2 Billion in 2100*, (Accessed December 20, 2023), https://www.un.org/en/desa/world-population-projected-reach-98-billion-2050-and-112-billion-2100
20. Meadows, Donella, Dennis Meadows, & Jorgen Randers, *Limits to Growth* (Chelsea, VT: Chelsea Green Publishing, 1972).
21. Krier, Leon, *Houses, Palaces, Cities* (London, UK: Architectural Design Editions, Ltd., 1984).
22. Tabb, Phillip, Biophilic Urbanism: Designing Resilient Communities for the Future (New York, NY: Routledge, 2021).
23. National Library of Medicine, (Accessed January 11, 2024), https://www.ncbi.nlm.nih.gov/pmc/articles/PMC3377942/
24. Harrington, Holly, *Is the 15 Minute City Having its 15 Minutes of Fame, or is it Here to Stay?* (Accessed December 10, 2023), https://studiopdp.com/think-blog/is-the-15-minute-city-having-its-15-minutes-of-fame
25. van Uffelen, Chris, *Pedestrian Zones: Car Free Spaces* (Salenstein, CH: Braun Publishing, 2015).
26. Hathaway, Billy, Fehr, & Peers, *On the Park Bench: A Public Square Conversion*, (Accessed July 18, 2023), https://www.youtube.com/playlist?list=PL8GKDNzoOfinu_7tkDgweBq-GHNZ8sP5v
27. *How Long Commutes Can Affect Spine Health*, (Accessed January 21, 2024), https://www.flexispot.com/spine-care-center/how-long-commutes-can-affect-spine-health
28. Acton, Brian, *The Negative Health Consequences of Commuting by Car*, (Accessed January 20, 2024), https://www.coreproducts.com/blogs/news/the-negative-health-consequences-of-commuting-by-car
29. Wei, Marlynn, *Commuting: "The Stress That Doesn't Pay,"* (Accessed January 21, 2024), https://www.psychologytoday.com/us/blog/urban-survival/201501/commuting-the-stress-that-doesnt-pay
30. Skenazy, Lenore, Free-Range Kids: How Parents and Teachers Can Let Go and Let Grow (New York, NY: Jossey-Bass, 2021).
31. Ardell, Donald, High Level Wellness: An Alternative to Doctors and Drugs, and Disease (Emmaus, PA: Rodale Press, 1977), pp. 20–24.
32. Kaplan, R. & S. Kaplan, *The Experience of Nature: A Psychological Perspective* (Cambridge, MA: Cambridge University Press, 1989).

33. Cohen, Mychal, Kimberly Burrows, & Peace Gwam, *Health Benefits of Parks and their Economic Impacts*, (Accessed October 10, 2023), https://www.urban.org/sites/default/files/2022-03/the-health-benefits-of-parks-and-their-economic-impacts_0.pdf
34. Nelson, Noelle, *How Urban Farming Can Help Reduce Poverty*, (Accessed March 25, 2023), https://borgenproject.org/urban-farming-can-help-reduce-poverty/
35. Pressman, Andy, Lydia Oberholtzer, & Carolyn Dimitri, *Urban Agriculture in the United States: Baseline Findings of a Nationwide Survey*, (Accessed April 21, 2023), https://attra.ncat.org/publication/urban-agriculture-in-the-united-states-baseline-findings-of-a-nationwide-survey/.
36. Massy, Charles, *Call of the Reed Warbler: A New Agriculture, A New Earth* (White River Junction, VT: Chelsea Green Publishing, 2018).
37. Ploeg, Michael Ver, Lisa Mancino, Jessica Todd, Dawn Clay, & Benjamin Scharadin, Where Do Americans Usually Shop for Food and How Do They Travel to Get There? Initial Findings from the National Household Food Acquisition and Purchase Survey, (Accessed November 17, 2023), https://www.ers.usda.gov/webdocs/publications/43953/eib138_erratasummary.pdf
38. Despommier, Dickson, *The Vertical Farm: Feeding the World in the 21st Century* (New York, NY: St. Martin's Press, 2010).
39. Duany, Andres & Brian Falk, *Transect Urbanism: Readings in Human Ecology* (San Francisco, CA: ORO Editions, 2020).
40. Thorburn, Andrew, "*Planning Villages*," Estates Gazette Limited, London, UK, 1971.
41. Putnam, Robert, Bowling Alone: The Collapse and Revival of American Community (New York, NY: Simon & Schuster, 2001)
42. DePuy, Gove & Phillip Tabb, "Chapter 3 Wellness Strategies," *Wellness Architecture and Design Pathways*, Global Wellness Institute, 2023.

4 WELLNESS ARCHITECTURE STRATEGIES

ARCHITECTURE SCALE STRATEGIES

Health and wellness strategies at the architectural scale involve a variety of design interventions. It should be noted that different locations, functions, building types, and scales require site- and project-specific design responses. They include the climate responsiveness of the building form and modulation in response to varying weather conditions, the characteristics and functions of the building envelope, the efficiency of conventional building systems and the incorporation of renewable technologies, the encouragement of increased indoor-outdoor relationships, and the inclusion of sacred placemaking strategies. According to Carol Venolia, healing environments stimulate positive awareness of ourselves, enhance our connections with nature, culture and people, allow for privacy, are safe and do us no physical harm, provide meaningful stimuli, encourage times of relaxation, allow for productive interactions, contain a balance between familiarity and flexibility, and are beautiful.[1] Health and wellness benefits from the strategies at this architectural scale range from improved comfort and respiratory function to stress reduction and improved mental health. They benefit in particular ways with physical, psychological, mental, social, spiritual, economic, and environmental outcomes. The architectural scale strategies in this section include climate-responsive form, building envelope and smart façades, healthy building systems, indoor-outdoor access to nature, nudge design strategies, healing water, passive survivability, and spiritual dimensions of wellness.

1. **Climate responsive architectural form**
   Climate change and environmental degradation are also the consequences of our contemporary condition, a situation the public has recently recognized. Climate neutrality and carbon neutrality promote the reduction of emissions-producing activities, improving efficiency, incorporating renewable energy technologies, and phasing out the use of fossil fuels. Design responses to climate can support sustainability and promote health and wellness outcomes.[2] Climatic responses to architecture take into consideration seasonality, sun direction (sun path and position), self-shading factors, and environmental factors, such as wind, rainfall, humidity, mildew and mold, under- and over-heating, and the destructive hazardous events and vulnerability caused by earthquakes, volcanic eruptions, tornados, cyclones, hurricanes, tsunami surges, drought, wildfires,

DOI: 10.4324/9781003472902-4

avalanches, monsoons, and flooding. Natural disasters occur globally while often regionally distributed affecting vulnerable populations. Human populations are distributed throughout all climatic locations. The majority of global populations live within temperate climate zones and urban areas. There are 40% living in low-elevation coastal areas. Therefore, climatic design approaches should especially address temperate, urban, and coastal areas where most people live. Location, resiliency, preparedness, and climatic design responses are necessary for the protection of human life. According to the UN Department of Economic and Social Affairs, close to three in five cities worldwide with at least 500,000 inhabitants are at high risk of a natural disaster.[3] Refer to Figure 4.1 for contemporary climatic designs in contrasting polar, hot-humid, and temperate climatic regions.

Climatic design considerations at the architectural scale focus on siting, orientation, primary, secondary and tertiary building form responses, spatial arrangements, circulation, and material choices. Siting is usually in response to topography, sun orientation, exposure to prevailing winds, and the types and amounts of precipitation. Over- and under-heating contexts will influence the degree of compactness for the conservation of heat or the open fragmentation encouraging natural ventilation. Orientation plays an important role in solar energy gain and solar protection. The roof design is important for self-shading in hot climates and solar access in cold climates. The secondary and tertiary responses typically address fenestration shading and protection, and envelope material choices are particularly important where moisture is prevalent and there is a need for fire protection. Wellness is affected by the degree to which the building encourages the biophilic effect and indoor-outdoor flows, access to daylight and solar control especially for glare, indoor thermal comfort, reduction of carbon emissions, and reduction of climate anxiety to the locus of climate and weather disasters and climate change.[4]

The Borgafjall Hotel, built between 1948 and 1950 and designed by architect Ralph Erskine, is located in Borgafjall, Sweden. It represents an example of a climate-driven design for an extreme cold context. The roof forms of the building provide wind and snow protection while the southern façade opens up for passive solar heating. In contrast, Renzo Piano designed the Jean-Marie Tjibaou Cultural Centre in New Caledonia, which was built in 1998. The design identifies the Kanak culture links between the landscape and built structures. Located within a subtropical climate zone, the wind-generated forms present a functional, yet symbolic and historic memory of the place. Architecturally, the design features a series of wooden pavilions aligning a ridge along the peninsula with well-defined concave inner spaces on the leeward sides, while simultaneously being protected by the convex curvature of the windward sides.[5] The 8 House in Ørestad in Copenhagen, Denmark was designed by the Bjarke Ingels Group and represents a temperate climate response to both over- and under-heating conditions. The combination of the U-shaped building form, abundant façade glazing, and balcony overhangs help encourage and control solar energy while encouraging indoor-outdoor relationships.

With a huge inventory of cities, infrastructures, and buildings already in place, it is difficult to turn back the clock and rechoose locations and spatial structures that are a more natural disaster and climate change free. However, for ongoing new development, safer and healthier choices can be made. Each year, worldwide, natural disasters force millions of people from their homes. Climate migration is occurring, and projections for 2050 predict there will be as many as 12 billion climate refugees.[6] So this influx of new development could redefine land reform in existing urban, suburban, and exurban locations with well-oriented planning and design considerations.

Wellness strategies include the creation of climate-responsive building forms appropriate in both under- and over-heating contexts and include form, orientation, fenestration schemes, and solar energy responses, as well as material choices in response to dynamic climatic and weather conditions. Wellness strategies also include responses to natural hazard mitigation and passive survivability designs. The health benefits are increased energy, mental clarity,

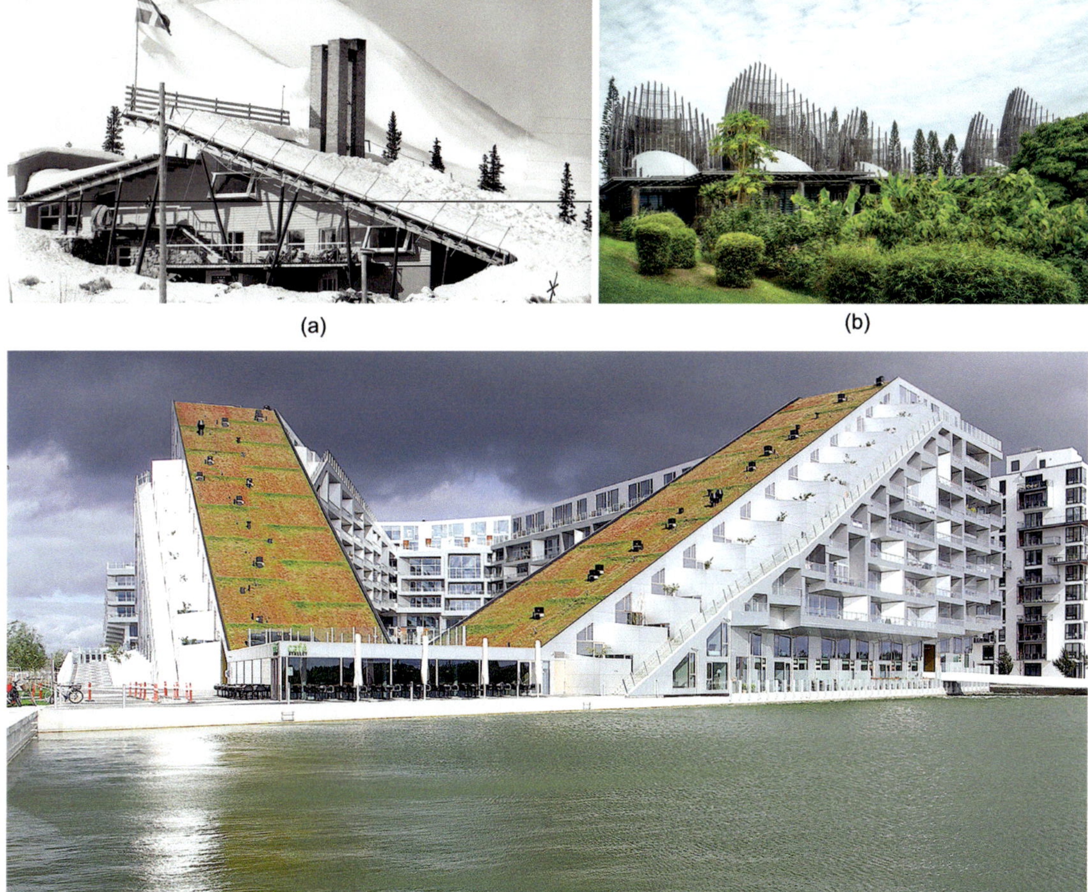

4.1 Climate Responsive Wellness Strategies a) Borgafjall Hotel Cold Climate, b) Tjibaou Cultural Center Hot-Humid Climate, c) The 8-House Temperate Climate

(Sources: Wikimedia Commons and Shutterstock)

(a) (b) (c)

decreased stress, lower blood pressure and heart rate, and increased positive moods. Environmental benefits include improved biodiversity, improved microclimate, use of local and historically significant materials, and increase in pro-social and pro-environmental behaviors.

2. **Building envelope and smart façades**

Façades are the interface between the interior and exterior of a building. They represent the face of the building and are their most striking and visible parts. Smart façades mediate both positive and negative environmental forces and include solar energy gain, heat gain/loss, access and use of natural light, ventilation and views to nature, reduction/elimination of unwanted air pollution, noise, high winds, intruders, and views. Key to a wellness-oriented facade is its ability to respond to natural elements and modulate both positive and negative environmental conditions. This happens through its components (passive or active), which adjust and adapt to different conditions, responding to changes that occur on the outside and inside of the building.

The Bosco Verticale, or Vertical Forest is a pair of residential towers completed in Milan, Italy in 2014, Figure 4.2a. Their heights are 364 feet (111 meters) and 249 feet (76 meters), respectively. Together they host 900 trees in planters and on terraces and balconies positioned around their façades. The towers were designed by Boeri Studio with consultations from horticulturalists and botanists. The buildings were conceptualized as a hope for trees that simultaneously house humans and birds. The buildings are self-sufficient by using renewable energy from solar photovoltaic panels and filtered wastewater to sustain the buildings' plant life. These green technology systems reduce the overall waste and carbon footprint of the towers and provide carbon sequestering. The Vertical Forest is a prototype design for an emerging format of architectural biodiversity and carbon sequestering. It creates a direct opportunity for interactions between humans and living species. The wellness strategies are its living and weather modulating façade and the positive consequences of human-nature interactions.

The Futurium is a building for exhibitions and events in the heart of Berlin, Figure 4.2b. The façade is made up of more than 8,000 panels (casted glass). The 70cm × 70cm large elements consist of varyingly folded metal reflectors and textured glass with a ceramic print. Under constantly shifting lighting conditions, they generate an ever-changing cloud image. The enclosing envelope and smart façade provide a mediating function with varying ambient conditions. Benefits include more responsive climate control, thermal comfort, increased productivity, and energy conservation. Using its geometrical shape, the roof collects the entire rainfall in the manner of a catch basin. The water is drained at the lowest point of the roof, collected in a cistern, and used for cooling down the building. Nearly the entire surface of the roof is covered in solar-energy panels for the photovoltaic (electricity) and solar thermal (heat) systems.[7] The health and wellness outcomes include climate change mitigation, use of natural resources, and encouragement of pro-environmental behaviors.

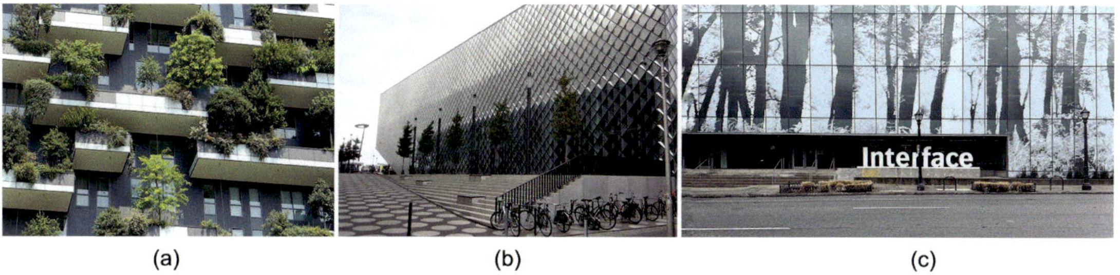

(a) (b) (c)

4.2
Building Envelope and Smart Façades Strategies a) Bosco Verticale, Milan, Italy, b) Futurium, Berlin, Germany, c) Interface Headquarters, Atlanta, Georgia

(*Sources: Wikimedia Commons and Phillip Tabb*)

The Interface Headquarters is a 40,000 square foot (3,716 square meter) renovation of the original 1960 office building completed in 2018, and is located in mid-town Atlanta, Georgia. It was designed by Perkins and Will, Figure 4.2c. It was conceived as a workplace forest, in which its façade is made with 307 glass panels sheathed in semi-transparent images of the nearby Piedmont Forest. In addition, the building features a green roof terrace fostering indoor-outdoor experiences, a 15,000-gallon rainwater collection and filtration system, high energy efficiency, and an open flexible floor plan allowing for abundant natural lighting. Inside are wellness and restorative rooms and community gathering spaces enhancing collaboration. This is a good example of a commercial application of biophilic and wellness-oriented design principles. It creates positive spaces for the people who use it, and benefits guests, employees, and the surrounding community.

Envelope strategies include the creation of smart modulating façades, filtering light, shading, views of nature, and creating privacy. They incorporate climate responsive building orientation, appropriate insulation levels, and vapor barriers. They avoid thermal bridging, and provide adequate means of egress and fire-rated materials. Smart façades avoid rain and water flow through the envelope, and they provide solar control, design for durability (especially ultraviolet degradation, material corrosion, and freeze/thaw), and provide views and access to the outdoors and nature. Benefits include safety and protection from inclement weather, improved comfort, CO_2 sequestering, improved indoor-outdoor access, stress reduction, and financial benefits from lower energy consumption, controlled interaction with exterior conditions, and comfort and hedonic subjective well-being.

3. Building systems

While most of our apparent concerns and efforts to improve the built environment were directed toward sustainability, they in fact focused upon correcting what John Ehrenfeld called "*unsustainability*" that is the unsustainable technologies, buildings and design practices, and continued consumer-oriented living styles. The term "*unsustainability*" refers to mainstream values and consumption patterns that continue to dominate the production, use, and disposal of goods, and are the proximate cause of the damage to the environment.[8] Since we spend most of our time within buildings, it is important to create environments that support wellness, and physical, psychological, and social health. Building systems typically moderate indoor air conditions and comfort, dispose of waste, and provide light, water, and energy. Initially, renewable technologies were introduced in architecture one system at a time, however now they are considered in a more wholistic way integrating systems including renewable solar and geothermal energy, energy storage, water collection and management, waste-to-resource systems, low-impact hydroelectricity, biogas, and high-yield organic agriculture. According to the Harvard School of Public Health, the nine evidence-based strategies that constitute heathy buildings are ventilation, air quality, thermal health, moisture protection, dust and pests, water quality, unwanted noise, natural light and views, and safety and security.[9]

Renewable systems include geothermal heating and cooling, photovoltaic electricity production, rainwater collection and filtering systems, solar thermal systems, and passive heating systems, Figures 4.3a/b. The wellness benefits of these natural resources and delivery systems include improved sustainability, increased resiliency, greenhouse gas reductions, reduced air pollution, improved atmospheric health, and improved human health (lung, throat and airway function, reduction of water-borne illnesses, and occupant comfort). In addition, clean water improves the productivity and nutritional value of urban agriculture and domestic food gardens. The combination of these systems contributes to passive survivability and the ability to maintain critical life-support systems during catastrophic events and power shortages. Conventional building heating and air conditioning systems, water supply and waste disposal, and electricity and artificial lighting can be made more efficient and responsive to human health and wellness.

The Kendeda Building in Atlanta, Georgia is considered a holistic green building receiving the first Living Building Challenge Certification in Georgia. The design prioritized occupant health and comfort. The building fosters regenerative systems, green design principles, and a concerted effort to relate humans with nature. By incorporating salvaged materials during construction, the building diverted more waste from landfills than it sent. Specific design attributes include efficient and renewable mechanical and electrical systems, rainwater collection, elimination of construction waste by using reclaimed and locally sourced materials, sunshading, daylighting, and the intentional expression of and interactions with nature and the renewable systems. The environmental benefits include the elimination of hazardous "Red List" chemicals, reduced energy consumption and CO_2 production, and encouragement of pro-environmental behaviors. The health benefits include increased energy, mental clarity and focused attention, decreased stress, lower blood pressure and heart rate, and increased positive moods. Refer to Figure 4.3c.

Passive survivability refers to the ability to maintain critical life-support conditions if those conditions have been shut off for an extended period of time. Passive survivability was introduced by Alex Wilson in the wake of Hurricane Katrina and was intended for houses, apartment buildings, and emergency shelters. Passive survivability is a building's ability to maintain critical life-support systems in the event of extended systems failures, especially for electricity, water, and heating fuel. The wellness system strategies provide a

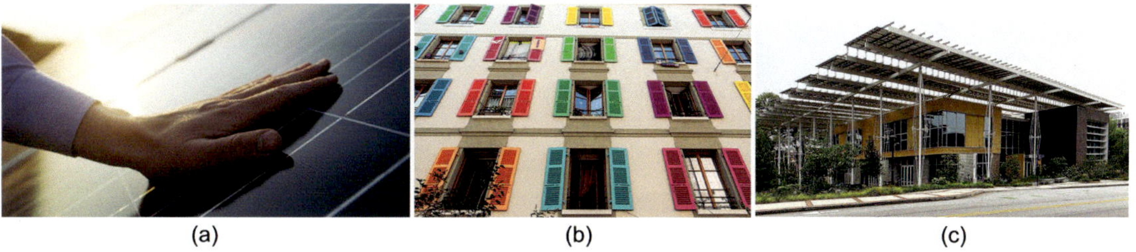

(a) (b) (c)

4.3
Healthy Building Systems Strategies
a) Solar System,
b) Shutters,
c) Kendeda Building

(Sources: Shutterstock and Phillip Tabb)

range of healthy, safe, and productive buildings during normal and catastrophic events. These systems are responsive to human health, comfort, and satisfaction, and to direct interactions with and control of them. In larger buildings this includes environmental sensors, controls and diagnostic services, and occupant engagement tools that support wellness and sustainability.

The strategies include climatic design response, abundant natural light, use of renewable resources and efficient building systems, reducing operational carbon, encouraging indoor-outdoor connections, occupant control of natural ventilation, and use of non-toxic materials. The wellness benefits include access to nature, stress reduction, noise reduction, enhanced cognitive function, increased pro-environmental education and behaviors, as well as financial benefits of increased productivity and lower resource and energy consumption. Further, they include healthy indoor air and water quality, ventilation, thermal health, moisture, dust and pest control, noise control, lighting and views, and safety and security.

4. Indoor-outdoor access to nature

According to the Environmental Protection Agency (2018), the average American spends as much as 93% of their time indoors with 87% of that time spent in buildings and 6% in automobiles.[10] According to Wayne Ott, the conclusion of his research on human activity found, "*We are basically an indoor species*."[11] The relationship between health and human activity reveals important distinctions. Too much time indoors can create physical health problems caused by inactivity and detachment from the natural world. This can have deleterious effects, such as breathing indoor polluted air, Seasonal Affective Disorder, depression, respiratory problems, and insufficient daylight causing mood swings, and lower levels of energy and alertness. In addition, circadian disorders can affect sleep cycles. Excessive indoor living increases instances of eye, nose, and throat irritation as well as higher levels of fatigue. And living in damp and moldy homes increases the risk of asthma by as much as 40%. We now are being considered an "indoor generation." The relationship between health and human activity can be encouraged with the provision of outdoor balconies, decks, barrier railing doors, patios, rooms, terraces, gardens, parks and/or plazas. Further, walls of glass, movable walls, operable windows, and French doors can encourage a more seamless visual and physical connection between indoors and outdoors. Interstitial space occurs in-between the two. A final strategy is including house pets which have proven to contribute to positive wellness benefits. The indoor-outdoor relationship is essential in biophilic design, which in turn provides both health and wellness outcomes.

The Church on the Water is located on the northern island of Hokkaido near the city of Tomamu, Japan. It was designed by architect Tadao Ando in 1988. This extraordinary architecture blurs the difference between inside and outside, and between human celebration of the sacred and the profound experience of nature. It is an expression of the Celtic notion of a "thin place." The pond and clearing of beech trees form a perfect invitation and view of the serene environment, particularly the element of water. The wellness strategies are evident in the serene context and openness and direct access to the natural environment. Within the church, there is an experience of silence and serenity. The health benefits include increased energy, mental clarity, decreased stress, lower blood pressure and heart rate, and increased positive moods. Refer to Figure 4.4a which shows the open-air connection between the worship space and the pond.

Farm-to-table is another opportunity to connect indoors and outdoors, but more importantly it connects us to healthy organic nutrition. Grocery stores, food markets, and farm-to-table restaurants are often an overlooked building type when considering wellness architecture models. Farm-to-table also functions within school cafeterias, faith community activities, and certain corporate environments. Farm-to-table concepts offer great wellness benefits including improved nutritional value containing no preservatives, less sugar, fats, calories, and carbohydrates. They suggest both a direct and indirect connection to nature through all the senses, and they typically have fresh flavors. Other benefits include support for the local community and economy, lower and possibly no transport costs, and close or adjacent farms produce CO_2 sequestering and oxygen production in the ambient atmosphere.

The design strategies for encouraging indoor and outdoor connections include creating large openings, opening up room corners, creating outdoor rooms or compelling places in which to engage, connecting indoor and outdoor rooms, providing carry-through openings, providing carry-through materials for floors, walls and ceilings, and providing patio doors, nana walls, and sliding glass walls. Outdoor rooms can assume a variety of sizes, functions, and qualities from walled-in gardens to conditioned outdoor living spaces replete with bars and outdoor kitchens, Figure 4.4b. In Europe, the conservatory, somewhat like a greenhouse, is attached to the main house and functions to mediate seasonal outdoor temperatures and to accommodate certain domestic activities. These strategies lend to potentially greater interactions with nature leading to sensory interactions (visual, auditory, haptic, and olfactory) that might normally be sealed off from daily experience. The dining setup for the Serenbe ArtFarm features an outdoor farm-to-table culinary experience (Figure 4.4c). Leaving windows and doors open to the outdoor air oxygenates interior spaces, and when adjacent to natural landscapes they bring in sounds and fragrances from the outdoors. The benefits include improved respiratory system, stress reduction, increased activity, encouragement of social interactions,

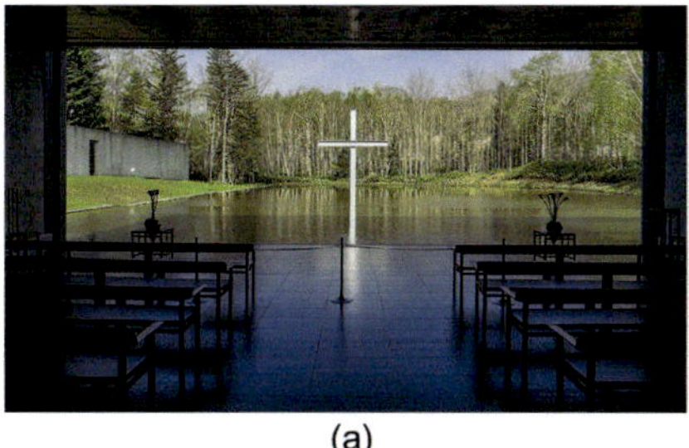
(a)

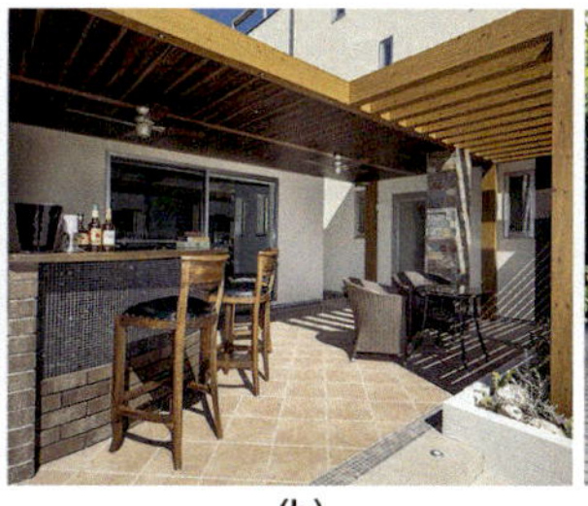
(b)

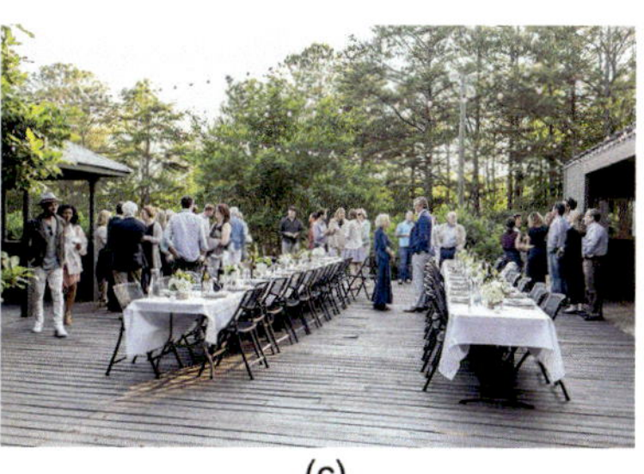
(c)

4.4 Indoor-Outdoor Access to Nature Strategies
a) Church on the Water, b) Outdoor Room, c) Serenbe Farm-to-Table Luncheon

(Sources: Shutterstock and Serenbe Community)

enhanced spiritual connection to place, and encouragement of pro-social and pro-environmental behaviors.

5. **Nudge design and choice architecture**

Nudge theory is about subtly influencing actions and ideas. While nudging tends to steer people in particular directions, it allows them to go their own way. Nudge theory was popularized by Richard Thaler and Cass Sunstein in their 2008 book titled "Nudge: Improving Decisions About Health, Wealth, and Happiness."[12] In architecture, it refers to what is called "*choice architecture*," making behavioral choices relative to building form language, design elements, spatial order, circulation, and wayfinding. It suggests that the choices we make while navigating and/or experiencing a building can affect our wellness. The concept of choice architecture is closely linked to nudging where positive reinforcement and implicit suggestions affect decisions influenced by the way that choices are presented. For the planner or designer, it involves the arrangement of design elements in such a way that choices toward wellness are emphasized. For example, choosing stairs over an elevator or escalator for navigating floors of a building. This depends upon the number of floors in a building. Other wellness-oriented nudges may include encouraging views to nature through well-placed windows, more movement inside and out, interactions with climate-related technologies, encouragement of energy conscious behaviors, and providing wayfinding during emergencies.

Building designs and design elements can possess incentives or elicitors that influence a particular choice. It is a nudge. Nudge designs can be either overt or subtle. According to Industrial Designer Ed Mitchell, a paper towel dispenser by Saatchi and Saatchi is an example of an overt nudge. It integrates an environmental message into a paper towel dispenser, which has a cut-out in the shape of South America. It's filled with green paper towels, which illustrate the continent's green rainforest canopy. As paper towels are dispensed, the user sees the continent drained of its greenness. Other examples include traffic calming with speed bumps, narrow streets, and mixes of modes, or circulation in cafeterias and retail stores. Admission to theatres, museums, sports facilities, hospitals, transportation hubs, and sidewalk or subway escalator etiquette use nudging techniques to help in public circulation, mapping, and destination information.

Cues in architecture and our environment have always influenced our actions or the altering of certain outcomes. Nudge examples and choice architecture mean that our decision choices are influenced by the way that choices are presented. Architecture becomes like a gesture, and nudges help redesign the choice environment by using deliberate and predictable cues that activate unconscious processes of thought in decision making. During COVID-19, for example, nudges were commonly employed to facilitate social distancing. Nudge designs can be divisive and therefore should be carefully employed. According to a *New York Times* article, nudging should include the following conditions:[13]

- All nudging should be transparent and never misleading.
- Nudging should be as easy as possible to opt-out.
- It should be obvious that the nudging is designed to improve welfare.

For wellness design interventions, nudging is presumed to provide choices that may lead to wellness behaviors providing health benefits. The most obvious nudging strategies are aimed at increasing physical activity, safety, social interaction, wayfinding, reducing overconsumption, and creating environmental sensitivity. The desired possible wellness benefit is paired with specific choice architectural languages and devices. The narrow street, tree buffer, and roundabout slow traffic and protect pedestrian movement on the adjacent sidewalks, Figure 4.5a. In the three-story One Mado Building located in Serenbe Community and further discussed in Chapter 7, a protected elevator is located and partly hidden outdoors behind a partial wall along with inviting large spiral stairs in the foreground. The intended nudge is to present the use of the stairs first and overtly, but, if need be, the partially hidden elevator is available subtly behind for those who need it, Figure 4.5b. The double-loaded corridor that connects the various businesses and offices is also outdoor and protected from the elements and provides good views of the nearby natural areas. Nudge and choice architecture can be applied to individual, social, and environmental behaviors.

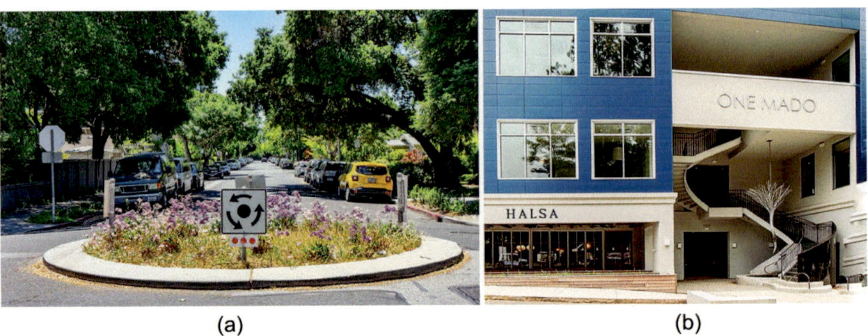

4.5 Architectural Nudging Strategies a) Neighborhood Roundabout Traffic Calming, b) One Mado Building Stair, Serenbe, Georgia

(Sources: Shutterstock and Phillip Tabb)

6. Healing water

Water is indicative of life's beginning and inception and is prominent in creation stories. According to Celeste Ray, "*Fresh waters are not only sites of creation, but are prototypical symbols of renewal during life*."[14] Water is the most abundant molecule and is necessary for life. According to Abby Phon, the health benefits of water for the human body include increasing energy, flushing out toxins, promoting weight loss, improving skin complexion, maintaining regularity, boosting the immune system, and preventing cramps and sprains.[15] Our bodies are made up of 60% water and as such, have a resonance with other water sources. Water's phases are also a fascination with its mesmerizing quality from moving clouds, snowflakes, ice cycles, and rippling streams to huge bodies like ponds, lakes, glaciers, and oceans. Water is needed extensively for commercial, industrial, agricultural, electrical production, and domestic uses. Water in architecture usually occurs for plant health, evaporative cooling, healing, biophilic, and aesthetic purposes. As a concern, microbial contamination is by far the largest contributor to the global burden of waterborne disease-transmitting pathogens (cholera, dysentery, typhoid, and polio). Historic examples of healing water are natural springs, Roman baths, baptisms, oracle voices of the "otherworld," and the healing and nourishing effects of Holy well water.

Therme Vals is a destination spa and hotel located in the hamlet of Leis in Vals, Switzerland. It was designed by Peter Zumthor, with Marc Lowliger, Thomas Durish, and Rainer Weitchies, and opened in 1996. Peter Zumthor and his wife lived in the village for 20 years and the spa was intended to be a community facility. The design concept was to create a cave or quarry-like structure working with the natural surrounding Adula Mountains and comprised 60,000 local Valser quartzite slabs placed in layers.[16] While the use of stone, concrete, and earthen roofs express the solidarity and density of the element earth, the multiple gaps between the units create a light and open feeling that is further complemented by the ubiquitous presence of water. The bathing rooms and spas are half buried into the hillside offering a peaceful experience. Water for the spas comes from the Graubünden thermal mineral source beneath the ground. Going to the spa from the hotel occurs through an underground tunnel that leads to a reception space. Beyond that, you enter into another corridor made of stone with periodic fountains, which have stained the walls with their iron mineral contents. Then going through a small passage, you enter the spas of varying sizes and levels of intimacy. The pools provide a variety of the ancient benefits of bathing.

The National September 11 Memorial and Museum and the One World Trade Center in New York City together are another good example of a thin place working in tandem. The tower is currently the tallest building in the US and is *uplifting* and *optimistic* functioning as a historic place marker and an expression of verticality. The two pools, echoing the Twin Towers, are in direct contrast to the levity of the One World Trade Center building, with the grounding and reverent soulful descent of water in the pool. The 30-foot granite pool walls and waterfalls form a boundary for the disappearing water. Designed by

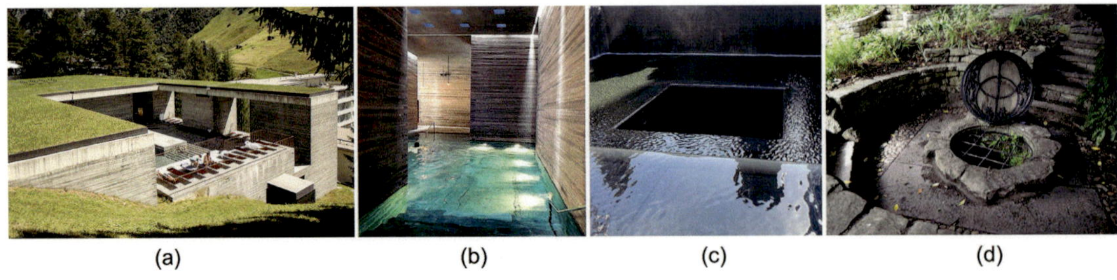

(a) (b) (c) (d)

4.6
Healing Water Strategies
a) Therme Vals Outside, b) Therme Vals Inside Pool, c) 911 Memorial Pool, d) Glastonbury Chalice Well

(Sources: Shutterstock and Phillip Tabb)

Michael Arad and Peter Walker, they conceptualized the design as "*reflecting absence*."[17] The emotional effects are known for its concept of hope, its beautiful and inspiring form and space, and its respect for the victims of the 9/11 tragedy. In the past, a Holy well was a community center for not only the necessary access to fresh water, but also ascribed certain rituals, guardian spirits, saints, and votive offerings. While well water is mysterious, it is transforming, life-giving, refreshing, pure, and constantly in motion.

On a more intimate scale another example is Glastonbury Tor in Somerset, England is a hill with the Chalice Well near its summit, situated within its small stone surround and movable wood and iron opening. Archeological evidence suggests that the Well has been in constant use for more than 2,000 years. Glastonbury Chalice Well is considered one of the most spiritual places in England.

The wellness strategies for healing water include design for curative water, waterfront places, holy wells, and water movement that can lead to hydrological consciousness.[18] Designs for rainwater collection, gutters and rainchains and retention pools, birdbaths, fountains, wells, and reflecting pools, daylit stormwater systems, and sacred rivers (such as the Urubamba River, Jordan River, Ganges River, and the Columbia River) contribute to this hydrological awareness and appreciation. Healing wells and divine waters have long been a focus of community life, spiritual renewal, and a reminder of our origins. Today healing waters are most likely to be found inside temples and compounds, health spas, thermal baths, and wellness retreats. Refer to the two pools in Figure 4.6 for the Therme Vals, 911 Memorial Pool, and the Chalice Well. The wellness strategies further include the use of clean, natural or filtered water, natural ventilation through breezeways, indoor-outdoor connections, and nature views. The benefits derive from the physical, emotional, mental, social, spiritual, and environmental pillars, and include access to nature, reduced stress, lower heart rate and blood pressure, increased feelings of tranquility, positive emotional responsiveness, improved concentration, perception, and memory.

7. Passive survivability

Passive survivability is an applicable strategy for both natural disasters and climate change resiliency. In the event of increases in the duration, frequency, and intensity of disasters and the consequences of climate change, passive survivability involves the ability of a community or building to continue sheltering inhabitants for an extended period. The term, *passive survivability*, was coined by Alex Wilson in 2005 in the wake of Hurricane Katrina. According to Wilson, "*Passive survivability can be achieved by incorporating the sustainable design features that have been so actively promoted by the green building community: such design features include cooling-load avoidance strategies, capabilities for natural ventilation, a highly efficient thermal envelope, passive solar gain, and natural daylighting.*"[19] Strategies aligned with survivability include the provision of electricity for the running of critical appliances, lighting, water supplies, access to food, and sustained access to the Internet. Specific technologies include passive solar heating and cooling, photovoltaic electricity and/or backup power production, rainwater harvesting, and storage of food supplies. These systems can be designed at both the community and individual building scales.

Houses, apartment buildings, and public buildings, especially schools and civic buildings that could be used as emergency shelters, should incorporate design features that will maintain livable conditions in the event of extended loss of power, heat, or water. Passive survivability can be achieved by incorporating the sustainable design features that have been promoted so actively by the green building community and alliances. Indeed, these measures are so important that they may need to be incorporated into building codes. Buildings can go even further with features such as generating and storing photovoltaic electricity and collecting and storing rainwater, but the aforementioned passive survivability measures are most important.[20]

Passive survivability promotes resilience by enhancing buildings that optimize a power grid, that can help reduce and shift loads, and are designed and operated to be resilient to impacts to the power and water systems. Passive survivability is safe and provides a reasonable level of functionality during extended power outages, and loss of heating fuel or water. Further, systems are responsive to storm events and flooding, and reduce reliance on electricity-driven elevators and air-conditioning. Furthermore, they are designed with high-performing envelope features including daylighting, minimized cooling loads, the ability for natural ventilation, and protection from storm surges. The provision of generators, solar water heating and photovoltaic power, on-site clean water storage, and provision for the potential of on-site food production are also important. Passive survivability wellness manifests in the forms of building safety and provision of critical life-support systems during and after disaster events. Mitigation strategies for disaster-prone building designs include a variety of building types, components, construction details, and renewable building systems. Several design measures follow:

- Adequate anchoring to prevent flotation, collapse, and lateral movement.
- Flood-resistant foundations and lower elevation materials.
- Building systems which incorporate exclusion technologies and be isolated from water exposure and accumulation.
- Detachable or retractable secondary building elements like porches, overhangs, and eaves.
- Foundations deeply and securely connected to the ground, and resistant to high winds.

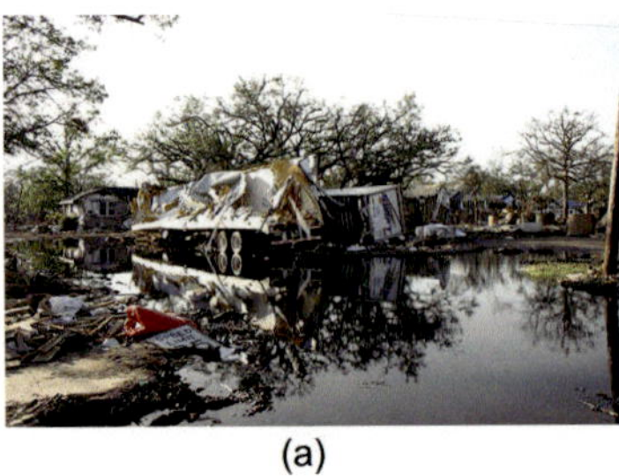
(a)

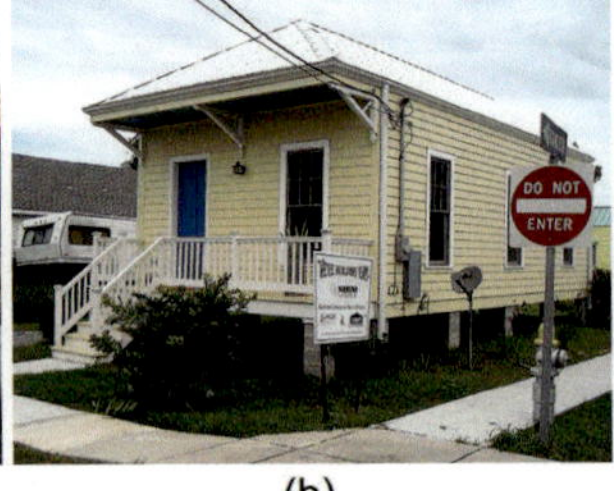

(b)

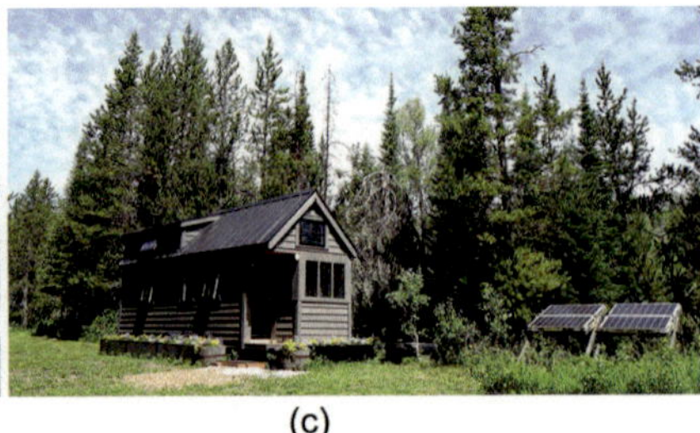
(c)

4.7 Passive Survivability a) Hurricane Katrina, b) Disaster Mitigating Design, c) Off-Grid Cottage

(Sources: Shutterstock and Wikimedia Commons)

- Avoidance technologies which include connection details are crucial for foundations, structural frames, roofs, and sheathing.
- Impact-resistant windows, doors, and other fenestrations.
- Passive building systems for water, heat, electricity, and food.
- Elevated and protected service equipment.

Extreme weather inherently poses risks, however, because of the rarity of occurrence means systems are less likely to be designed to function in such conditions. Climate change is projected to cause a range of impacts, including an increase in the duration, frequency, and intensity of extreme weather events. Disasters, both natural and human-made, are an important public health issue. Mitigation practices can lessen the adverse impacts and harm on physical health, social disruption, property, economies, and the environment. Another benefit of designing buildings for passive survivability is a possible return to the regional diversity and the inborne sustainable characteristics of vernacular architecture assuming they derive from sustainable practices and the needs of contemporary culture and technologies. Figure 4.7a shows the aftermath of Category 5 Hurricane Katrina which caused 1,836 fatalities and unfathomable damage. Figures 4.7b/c show weather mitigating and off-grid designs for affordable homes with passive survivability.

8. Spiritual dimensions of architecture

Spirituality is now recognized as a health and wellness benefit. A spiritual experience goes beyond the ordinary and can be mystical or euphoric, where there is an awareness of synchronicity, the presence of intuitive thoughts, a sense of ultimate peace and well-being, and a degree of surrender. This includes questions about the meaning and purpose of life, such as whether there is life after death, what are our origins, to where is humanity evolving, what is grace, and is there a God or a higher Deity. To Lionel Corbett, the sacred experience is broad encompassing much from a sense of a presence to a sense of mutuality and to the union of the soul with the divine.[21] These experiences can be noetic, carrying information or knowledge that later can be assessed and assimilated. Sacred architecture employs design devices to accomplish this, typically with uses of form and geometry, orientation, gestures reaching upward (heavenward), expressed structural systems (biomorphic), generous and impressive interior spaces, discriminating views (use of stained glass), abundant natural light, symbolic content, and ritual practice through active participation. While extraordinary sacred spaces can be created, ordinary sacred space is also important and, according to Dacher Keltner, "*The wonders of life are so often nearby.*"[22]

While sacred spaces are usually associated with religious traditions and used for worship, prayer, meditation, and rituals, more contemporaneously they serve awe and serene emotional experiences, spiritual renewal, and health and wellness functions. The wellness benefits of sacred spaces and the therapeutic functions they support include stress reduction, lower blood pressure, and improved attention span through the experience of calm spaces and meditation.[23] These experiences are often accompanied by a reduction in John Steele's "*temporal density*," where any given interval of time is filled and saturated with a myriad of events, processes, information, and thoughts.[24] Sacred places can help reduce this density, ground us, support improved self-image and a more positive outlook on life, and generate kindness. Sacred space can inspire hope for the alleviation of pain and a return to wholeness. Natural sacred sites and strategies for sacred space design include individual and cultural benefits. These are places set apart from profane and secular contexts that are attributed to transcendent experiences of the unknown, divine, or a higher power. Sacred buildings can also embody cognitive meaning through geometry and symbols. Wellness occurs through mediation between the biophysical nature of people and the social-cultural meanings associated with particular symbols, geometries, orientations, colors, and iconographic images.

The work of architect Erik Asmussen, particularly at the Vidar Clinic in Jarna, Sweden, illustrates the supporting role of architecture in the recovery process. The community is located about 32 miles (50 km) south of Stockholm near the Baltic Sea and surrounded by biodynamic farms. The Vidar Clinic is a nontraditional and anthroposophical hospital that was opened in 1985. Until 2019, it functioned with a focus on anthroposophic medicine based on Rudolf Steiner when it changed from a hospital to a retreat. According to Gary Coates, the courtyard affords a wind-protected, sunny outdoor setting for a variety of activities, Figures 4.8c/d. Thus, the courtyard serves both biophilic, social, and ceremonial functions that can be considered to serve sacred or spiritual wellness. On the upper level of the clinic, patients and staff can move from one wing of the clinic to the other either by an indoor passageway or by using the outdoor bridge. The upper bridge passage is framed by a railing that rhythmically moves upward and downward echoing tree branches.

The StarHouse is a community-oriented building constructed in the mid-1990s in the foothills of the Rocky Mountains outside of Boulder, Colorado. Designed by architect Phillip Tabb, it is a non-toxic, sustainable building based upon sacred and astronomical geometrical principles. The StarHouse is particularly interesting as a thin place because of the intentional nature of the design, the ceremonial quality of the construction process, and its seasoning through continued use. The structure is primarily constructed with natural materials, stone, wood, tree posts from the site, and copper roof. The building was constructed on the basis of non-toxic materials that were available at that time. The structure did not have any plumbing or electricity rendering the interior space as "energetically clean." The building is used for meditation, dance, music, theater, weddings, lectures, courses, workshops, and seasonal ceremonies

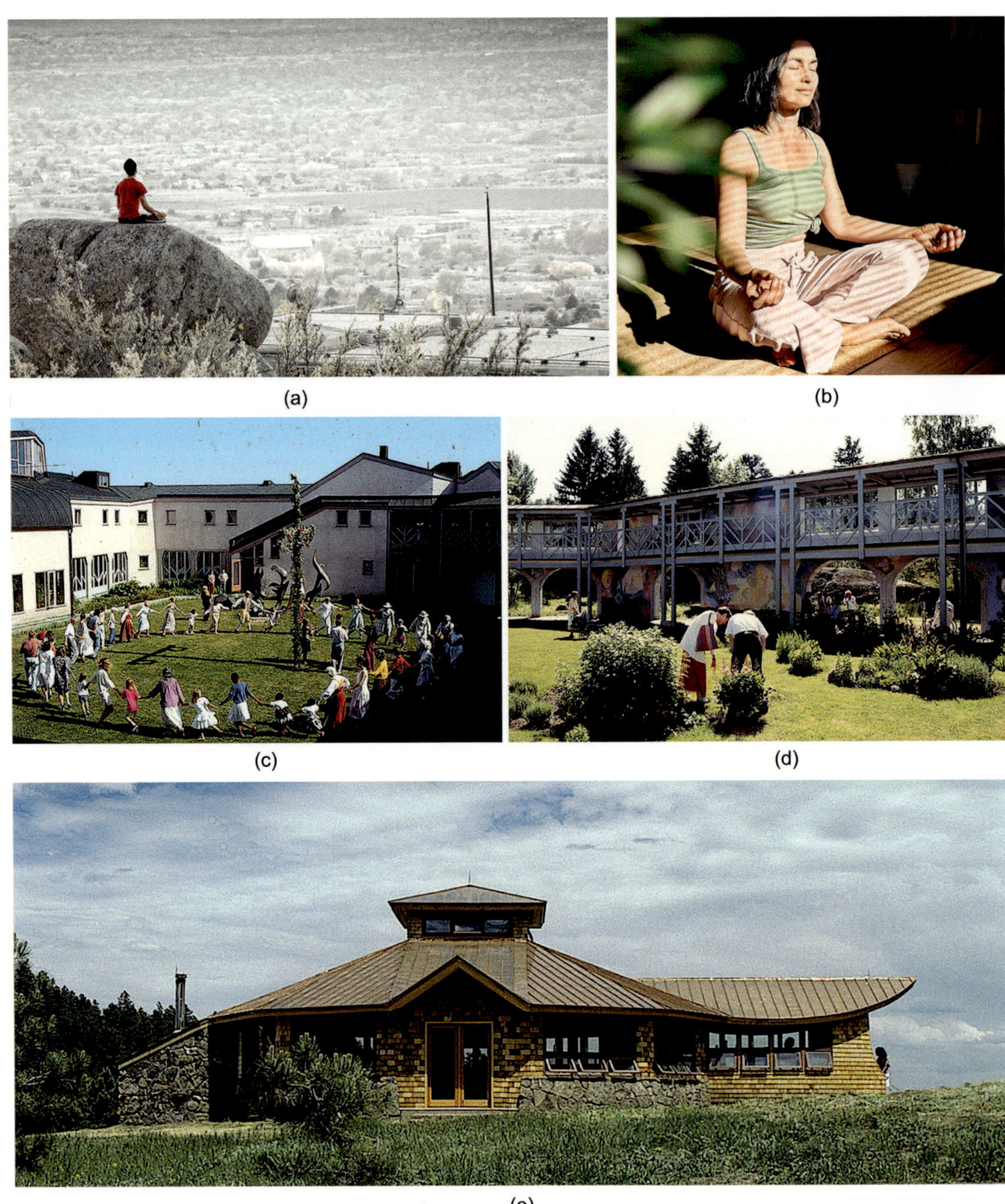

(a) (b) (c) (d) (e)

4.8
Spiritual Dimensions of Wellness Strategies a) Outdoor Meditation, b) Indoor Meditation, c) Vidar Clinic Maypole Celebration, d) Vidar Clinic Courtyard Bridge, e) StarHouse Photograph

(Sources: Wikimedia Commons, Shutterstock, Gary Coates, and Phillip Tabb)

and celebrations. The StarHouse fosters social and symbolic wellness through its focus on overall form, significant numbers, cardinal orientation, and celestial geometry. Ritual meaning can be derived through movement and participation in dance, theatrical performances, and music within the space. Refer to the outdoor meditation spaces and the image for the StarHouse in Boulder, Colorado in Figure 4.8e.

For the StarHouse, the wellness strategies include sacred space design, use of significant numbers and sacred geometry, use of natural and non-toxic materials, natural light and ventilation, creation of a positive social climate, and views of celestial phenomena. The benefits include physical, emotional, mental, social, spiritual, and environmental benefits, access to nature, stress reduction, improvements in mood, encouragement of pro-social and pro-environmental behaviors, encouragement of social interactions, cultural and spiritual connection to place, and improved life satisfaction.

9. Wayfinding

Dementia, a relatively newly recognized health condition, represents overarching forms of Alzheimer's, Vascular, Lewy Body, and Frontotemporal Dementia. They involve memory loss, visual and information processing errors, and experiences of declines in coordination and response time.[25] Wayfinding is an intentional strategy in response to these conditions aided by space, form, color, signage, and other design elements to help occupants navigate space. Wayfinding can be an effective tool to intentionally manage the movement and flow of people, encourage social distancing, improve user experience, and contribute to a sense of well-being and security. This is an important design consideration for complexes, campuses, very large buildings, hospitals, airports, subways, transportation hubs, and other institutional facilities. Poor wayfinding results in getting lost, confused, or frustrated while en route to campus or an interior destination. Emergency wayfinding is critical for indoor evacuation of buildings, especially during fire or other disasters. Effective wayfinding can lead to safe and efficient evacuation while poor emergency wayfinding can lead to confusion and prolonged evacuation times.[26] Also important is wayfinding evacuation during extreme weather emergencies. It is also a common activity in daily life as we move through our cities, neighborhoods, and buildings, especially hospitals, schools, libraries, shopping malls, and airports.

The strategies for effective wayfinding include creating identities at all destinations (differing visual characters), using landmarks, identifying markers and cues to provide orientation, spatial clarity and structured circulation, and eliminating complexity, ambiguity and too many navigational choices. Wayfinding may not be critical in certain non-health related circumstances, where wonder, mystery, and uncertainty might be desirable (amusement parks, labyrinths, and mazes), Figure 4.9a. However, wayfinding is generally an efficient and easier way of navigating space, especially unfamiliar spaces, and as such can reduce disorientation, stress and anxiety, and improve confidence, productivity and safety, improved moods and satisfaction for users, healthcare (especially in dementia patients), and concerned families.[27] Social and physical distancing, especially during pandemic conditions, are other off-shoots of wayfinding designed to protect people from the spread of communicable diseases such as COVID-19, and the wayfinding markers on floors served to enable proper distancing, Figure 4.9b.

Wayfinding strategies for people with dementia include correct lighting, space, and use of artificial cues, such as signs, landmarks, and include mobile augmented reality wayfinding devices. According to Dac Kopec, creative designs for dementia disorders and Alzheimer's disease should follow the *serial position effect* that supports rote memory.[28] This includes space sequencing, architectural element rhythms, and color clusters. For patients in healthcare settings, wayfinding serves confused patients and provides ways to visualize space, separates patients and staff, provides faster emergency assistance, and clears congested hallways. For streamlined circulation flows there is limited contact and risk of infection and contagion. Identifiable places form the building blocks of our cognitive mapping and corridor attributes (width, light, and directionality) are also important in the wayfinding process. Patients need to know where they are in a space (navigation origin and identity), whether the route is clear (navigation is well structured, legible, and coherent), and finally if the destination is apparent (destination recognition and anchors).[29]

There are benefits to retail wayfinding such as optimizing store layouts and product placements for visual and physical access, and ensuring safety and security in the event of emergencies. For normal navigation of space, wayfinding is a prerequisite for the successful use of buildings. Wayfinding can be created with removal of clutter, identification of clear entries and decision points, reduction of interference, confusion and ambiguity, provision of aiming strategies or strategic positioning (sight lines and target-directed circulation), creation of consistency (hierarchy and contrast), and provision of clear and understandable signage. Wayfinding can be encouraged with light-level gradients toward a destination. Landmarks at the interior scale are identifiable markers, cues, or anchor points made visible from a distance. These markers include sculptures, totems, maps, color and color scheming, digital guides, and signage. Indoor digital navigation technology is another wayfinding strategy in smart buildings. Wayfinding benefits include reduction of stress, improvement of moods and satisfaction, increases in physical activity (walking), and operational efficiency.

4.9 Wayfinding Strategies a) Wayfinding Cues, b) Physical Distancing

(Source: Shutterstock)

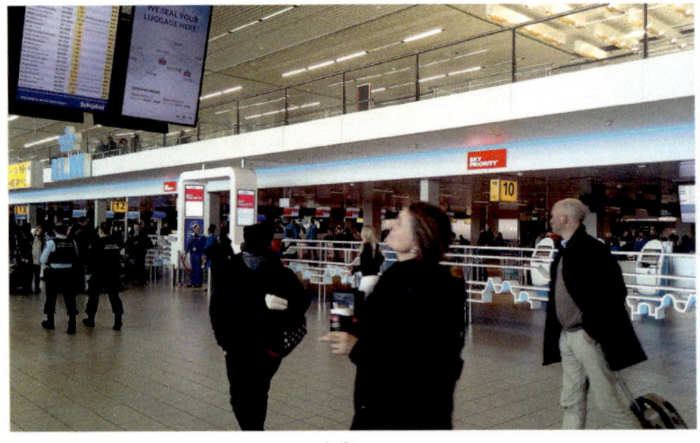

(a)

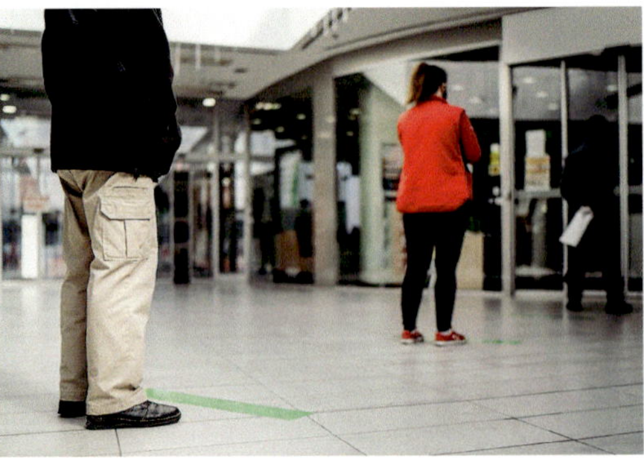

(b)

Architecture scale summary

The architectural scale offers a multitude of opportunities for specific design strategies to incorporate health and wellness benefits that range from the site planning and building envelope design to the promotion of natural light, ventilation, renewable energy, and access to nature. This scale offers opportunities for financial benefits through functional space planning, climatic form responses, use of renewable resources, and building systems efficiencies. Further, spiritual qualities are possible creating the benefit of enhanced stewardship, place reverence, and high-level wellness. This architecture scale certainly sets the context for the interior scale strategies that follow. The material aspect of architecture, covered herein, is more fully addressed in the next chapter on interior wellness under wellness-oriented materiality. Wellness outcomes at the architectural scale contribute to pro-individual benefits through interactive building wellness strategies, contribute to pro-social benefits through fostering social interactions and healthy public spaces, and contribute to pro-environmental benefits through protection from negative climatic effects and positive interactions with nature. It must be noted that implementation of these wellness design strategies does not guarantee the positive health outcomes discussed herein but they can provide greater opportunities for them to occur. Wellness in the context of this work does not include the important health-oriented design determinants for healthcare facilities and hospitals. Table 4.1 was originally developed by Gove Depuy and Phillip Tabb.

ARCHITECTURE SCALE STRATEGIES

1. Climate-responsive architectural form.
2. Building envelope and smart façades.
3. Building systems.
4. Indoor-outdoor access to nature.
5. Nudge design strategies.
6. Healing water.
7. Passive survivability.
8. Spiritual dimensions of architecture.
9. Wayfinding.

STRATEGY	DESIGN INTENTIONS	WELLNESS STRATEGIES	WELLNESS OUTCOMES	REFERENCES
Climate-Responsive Form	To design to mitigate extreme weather and climatic conditions, taking advantage of on-site renewable resources, and providing safe and comfortable spaces celebrating the changes of seasons.	Form and material responses to varying climate and weather conditions, especially sun, wind and precipitation, and to earthquakes, hurricanes and storm surges, designs for bioclimatic sustainable.	Occupant safety, thermal comfort, lower energy consumption, reduced greenhouse gasses, disaster mitigation, improved biodiversity and pro-environmental behaviors.	https://webstor.srmist.edu.in/web_assets/srm_mainsite/files/downloads/climateresponsivearch.pdf

Envelope & Smart Facades	Building envelopes are the first line against the negative external forces as well as mediating positive interactions with nature and the elements. Intentions are to protect and to modulate the interactions and reinforce the biophilic effect.	Design for envelope modulation for daylight, sunshading, natural ventilation, and thermal comfort. Design for maximum water and moisture protection, design for hazards mitigation. Provide views to nature.	Occupant safety and comfort, lower risks to natural disasters, modulation for immediate responses, reduction of glare, improved indoor air quality, lower energy consumption, and stress reduction.	https://quarryviewbuildinggroup.com/how-building-envelopes-impact-your-health/ https://www.scnsoft.com/blog/smart-buildings
Building Systems	Design for efficient HVAC and renewable energy systems, water collection and filtration, clean air and ventilation distribution, and efficient and non-toxic mechanical systems. Design for daylighting.	Integrating passive solar heating, ventilation and ample daylighting, renewable energy systems, planning for passive survivability, providing smart sensors, optimizers and controls, encouraging occupant interactions with systems.	Improved thermal comfort and the ability to fine tune, reducing energy consumption, reaching carbon neutrality, increasing building value, improved mood and less stress, and providing physical safety.	https://www.csemag.com/articles/how-smart-buildings-combat-health-concerns/
Nudging and Choice Architecture	To provide nudge designs and choice architecture that are intended to influence the way in which choices are presented especially those that effect wellness.	To suggest behavioral choices that support wellness attributes, especially increase physical activity, social interactions. Making circulation and wayfinding choices.	Outcomes are particular to specific nudges, but generally are physical, social and environmental. They often provide safety and wayfinding.	https://www.delve.com/insights/whats-a-nudge-in-product-design https://www.nytimes.com/2015/11/01/upshot/the-power-of-nudges-for-good-and-bad.html
Indoor-Outdoor Access to Nature	To design for indoor-outdoor connections facilitating positive interactions with nature (views, haptic, auditory, olfactory) and eliminate negative factors (climate, weather, pests, insects, and intruders).	Multiple indoor-outdoor passages, operable windows, providing outdoor rooms (balconies, terraces and courtyards), providing windows with views to nature.	Increase activity, reduce obesity, reduce stress, improve mood, improves cognitive function, restores attention, increases biophilic effect, and promotes pro-environmental behaviors.	https://www.apa.org/monitor/2020/04/nurtured-nature
Passive Survivability	To provide critical life-support resources and functions during severe weather events, natural disasters and other power outages. Provide safety.	Incorporate off-grid technologies for on-site water collection and storage, electricity production and thermal comfort. If possible provision of on-site food production.	Provision of clean water, warmth shelter from the elements. Provides cognitive and emotional security. Provides physical safety.	www.buildinggreen.com/feature/passive-survivability-new-design-criterion-buildings

Healing Water	Designs for blue spaces, aquatic environments, and to preserve and create healing places featuring natural springs, rivers, ponds and ocean fronts and built wells, fountains and water features.	Design for and include holy wells, curative water features, spas, thermal baths, cold plunges, sweat lodges, views of natural water bodies, and provide for rainwater collection and purification.	Improved physical, mental and emotional wellness, increase tranquility, concen-tration and memory, boosts energy, removes toxins, encourage social interaction, and reduced stress.	https://www.webmd.com/diet/ss/slideshow-water-health https://www.cdc.gov/healthy places/healthtopics/parks_resources.htm#green
Spiritual Dimensions	To design for spiritual renewal, transformative and sanctuary experiences, provide opportunities for recharge, self-reflection, connectedness to larger context. Designs that are ineffable and indescribable.	Designs with sense of entry, boundaries, central focus, often with significant geometry, with embodied symbolism, living color, with light and luminosity. Spaces that are safe and noise-free. Spaces that invite participation.	Creates calm and contentment, self-empowerment, stress reduction, improved mood, reduction of temporal density, facilitates meaningful social connections, addresses existential questions of life, and increase life satisfaction.	https://greatergood.berkeley.edu/dacher keltner/docs/shiota.2007.pdf https://www.researchgate.net/publication/15347724_Development_of_the_Serenity_Scale
Wayfinding	Providing clear and structured flow for functional circulation an emergency exiting. Providing clear spatial distancing during pandemics.	Clear spatial definitions, direction, correct lighting, use of visible cues such as landmarks and signs, and removable of obstructions.	Reduced stress, improved moods and satisfaction, increase physical activity, and internal operational efficiency.	https://www.sciencedirect.com/science/article/abs/pii/S235271022302034X http://www.ai.mit.edu/projects/infoarch/publications/mfoltz-thesis/node8.html

Table 4.1
Architectural Scale Strategies

NOTES

1. Venolia, Carol, *Healing Environments* (Berkely, CA: Celestial Arts, 2008), p. 11.
2. Olgyay, Victor, *Design with Climate: Bioclimatic Approach to Architectural Regionalism* (Princeton, NJ: Princeton University Press, 1963).
3. *Majority of the World's Cities Highly Exposed to Disasters*, (Accessed March 15, 2023), https://www.un.org/development/desa/en/news/population/world-cities-day-2018.html
4. *Eco-anxiety: The Psychological Aftermath of the Climate Crisis*, (Accessed March 15, 2023), https://www.iberdrola.com/social-commitment/what-is-ecoanxiety
5. Tabb, Phillip James, *Elemental Architecture: Temperaments of Sustainability* (London, UK: Routledge, 2019), pp. 129–130.
6. McAllister, Sean, *There Could be 12 Billion Climate Refugees by 2050. Here's What You Need to Know*, (Accessed July 19, 2023), https://www.zurich.com/en/media/magazine/2022/there-could-be-1–2-billion-climate-refugees-by-2050-here-s-what-you-need-to-know
7. Futurium, *House of Futures*, (Accessed October 20, 2022), https://futurium.de/en/about-us/architecture

8. Ehrenfeld, John R., *Sustainability by Design* (New Haven, CT: Yale University Press, 2008).
9. Harvard School for Public Health, *Building Evidence for Health: The 9 Foundations of a Healthy Building*, (Accessed February 20, 2023), https://forhealth.org/Harvard.Building_Evidence_for_Health.the_9_Foundations.pdf
10. World Health Organization, *Bulletin of the World Health Organization, Urbanization and Health*, (Accessed September 28, 2022), http://www.who.int/bulletin/volumes/88/4/10–010410/en/
11. Ott, W.R., Human Activity Patterns: A Review of the Literature for Estimating Time Spent Indoors, Out-doors, and in Transit. In: *Proceedings of the Research Planning Conference on Human Activity Patterns* (Las Vegas, NE: EPA).
12. Thaler, Richard H., *The Power of Nudges, for Good and Bad*, (Accessed August 15, 2023), https://www.nytimes.com/2015/11/01/upshot/the-power-of-nudges-for-good-and-bad.html
13. Mitchell, Ed., *What's a Nudge in Product Design?* (Accessed August 15, 2023), https://www.delve.com/insights/whats-a-nudge-in-product-design
14. Ray, Celeste (Ed.), *Sacred Waters: A Cross-Cultural Compendium of Hallowed Springs and Holy Wells* (London, UK: Routledge, 2020), pp. 2–3.
15. Phon, Abby, *10 Reasons Why You Should Drink More Water*, March 20, 2012, (Accessed November 22, 2022), https://www.mindbodygreen.com/0–4287/10-Reasons-Why-You-Should-Drink-More-Water.html
16. Tabb, Phillip, *Thin Place Design: Architecture of the Numinous* (New York, NY: Routledge, 2024).
17. Ibid.
18. Ray, Celeste (Ed.), *Sacred Waters: Cross-Cultural Compendium of Hollowed Springs and Holy Wells* (London, UK: Routledge, 2020).
19. Wilson, Alex, (Accessed January 12, 2020), https://www.buildinggreen.com/feature/passive-survivability-new-design-criterion-buildings
20. *Passive Survivability: How LEED Helps When the Power Goes Out*, (Accessed October 4, 2023), https://www.usgbc.org/articles/passive-survivability-how-leed-helps-when-power-goes-out
21. Corbett, Lionel, *The Sacred Cauldron: Psychotherapy as a Spiritual Practice* (Ashville, NC: Chiron Publications, 2015).
22. Keltner, Dacher, *Awe: The New Science of Everyday Wonder and How it Can Transform Our Lives* (New York, NY: Penguin Press, 2023).
23. Gesler, Wilbert M., *Healing Places* (Lanham, MD: Rowman & Littlefield Publishers, 2003).
24. Steele, John, *Geomancy: Consciousness and Sacred Sites* (New York, NY: Trigon Communications, 1985).
25. Kopec, Dac, *Person-Centered Health Care Design* (New York, NY: Routledge, 2021), pp. 199–204.
26. Fu, Meiqing, Rui Liu, & Qipeng Liu, *How Individuals Sense Environments During Indoor Emergency Wayfinding: An Eye-tracking Investigation*, (Accessed December 14, 2023), https://www.sciencedirect.com/science/article/abs/pii/S235271022302034X
27. Clifton, Dave, *12 Benefits of Wayfinding for Campus Environments*, (Accessed December 12, 2023), https://spaceiq.com/blog/benefits-of-wayfinding/
28. Kopec, Dac, *Person-Centered Health Care Design* (New York, NY: Routledge, 2021), p. 229.
29. Massecuites Institute of Technology, *Design Principles for Wayfinding*, (Accessed December 15, 2023), http://www.ai.mit.edu/projects/infoarch/publications/mfoltz-thesis/node8.html

5 WELLNESS INTERIOR STRATEGIES

INTERIOR SCALE STRATEGIES

Wellness strategies that are directly related to place have numerous opportunities with the design of interior spaces in buildings. On average, Americans spend nearly 90%of their time indoors.[1] This was never more evident than during the COVID-19 pandemic when stay-at-home, lockdowns, isolation, and quarantine were widespread throughout the world. Modern amenities, emergent technologies, more humane workspaces, and larger domestic dwellings have undoubtedly made contemporary life easier. However, there are health risks associated with too much indoor living. They include the reduction of physical activity, exposure to indoor air pollution and dampness, decreased exposure to daylight and fresh air, and the reduction of access to nature. Health and wellness strategies at the interior design scale involve a variety of design interventions that address these issues. They are the inclusion of biophilic principles and nature within interior spaces, provision of gathering places that foster social healing, plentiful daylighting strategies, incorporation of natural ventilation and access to fresh air, the use of natural and non-toxic materials and finishes, strategic introduction of healing color, and the design of thin place principles and inclusion of sanctuary spaces. Health and wellness benefits from the strategies at this scale range from reduced contamination and respiratory ailments to mental clarity and improved circadian rhythms. They benefit in particular ways as discussed in Chapter 2 with physical, psychological, mental, social, spiritual, economic, environmental, and spiritual outcomes. The interior scale strategies in this section include incorporating nature within, daylighting strategies, natural ventilation strategies, wellness-oriented materiality, living color, and thin place sanctuary spaces.

1. **Incorporating nature within**
   Incorporating nature in architecture has strong ties to the biophilic effect, and within thin places it is often one of the most powerful elicitors of health and wellness. Nature provides positive health and wellness outcomes. Nature within includes views to places of natural scenery – vast, unusual, colorful, and beautiful landscapes, places that are compellingly serene – intimate, personable, familiar, and small-scale spaces, and places of memory, that are historic landscapes, important landmarks, and places of cultural significance. While nature has both beneficial and destructive effects, for interior places nature

DOI: 10.4324/9781003472902-5

is safe, welcomed, and beautiful. Examples are views to flora and fauna, the geology of a region, water features (streams, rivers, ponds, lakes, and oceans), and celestial phenomena. There are two major causes of decreasing contact with nature especially in urban and interior environments. The first is the diminishment of natural land in which to view nature, and the other is the increasingly limited access to the remaining urban parks and landscape gardens. The experience of nature is a health and wellness benefit and for nature to be incorporated indoors increases daily access to it.

The Eden Project is located in Cornwall, UK and was designed by Nicholas Grimshaw and completed in 2000. It features two large biodomes that cluster with smaller domes. The biomes are enclosed within hexagonal and pentagonal plastic cells that can be inflated or deflated to adjust the insulation levels responding to fluctuating outside temperatures. They enclose multiple complexes covering more than 3.9 acres (1.56 ha) of land, and housing over 100,000 plants. The tectonic form language is biomorphic and encloses the world's largest man-made rainforest. The goal of the project was to restore the human-nature bond. The biophilic features include access to nature, water, plants, the earth, sensory connections, refuge, living color, natural light, and numinous experiences. The Tropical Biome was the world's largest enclosed greenhouse covering more than four acres of land, with over 100,000 representing 5,000 species from many of the climate zones of the world. The Eden Project is an immersive experience, sustainability model, teaching tool, and protector of nature. While the interior was specifically programmed for flora and fauna, it represents an exaggerated example of the interior power and beauty of nature.

The dwelling shown in Figures 5.1c/d has been designed for health and wellness and was designed by architect Phillip Tabb. It has a small footprint with minimal impact on the site and has a total of 1,650 square feet (153 m^2) of enclosed space. The primary functions occur on the main level which is surrounded by coniferous and deciduous trees. With its 10.5-kW/h photovoltaic system (35 panels) and Tesla battery wall, it can function at net zero. The south-facing living spaces are passively solar heated in winter. The walled-in garden serves as a natural focus with its peach trees, flowers, edible plants, and reflecting pool. The design reinforces direct views with year-around access to the garden.

The wellness strategies for integrating nature inside buildings include providing abundant views outside to natural settings and the garden, introducing sunlight for daylighting and triggering circadian rhythms, providing natural fresh airflow especially to stimulate olfactory senses, viewing and hearing the presence of water, providing continuity with nature's colors and material connections, and including indoor vegetation. This scale also encourages bringing the outdoors inside for direct experiences. The walled-in garden also serves as a sanctuary, contemplative, and thin place.

The health benefits of the strategy of nature within are increased energy, mental clarity, decreased stress, lower blood pressure and heart rate, and increased positive moods. There are further benefits of the Eden Project with

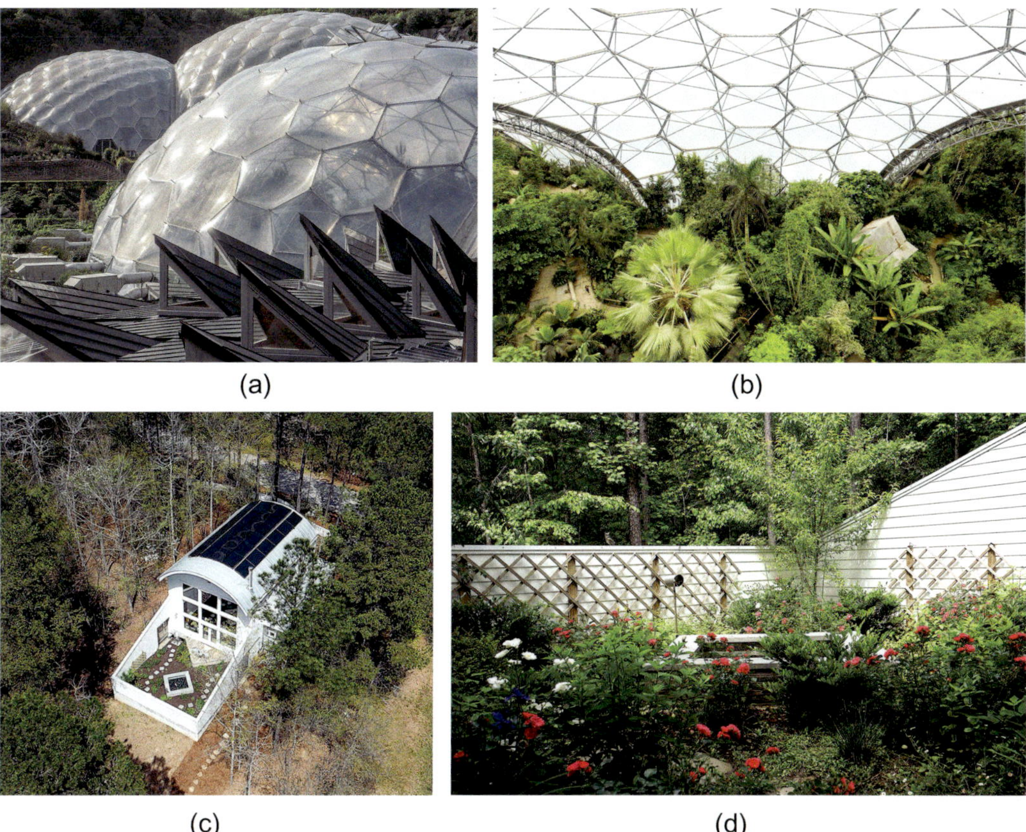

5.1 Incorporating Nature-Within Strategies a) The Eden Project Exterior, b) The Eden Project Interior, c) Tabb Residence Aerial View, d) Tabb Residence Walled-in Garden

(Sources: Wikimedia Commons, Shutterstock, and Phillip Tabb)

its positive financial contributions to the local economy. Environmental benefits include improved biodiversity, improved microclimate, and increased pro-environmental behaviors. In addition, nature and plants experienced within indoor spaces improve indoor air quality due to "phytoremediation" or contaminant scrubbing from indoor air. However, care should be taken regarding pest infestations and possible allergies. There is also evidence that bonds between people and their pets are linked to health benefits, including increased longevity. Animals can serve as a source of comfort and support, and research is showing that connections with animals can build a bridge for social interactions.[2] And finally, plants may improve one's outlook on life and boost feelings of being more alive and active. There is evidence that indicates making nature more visible within a building elevates the spirit.

2. Daylighting strategies

Natural and artificial lighting create ambiance, enhancing colors and textures, and highlighting architectural features. Light impacts health and performance, and is expressed in many forms related to luminosity, inspiration, the ethereal, and the numinous. Fluid luminosity refers to the changing qualities of light, whether it is due to fluctuating conditions, differing sources, color, or architectural design. Natural light affects both our eye function and our inherent circadian rhythms.

It is natural, dynamic, and can be direct, filtered, diffused, or reflected. It can form pools of light, define shapes, and provide warmth. Daylighting provides the full spectrum of natural light, and natural daylighting reduces AC and electricity demands. Natural light can reduce mildew and mold build-up. It is also linked to an increase in work satisfaction. The positive health outcomes include boosting vitamin D, warding off seasonal depression, improving sleep, producing serotonin, reducing eye strain, and expediting healing. Light is expressed in many forms and is related to luminosity, the ethereal, inspiration, and the numinous. Considering daylight, it can be facilitated through the use of windows, transparent doors, skylights, light shelves, dormers and roof lanterns, skyspaces, and glass roofs. According to Louis I. Kahn, silence is immeasurable while light is the giver of presence.[3]

Light brings visibility to interior spaces. It manifests in multiple ways including naturally filtered, diffused, or directed to illuminate significant places as well as artificial lighting. The night sky is mysterious and thought provoking. Light also marks the passage of time from the changes of seasons to the hours of the day. Both the quantity and quality of light are in effect. Light in concert with shadow gives definition giving cues about depth and position. Light elicits both awe and serene emotions often in very differing ways through its different qualities. Light ranges from the more stimulating sunlight and storm light to moonlight and starlight. Light, color, and temperature can affect emotions and relaxation, and help improve sleep and regulate blood pressure.[4] Properly designed sunshading devices will not only reduce heat gain in summer but will help prevent exposure to harmful UV light. Great care should be given to the relationship between access to daylight and the density of built form. As our need for accommodating greater populations, and as we spend most of our time indoors, daylight is not only required by codes, but is necessary for wellness. Poor lighting can create glare, headaches, eyestrain, fatigue and eye damage, and affects sleep quality and circadian rhythms, vitamin D deficiencies, physical safety, and human psychology including stress and moods.

The work of architect Erik Asmussen, particularly at the Jarna Community in Sweden, illustrates the artistic use of natural light and shading patterns. The corridor leading into the Vidar Clinic dining room is partly defined by a wall of windows with a biophilic, rhythmic pattern on the floor (tree branch-like), Figure 5.2c. Asumssen utilizes another wonderful daylighting strategy for indoor double-loaded corridors by providing periodic public open spaces adjacent to the passageway and connecting to the outdoors, thereby providing natural light inside. The Oculus Building in New York City houses the World Trade Center Transportation Hub and is another inspiring use of daylight, Figure 5.2d. It is an excellent example of the illuminating qualities of natural light. The transparency of the structure allows light to flood through into the grey and white marble floors below, and a retractable skylight that runs the length of the Oculus' spine will open each September 11 to honor the memory of the victims. The operable skylights or roof windows at the top of the spine help facilitate the stack effect. Natural light reduces the need for electrical energy for lighting and in

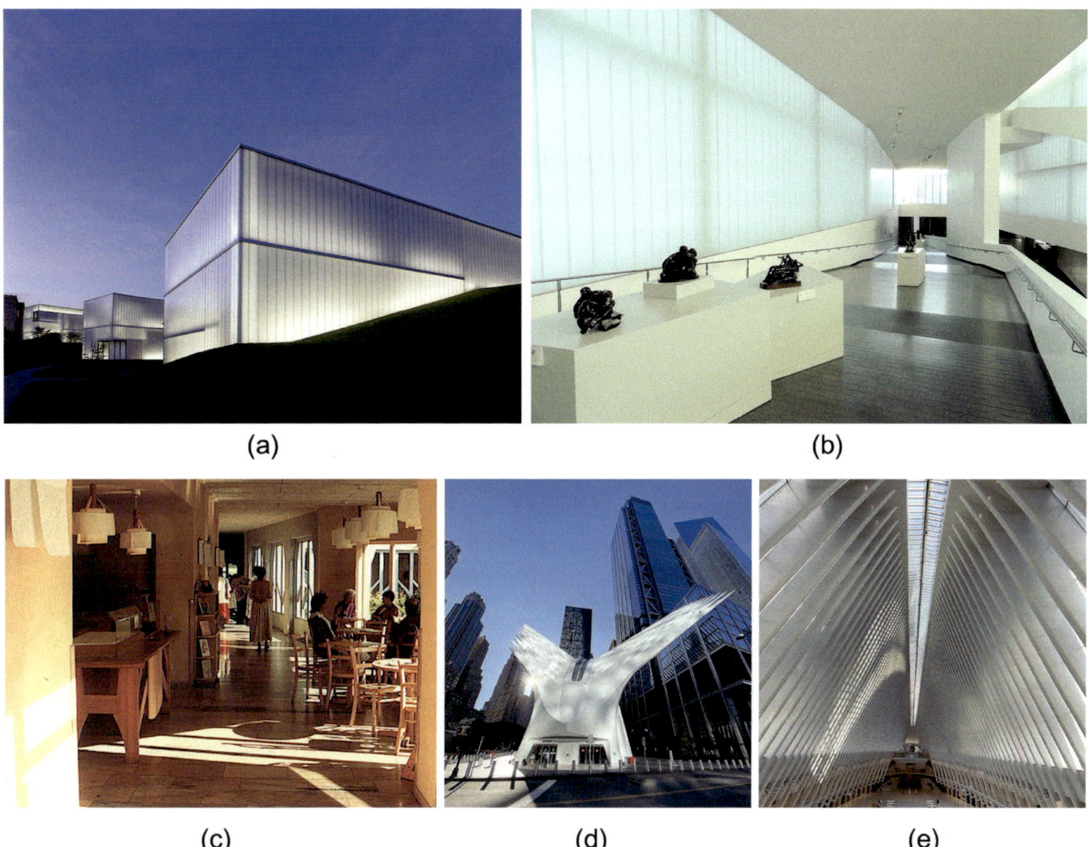

5.2
Daylighting Strategies
a) Nelson-Atkins Museum Exterior, b) Nelson-Atkins Museum Interior, c) Main Dining Corridor at the Vidar Clinic, d) Oculus Exterior, e) Oculus Interior

(Sources: Wikimedia Commons, Gary Coates, and Phillip Tabb)

part functions to illuminate the elliptical floor and space for the movement of 200,000–250,000 commuters per day to 13 subway lines. Refer to Figure 5.2e.

The Nelson-Atkins Museum of Art, designed by Steven Holl and located in Kansas City, Missouri originally opened in 1933, and now houses more than 40,000 works of art, Figures 5.2a/b. The museum features Asian art, Chinese landscape paintings, Chinese ceramics, African works, Egyptian sculpture, European Renaissance paintings, and Native American art. The curtain wall insertion creates an experiential environment of discovery and luminosity. The new building is covered by glass forms or lenses bringing light to the galleries. The layers of translucent glass that make up the lenses gather, diffuse, and refract light, and glow as if from another world. The wellness benefits include vision benefits, improving physiological well-being, improving mood, reduction of stress and anxiety, enhancing the quality of experience, improving attendance for students, and preventing the growth of fungi.

According to Lisa Heschong, daylighting strategies include increased glazing levels along with solar control, incorporating apertures like skylights, clerestories, and light shelves, use of high-performance glazing, tapering light levels, provision of reflective interior surfaces to distribute the light, and provision of measures to minimize glare.[5] The health benefits of daylighting are reduced eyestrain, increased Vitamin D production, improved circadian rhythms and sleep patterns, forestalled seasonal depression, enhanced mental clarity, increased focus and productivity, and increased positive moods. Further, they boost the immune system, prevents SAD, improves sleep and circadian rhythms, improves mood, enhances the spirit of place, have financial benefits via the Central Place Theory of light, function, and place, and offer historic and symbolic significance by contributing to the experience of awe.

3. **Natural ventilation strategies**

Ventilation in buildings is required to bring fresh air in from outside and dilute or remove occupant-generated pollutants. While air can be extremely destructive to buildings, it is also life-giving to people. The oxygen in the air is necessary for our survival. It is important for a building to function by repelling polluted air from building exteriors, expelling unwanted interior air to the outside, and permitting only healthy fresh air into and through the building. Air is also important in mitigating temperature differences affecting comfort. Experience of outdoor air can enhance sensory connections to nature and the elements. Climate-positive outcomes include carbon sequestering and oxygen production with abundant forested lands. Sustainability can be improved with the efficiency of fresh air, natural ventilation, and the use of internal filtering systems to reduce the need for outside make-up air.

Some of the benefits of healthy fresh air include boosting the immune system, providing fresh oxygen, increasing energy, and improving cognitive function. It is good for digestion, it cleans out the lungs, and it sharpens the mind.[6] Natural ventilation is one of the oldest indoor environmental strategies, especially when used to stoke firepits and remove smoke. Wall openings and later windows became ways of providing fresh air, and increased ventilation rates are critical in larger buildings. The positive qualities of air come from its low density and its subtlety. Therefore, its influence on architecture is also dispersed and subtle. Christopher Alexander and his colleagues in their seminal work "*A Pattern Language*," spoke of certain patterns that promote air circulation, such as patterns: #131 flow through rooms, #159 light on two sides of a room, #163 outdoor room, #180 window places, #194 inside windows, #221 natural doors and windows, and #236 windows that open wide.[7] Seemingly simple design considerations, contribute greatly to the health and quality of experience in interior spaces, especially in residential design.

Wind-catchers were a traditional method in North Africa and West Asia for capturing prevailing wind and redirecting it inward to a building's interior. Completed in 1993, the Queen's Building is arguably the best-known example of the work of Alan Short and Brian Ford in their pioneering efforts to reintroduce the use of natural ventilation into the design of large buildings. Important functions for natural well-ventilated spaces include the idea of "zone-coupling" where fresh air obtained from the perimeter of a building is connected to deeper interior spaces, and that unwanted air and sick building syndrome symptoms can be isolated and exhausted out of the building.[8] Efficient mechanical air handling systems also contribute to wellness by replenishing oxygen levels, removing dust and other particles, and adjusting temperature and humidity within the indoor air. Having multiple zones within a building allows for adjustments to the air quality and temperature based upon dynamic space orientation responses to the sun, types of activities, and differing 24-hour use.

The Marika Alderson House, Figure 5.3a, is located in the Northern Territory of Australia and was designed in 1994 by architect Glenn Murcutt. It features open and operable façades and fins that facilitate natural ventilation and indoor-outdoor connections. The vertical fins or blades funnel the horizontal direction of the breezes into the space while the roof overhangs trap the breezes. The blades also offer privacy. Openings on all sides of the building facilitate air movement within and through the space especially along windward façades. The large roof overhangs and fins provide sun and rain protection especially for the façades and openings. The shelter effect is important in contexts with hot and cold winds. The structure is lifted above the ground on a timber platform allowing for natural ventilation beneath the building. Elongated building shape and aspect ratio in warm-humid climate zones can enhance natural ventilation due to the increase of wind-exposed façades.

There are several strategies for natural ventilation. They are stack ventilation (utilizing temperature differences to generate air movement), top-down ventilation, single-side ventilation, and cross ventilation (with two or more

5.3
Natural Ventilation Strategies
a) Marika Alderson House, b) Operable Window,
c) Traditional Wind Towers, d) Modern Exhaust Fans

(Sources: Wikimedia Commons and Shutterstock)

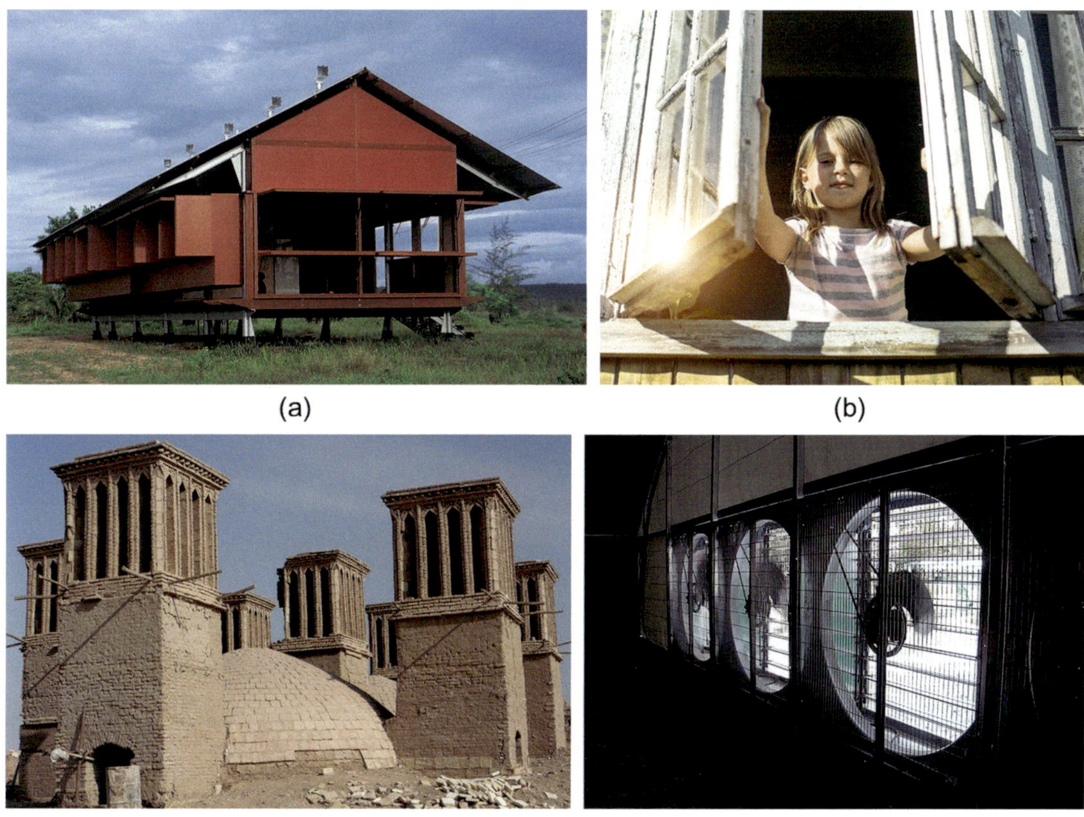

operable windows per room). These strategies can be directed or operationalized with opening windows, louvers, and the stack effect. Wind towers, windcatchers, and wind scoops are used to collect and direct wind inside buildings for ventilation and evaporative cooling. Natural ventilation can be augmented with mechanical fans and exhaust and supply (utilizing pressure differences between outside and inside air) ventilation. Window deflectors can be employed to provide sun control and breeze venting. Protection from excessive wind occurs with storm panels and roll-down shutters. Dynamic interior air movement versus static air conditions has been shown to produce positive health effects. The health benefits are increased energy, mental clarity, decreased stress, lower blood pressure and heart rate, reductions in respiratory illness, increased positive moods, increased productivity, lower CO_2 emissions, and increased pro-social behaviors.

4. **Prospect and refuge strategies**
The Prospect-Refuge Theory was developed by Jay Appleton theorizing that our innate desire for nature has prospects or critical viewing, while at the same time enjoying safety (refuge).[9] To Konrad Lorenz prospect-refuge means, one can "*see*, while not being *seen*."[10] Prospect creates discerning views of distant objects, changes in weather, intruders, and potential sources of danger. Refuge provides a secure, safe, and protected setting at both the urban design and architectural scales. While the theory is new, humans gravitated to survival-advantaged landscapes, like the East Africa Savannah during the Pleistocene Period (1.8 million years ago) where periodic trees offered safe views to surrounding grasslands, Figure 5.4a. While fight or flight are hard-wired into human nature, prospect and refuge seem intrinsically a part of us as well. Called "*a womb with a view*" by David Buss, prospect and refuge are preferred habitats.[11] It is clear that ancestral conditions are different today and that concepts of prospect and refuge have evolved quite differently. Modern security occurs not only with planning interventions and architectural designs, but also with the use of technology. In restaurants, cozy nooks and intimate settings are desirable. Refuge can also occur at the community level where residents can observe suspicious activity. In urban contexts, this includes the provision of dynamic public places with naturally occurring social surveillance opportunities. This strategy implies creating a safe refuge within community commercial and cultural destinations with natural street and place surveillance. Appropriate measures for refuge include home sheltering, possibly the need for isolation, and designs for passive survivability.

Prospect design strategies simply include the provision of windows, outdoor spaces, and entryways facing sidewalks, driveways, streets, and neighborhoods. Porches, decks, courtyards, terraces, and outdoor rooms also serve as prospect spaces. With new technologies, visual surveillance can be augmented by digital means and home security systems, such as ADT, Google Home, SimpliCam, Vivint, and Ring to name but a few. Passive survivability refers to the ability to maintain critical life-support conditions if those conditions have been shut off for an extended period. Passive survivability was introduced by Alex Wilson in the wake of Hurricane Katrina and was discussed in the last chapter.[12] Essential services include shelter from the elements, electricity, clean water, and food storage and access to the Internet. Prospect and refuge are important strategies for passive survivability with ability to see and respond to extreme weather events and to find safe spaces for refuge. This is a compelling idea in the face of climate change, natural disasters, and increased extreme weather events, including inhospitable temperatures, drought, and even terrorist's threats. Passive survivability design strategies are context-driven and would include the use of on-site renewable energy sources, daylighting, natural ventilation, passive solar heating or heat avoidance, rainwater harvesting or emergency water storage, and backup power sources.

The rapid emergence of the coronavirus was alarming and appropriate mitigation strategies were evolving along with it. Prospect and refuge emerged as attributes that could contribute to visual, safe, and supporting settings that connect to nature. Prospect allows for surveillance and the identification of danger. The sustainability outcomes occur in the form of passive survivability potentials when coupled with refuge spaces. Together these strategies produce positive health and wellness outcomes, including peace of mind, emotional security, stress reduction, and reduced boredom. Refuge also provides safety from potential intruders and suspicious activity, and protection from inclement weather. Furthermore, refuge spaces can provide solitude, quiet, and peace when processing stressful or emotional issues.

According to Steven Kellert, prospect and refuge designs provide comforting and nurturing interior spaces.[13] During the coronavirus pandemic, as throughout most of the world, residents sheltered in place, and in some instances, residents were able to safely engage with the natural surroundings without direct contact with other residents. The wellness strategies of prospect and refuge were important during the COVID-19 pandemic, but they also are important during natural disasters offering a safe haven from danger. According to David Buss, the evolutionary-inspired epiphanies afforded the Savannah ancestors while far less frequent, are still desired. It is within our power today to recreate through design some of the desirable conditions, such as the prospect of surveillance and beneficial views of nature, and refuge for comfort and safety.[14] Refer to Figure 5.4a.

The southern Aegean island of Santorini is a striking natural example of the interaction between the four terrestrial elements and architectural and urban forms. While Santorini is beautiful and picturesque, it is an expression of a very long struggle for survival in an isolated and adverse environment.[15] And so, it is not surprising that prospect and refuge play an important part in their "womb-like" designs. Figures 5.4b/c show the exterior of the south-facing dwellings (prospect) that seek warm sunlight with views to the Aegean Sea, and in more historic time views of intruders to the island. The interiors of a majority of the dwellings use a barrel-vaulted design that is comfortable and safe. The cave-like dwelling form is protected on three sides and supports

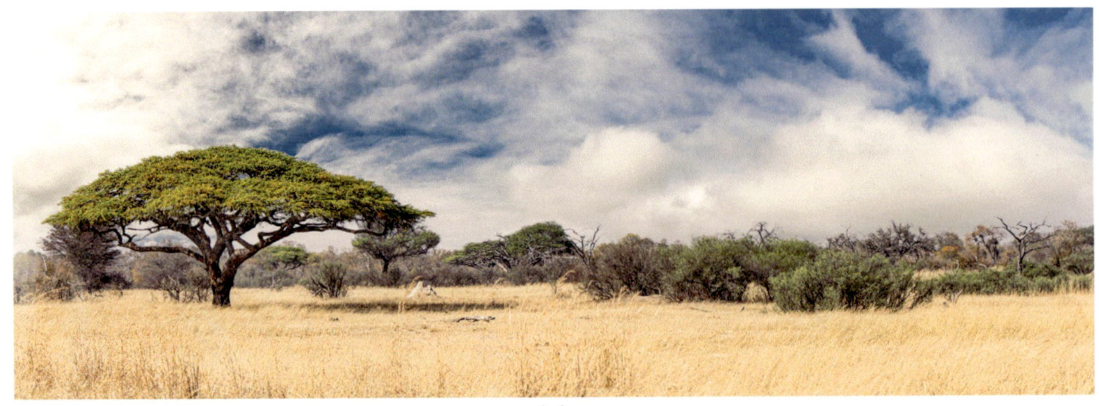

(a)

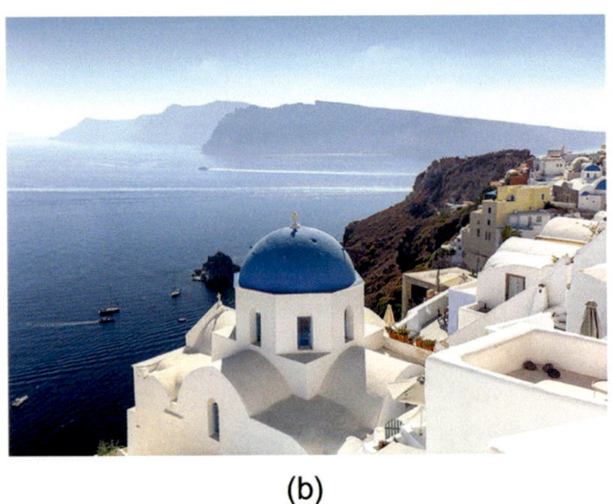

(b)

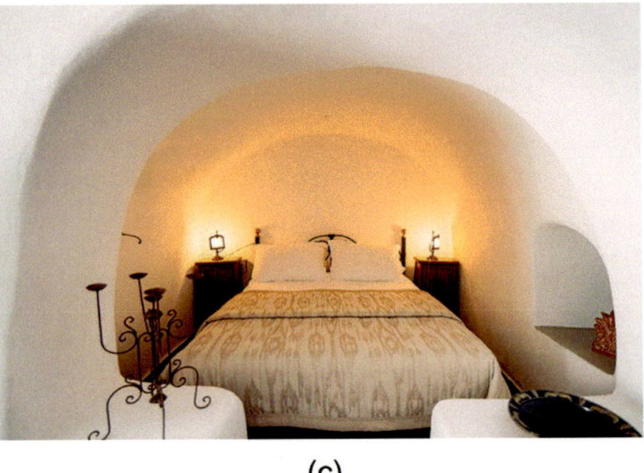

(c)

5.4
Prospect and Refuge a) East African Savanna, b) Santorini Prospect, c) Santorini Refuge
(*Source: Shutterstock*)

refuge. The wellness benefits are awareness, perception and protection from external threats (well-being), and feelings of safety, support, and protection (physical, emotional, and psychological well-being).

5. **Wellness-oriented materiality**
   The common definition of pollution is the introduction of contaminants into the environment, both natural and human-made, that cause disease, harm, instability, and destruction. Pollutants usually affect the elemental substances including the earth, water, and air, and can manifest in the very places we live – our homes, schools, places of work, and our communities. Building materials can produce indoor pollution and, fairly recently, the incorporation of non-toxic materials has been shown to reduce the negative health effects and improve wellness. Natural materials usually come directly from the environment as opposed to artificial materials that are man-made or created through industrialized processes. Natural materiality expresses non-objective, nonlinear, and random patterns, and experiencing them creates a semiotic narrative back to a living source.[16] For example, the use of natural wood in interiors (floors, ceilings, structure, walls, doors, windows, and furniture) reduces the carbon footprint, possesses an aesthetic appeal, and provides a connection to the living qualities of the trees from which they were harvested. By extension, this

wood-derived stimulation can have the physiological and wellness effects of forest bathing. Research has shown that olfactory stimulation is present with contact with natural materials.[17]

Non-toxic materials are incredibly important in wellness design as they are environmentally friendly, sustainable, safe, and can produce wellness outcomes. The physiological reaction from exposure to chemicals is called "*idiopathic environmental intolerance*," and can result in headaches, dizziness, poor memory, changes in cognition, breathing difficulties, chronic coughs, physical pain, and digestive issues.[18] Care should be given to ensure toxic out-gassing of radon, asbestos, formaldehyde, phtalates, and carbon monoxide. Natural materials include, but are not limited to, wood, clay brick, tile, stone, wool, bamboo, AshCrete, straw bale, living roofs, smart glass, eco-paints, and recycled steel and plastic. Glass functions to frame views, admit solar radiation, facilitate the greenhouse effect, and prevent internal heat loss.

In 1980, architect E. Fay Jones designed the Thorncrown Chapel in Eureka Springs, Arkansas, Figure 5.5a. Set in the Ozark Mountains, the chapel is placed among majestic rock bluffs, stone outcrops, and a densely wooded forest of oak, pine, and maple trees. The chapel is 24 feet (7.4 meters) wide, 60 feet (18 meters) in length, and 48 feet (14.6 meters) high. Jones described the chapel as displaying an authentic "Ozark Gothic" architectural language. Thorncrown Chapel was inspired by the light-filled interior of the 13th-century royal Sainte Chappelle, Paris's light-filled Gothic chapel. This Thorncrown Chapel is constructed mainly of indigenous wood from northwestern Arkansas. Materials needed to be carried to the construction site by two people, consequently the main structure was made from 2 × 4s, 2 × 6s and 2 × 12s where the truss framing was assembled on site. All of the wood was hand-rubbed with a grayish stain to blend with the bark of the surrounding trees and stone. The chapel is glass-enclosed with 425 glass windows amounting to 6,000 square feet (557 m^2) of glass, and the space is air conditioned. The crisscrossing of the structural framing is the building's signature, as is true of other of Jones' works. As one approaches, enters, and progresses into the interior space, the play of light against the structure sparkles with the moving perspective. Another visual inspiration and part of the architectural experience is the way the chapel's transparency frames the surrounding forest.

Log cabins have an ancient history in Europe, and in America are often associated with the first-generation home buildings by settlers, however there is a romantic connection to the building type with its natural materials, humble origins, and scale. Log cabins are mostly constructed without the use of nails and thus derive their stability from simple stacking, with only a few dowel joints for reinforcement, Figure 5.5b. The La boiserie dell'Aula Baratto was designed by Venetian architect Carlo Scarpa in 1960. The wood-exposed interior structure and window framing project a warmth, as seen in Figure 5.5c. The clay tile roof also gives a warm feeling, an intimate scale, and use of a natural earth-borne material.

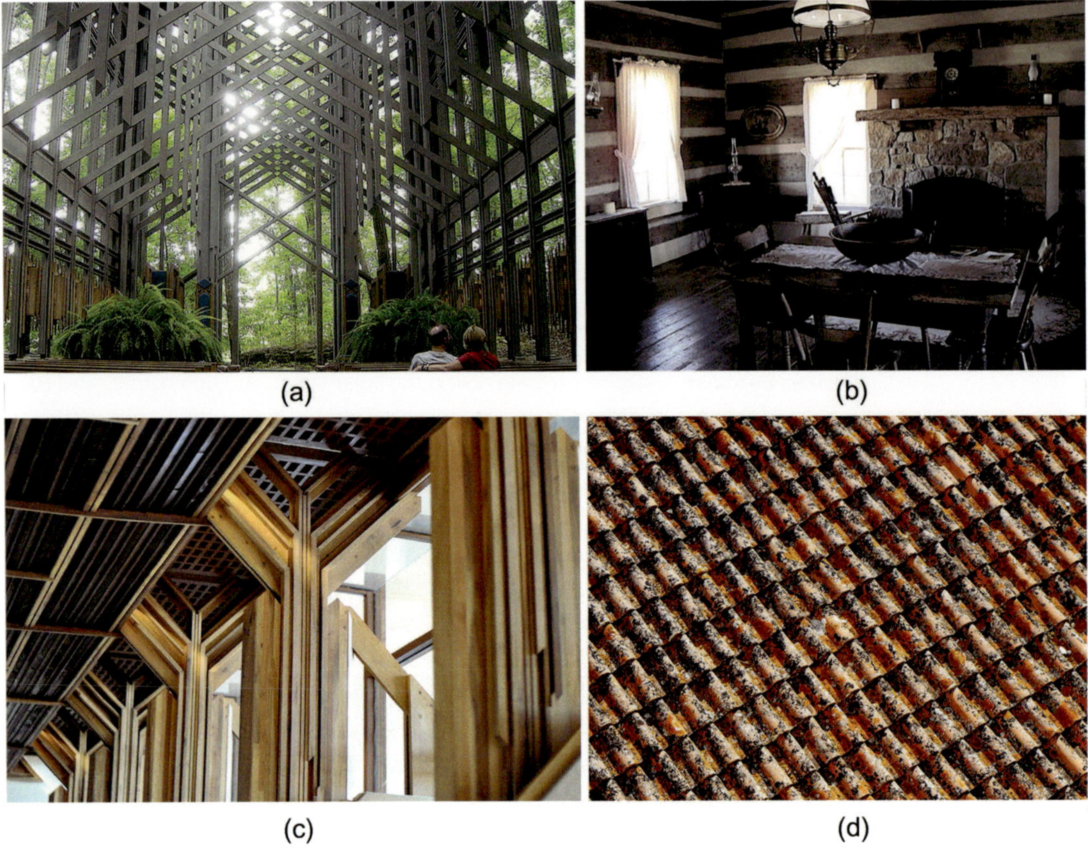
(a) (b) (c) (d)

5.5
Wellness Oriented Material Strategies a) Thorncrown Chapel, b) Log Cabin, c) Scarpa Wood Structure, d) Clay Tile Roof

(Source: Wikimedia Commons)

According to the US Environmental Protection Agency, indoor air can be as much as five times more contaminated than outdoor air.[19] This seems counterintuitive especially in urban and industrial areas. Building materials and chemicals considered to be harmful to human or environmental health have been collected and described in the Living Building Challenge's "*Red List*."[20] They are suggested to be phased out of use because of their toxicity, posing risks to human health and the greater ecosystem. Among materials on the red list are asbestos compounds, chlorinated polymers, formaldehyde, mercury, chromium, lead, other heavy metals, organotin compounds, creosote, pentachlorophenol, and volatile organic compounds (VOCs). Mold causes many health effects, including allergens, irritants, asthma, and in some cases, potentially toxic substances (mycotoxins). Generally, mold and fungi are brought indoors through roofs, windows, pipes, and where moisture has been allowed to seep inside. Key to mold prevention is moisture control by finding water sources, increasing ventilation especially spaces with water usage (bathrooms, kitchens, and washrooms), reducing or preventing condensation, and reducing humidity.[21]

The health benefits of natural materials are the experience of fresh air (little negative out-gassing), reduced respiratory ailments, mental clarity, improved circadian rhythms, and increased positive moods. Living in non-toxic environments can also slow down aging.[22] According to Bill Browning, wood materials are warm, comfortable, natural, inviting, and beautiful. Wood elicits visual, olfactory, and haptic experiences. The abundance of natural materials, and wood in particular, creates a strong connection or semantic process, back to the living and vital qualities of the trees and forests from which they came. This semantic processing ties our direct connection to the material thereby triggering a positive associative response.[23] Materials at the interior scale also include furnishing and furniture made from non-toxic materials that are durable, cleanable, bio-based and bio-compatible, and have low VOC levels and surface porosity. How carefully materials and products are used in construction, maintained and stored for internal use contributes to wellness.

6. Living color

Humans are visual creatures and as such color expresses a visible and vital element of life. Color plays a tremendous role in how we react and respond to things around us. It can affect the way we feel, how we think, and how we interact with one another. Colors, which enhance the beauty of nature connect the user to the outdoors and boosts health and well-being, subsequentially affecting a person physiologically and psychologically.[24] Color, which is natural and activated by varying qualities of light, can produce numinous experiences. It can be experienced as light and properties of surfaces, which change color over the course of a day. Colors also can have symbolic associations and elicit certain emotional responses, such as the color red representing passion and fire, blue with the calmness of the water, and green seen with abundant associations in nature and the plant world. Plant life within building interiors adds both vitality and living color. Indoor plantings, flower arrangements, living walls, greenhouses, and atriums provide direct access to the living world of plants and the colors they possess. Color and light perception changes with age usually beginning at age 40.

The healing benefits of color vary from color to color. While not all colors possess the same meaning and impact across cultures, they do have some overall emotional commonalities. The warmer colors tend to be more passionate and stimulate the senses and energy, while cooler colors calm the nervous system influencing mood and state of mind. Simply put, red is stimulating, orange is uplifting, yellow is cheerful, green is soothing, blue is calming, and purple is transforming. Color is used to raise awareness and for safety to alleviate physical hazards, such as danger, warnings, caution, and biological hazards. Color has been used extensively in Feng Shui as a notion of *living color* invoking a transcendent dimension with regenerative powers. The color goal of Feng Shui is to create balance and the correct color placement to improve vital energy. Colors, textures, lighting, and ambiance in physical spaces help define a sense of space and impact moods, thoughts, and productivity.

St. Gabriel's Parish Church in Toronto, Canada, according to architects Roberto Chiotti and Richard Vosko, is a meaningful expression of eco-theology, ritual-centeredness, the relevance of religious teachings in the world today, and active participation, Figure 5.6a. After its completion in 2006, the new church of St Gabriel's became the first church in Canada to receive Gold certification from

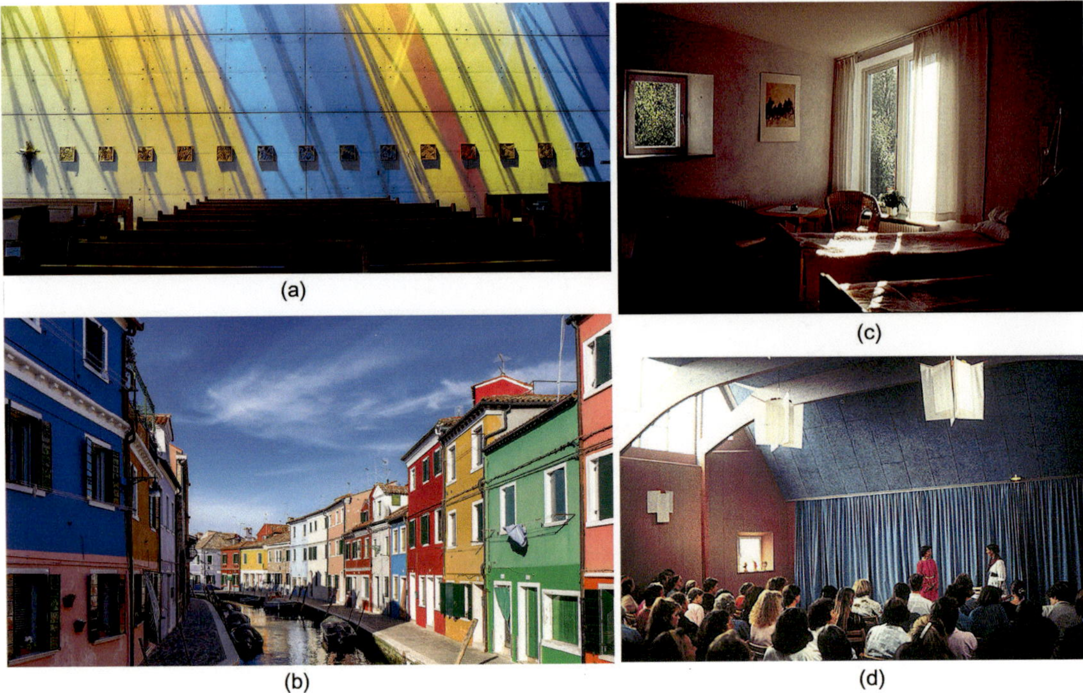

5.6
Living Color Strategies
a) St. Gabriel's Parish Church,
b) Burano Colorful Canal Street,
c) Vidar Clinic Recovery Room,
d) Vidar Clinic Auditorium

(Sources: Phillip Tabb, Wikimedia Commons, and Gary Coates)

the Leadership in Energy and Environmental Design (LEED™) Green Building Rating. Importantly the use of natural light and color expresses the splendor and constantly changing quality of time as the colored stripes move across the interior walls and over the Stations of the Cross throughout the day. This change marks the movement of the Earth turning on its axis. The warm colors of the yellow and the cool color of the blues are both stimulating and calming.

The incredibly colorful canal streetscapes in Burano, Italy, illustrated in Figure 5.6b are another example of the powerful use of color. It is written that originally color was introduced to the modest wooden homes in the 15th century as a wayfinding guide home from the lagoon seas for fishermen during misty and foggy weather. Another folktale suggests the reason for the diverse use of color was to distinguish one family home from another because so many shared common surnames thus creating individual family identity.[25] And because of the island's isolation and inbreeding, there were a lot of common names. Today, however, to visitors and tourists the colorful urban landscape is attractive, walkable, known for authentic lace, an accessible getaway a delightful half-hour vaporetto ride from Venice.

The work of architect Erik Asmussen, particularly at the Vidar Clinic in Jarna, Sweden, illustrates the subtle use of color. According to Gary Coates, the Vidar Clinic was designed specifically to function as a nurturing therapeutic environment.[26] Pigments were made with vegetable dyes within a beeswax medium as well as mineral dyes. The color quality in the most vulnerable patients' rooms, are the softest and most alive. According to the Vidar Clinic webpage, "A healing process has to encompass the wholeness of body, soul, social aspects and existential questions of meaning. Elements like presence, touch, conversation and participation of the patient are essential factors."[27] The soft colors and natural light illustrated in Figures 5.6c/d are of a typical recovery room in the Vidar Clinic and the small auditorium space.

The wellness strategies for living color are to introduce color through living plants and flowers within interior spaces, to provide ample views of outdoor nature and the color it possesses, and to introduce color pigments that are made from natural sources with zero volatile organic compounds, such as iron oxides, clay, crushed stone, and plant-based. Colors can relate to stimulating or calming effects by using warm and cool colors. The benefits derived from the electromagnetic wavelengths of the various colors produce positive wellness effects, including stimulation and calming of both mood and cognitive function. Colors also relate to the symbolic and connotative semantic associations coming through nature. Living color used in this way also contributes to a semantic associative process where there is an indirect relation between interior color and exterior living things.

7. Workplace innovation and wellness strategies

Although employment varies greatly, the average American spends just under eight hours a day or 40 hours a week at work.[28] This represents approximately 25% of our time. Despite the rise and interest in remote work, the majority of Americans (nearly 60%) still work in offices. According to the Pew Research Center, before the coronavirus outbreak, 20% of the workforce worked at home, during the outbreak that number increased to 71%, and after the outbreak more than 50% wanted to continue working from home.[29] Meanwhile, many companies have invested in innovative workplaces intended to enable employees at all levels to use and develop their skills, knowledge, experience, and creativity to the fullest while simultaneously enhancing business performance. Among these innovations is a focus on wellness. In research in the United Kingdom, key characteristics of an innovative workplace include the following:[30]

- The simultaneous achievement of high performance with quality of working life.
- Creation of a work environment built on fairness, job security, and advanced opportunities.
- Support of a systemic approach of job autonomy, self-management, and teamwork.
- Creation of a workplace culture of continuing engagement.
- Invitation flexibility in workplace time and place.
- Support of accountability, curiosity, creativity, coaching behaviors, and emotional intelligence.
- Inclusion of caregiving including paid time off and childcare.

Wellness within the workplace is defined by the Global Wellness Institute as the measure of employers' expenditures to improve wellness. These occur through services, products, and platforms that increase awareness, educational programs, incentives that address specific health risk factors, and encouragement of wellness lifestyles (workstyle practices). They address major challenges related to stress, burnout, work-life balance, and mental health. Workplace wellness programs target a wide range of employee behaviors (e.g., lack of exercise, poor eating habits, smoking, lack of sleep) and risk factors (e.g., chronic illness, obesity, addiction, depression, and stress).[31] Benefits of workplace innovation include attracting top talent, increasing efficiency, reducing waste, boosting employee engagement, strengthening customer relations, and increasing brand value. The major health and wellness benefits include stress reduction, improved mental health and emotional well-being, improved work-life balance, and financial well-being.

Examples of workplace innovation have occurred routinely within the Big Tech or information technology companies, such as Alphabet (Google), Amazon, Apple, Microsoft, and Meta (Facebook). Google Workspaces, for example, typically encourage "*casual collision*," there are abundant common areas for collaboration, unconventional workspace environments, an atmosphere of innovation, a dog-friendly attitude, with hackable (flexible and customizable) spaces. There is a commitment to wellness, so there is encouragement for exercise, use of recreational facilities, daycare for infants, provision of healthy food, and access to nature. Furthermore, there is a culture of work-life balance, which in addition to an emphasis on well-being, supports employee retention and long-term engagement, supportive leadership, and happiness impacts. In addition, the founders intended to promulgate features in the workspaces that promote efficiency, good feelings, and environmental awareness. The Googleplex (combining "Google" and "complex") in Mountain View, California is a complex of buildings that house 2,000,000 square feet (185,806 m^2) of office space, and the playful interiors were designed by architect Clive Wilkinson.

5.7
Google Workplace Wellness Strategies
a) Google Gymnasium,
b) Google Workstation

(Source: Shutterstock)

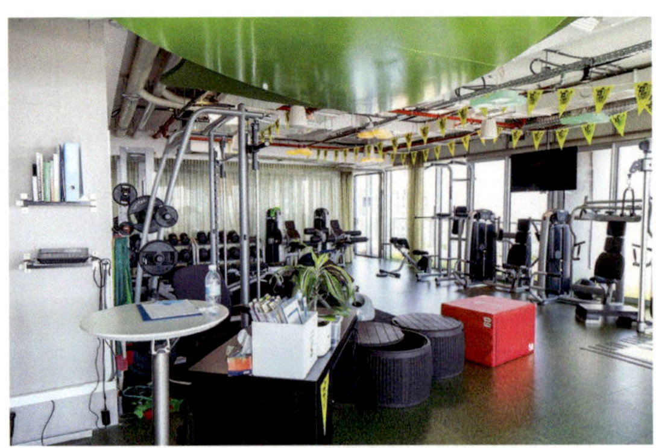

(a)

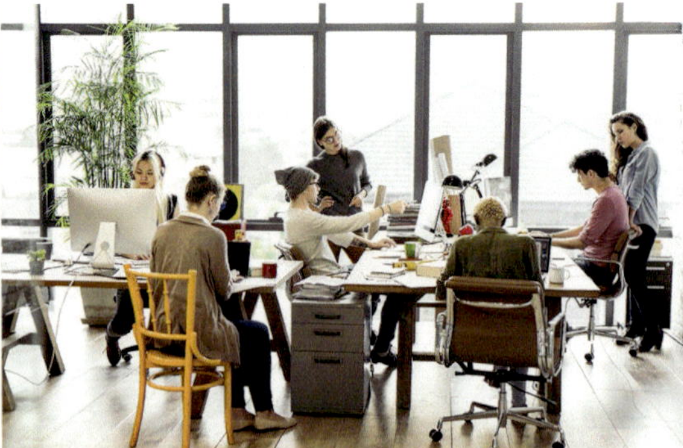

(b)

AI-powered workplace well-being tools, including *Reclaim.ai*, *Headspace*, *Welltory*, *Breathhh*, *Todoist*, and *MealMind*, are intended to monitor giving real-time feedback, to guide, and to optimize productivity.[32] Figures 5.7a/b show the Google gymnasium provided to encourage physical activity periodically throughout the workday, and a creative office space, which also serves as a group meeting place.

8. **Thin places and sanctuary spaces**

Thin places are locations or settings where a thin veil exists between the earthly world within which we live and the heavenly spiritual world that possesses a qualitatively different energy. Thin places are often referred to as sacred places, holy places, sanctuary places, vital places, soulful places, awe places, serene places, or charged places. Thin places suggest the connection between secular and sacred places which can produce strong wellness benefits, such as elicited by awe and serene emotional responses, inspirating experiences, and spiritual renewal. According to Dasher Keltner, awe emotions are characterized by perceived vastness and the need for accommodation (processing the experience).[33] And according to Kay Roberts, serene emotions are characterized by calm, contentment, belonging, and beneficence.[34] They possess certain energies and have characteristics guided by self-evident principles underlying the spiritual imagination and source experience whether found in nature or the built environment.[35] Sanctuary spaces foster stillness and peacefulness, and provide opportunities for emotional healing and access to deeper feelings. During the COVID-19 pandemic, spaces such as these were in high demand in order to quarantine and recover. In these spaces mitigating strategies occurred at three scales: 1) limiting person-to-person transmission through social distancing and sanitation protocols, 2) community suppression through suspension of mass gatherings and the isolation of high-risk settings, and 3) regional risk reduction by limiting public transportation and place-to-place travel.[36] Scientific research supports the relationship between inner peace (low-arousal, positive mental states) and well-being where one can experience life happenings with great clarity.

Sanctuary spaces can occur in varying forms, sizes, and locations from special alcoves in a bedroom or a home office space to a favorite hiding place in the woods or vacation spot. They can occur throughout everyday experiences or through special occasions. They are nurturing and personal. Children's treehouses or forts are a favorite sanctuary space allowing for intimacy, comradeship, creativity, and solitude. Places like Google are known for their unique and varying workspaces that serve to provide privacy, focus, connection, and recharge. Sanctuary spaces are also found in natural beauty spots, spiritual and thin places, therapeutic environments, and wellness retreats. During COVID-19, such spaces allowed for isolation and limited physical contact with fellow employees. The wellness benefits of such interesting environments include sources for renewal, relaxation, and quiet. Experiences within them can reduce stress and overstimulation, can strengthen the immune system, and can improve mood and positive feelings.

Steeple Dingle is the preservation, careful restoration, and interior renovation of the 150-year-old Kilmalkedar church overlooking the sea at Muirioch, Kerry, Ireland. The iconic traditional gable form with a steeple made of stone and slate is contrasted with the unique free-standing steel and glass structure inside which now serves as a private residence. It is the contrast between the new and the old, the church typology and residential function, and the vernacular and contemporary materials that render this a thin place. The new loft-style bedrooms are glazed separating them from the main church space and thereby creating two internal sanctuary spaces. In addition, the resident family erected a Hypedome sanctuary space next to it. Both the chapel-house and dome reflect wellness designs.

The Solar Egg Sauna is located within an Arctic climate outside of the northern city of Kiruna, Sweden, and was designed in 2017 by architects Bigert and Bergstrom. A new contemporary sauna, aptly named the "*Solar Egg*," has been constructed in northern Sweden and is an excellent example of the sanctuary, wellness, and thin place quality of the sauna. They elicit physical healing and social connectedness. In the center of the sauna is an iron heart-shaped wood-burning stove made of stones. With general precautions taken when in use, wellness benefits of saunas include stress reduction, improve heart health, detoxify heavy metals and chemicals, slow down temporal density providing contemplative moments.

The presence and importance of silence cannot be overstated. Silence facilitates deeper, more self-reflective, and peaceful moments in the context of a noisy world.[37] Moments of silence can be transitions to transcendent experiences of awe and serenity. The health benefits are mental clarity, decreased stress, lower blood pressure and heart rate, reduced cortisol, reduced insomnia, and increased focus and positive moods. Sanctuary spaces are places that are nurturing, comforting, therapeutic, and provide protection and a safe haven. They support social healing and can be sacred, these can include workshops, storm shelters, bedroom alcoves, treehouses, children's forts, bathtubs, and even baby cribs. Refer to Figure 5.8 for a view of various sanctuary spaces.

9. Spatial variety and quality

The spatial determinants of wellness are impacted by the immaterial essence of interior space. Spatial qualities are quite varied as defined by scale, horizontal dimensions, height, shape and configuration, openness, translucency, porosity, orientation to light, internal separations (columns, walls, furniture), function and use, indoor/outdoor relationships, entrances and thresholds, color, materiality, and other decorations.[38] A final spatial determinant of wellness is the planning for access to health and wellness services (healthcare facilities, hospitals), nutrition (urban agriculture, markets, grocery stores), and access to nature (parks, gardens, and playgrounds). Spatial quality affects space functioning,

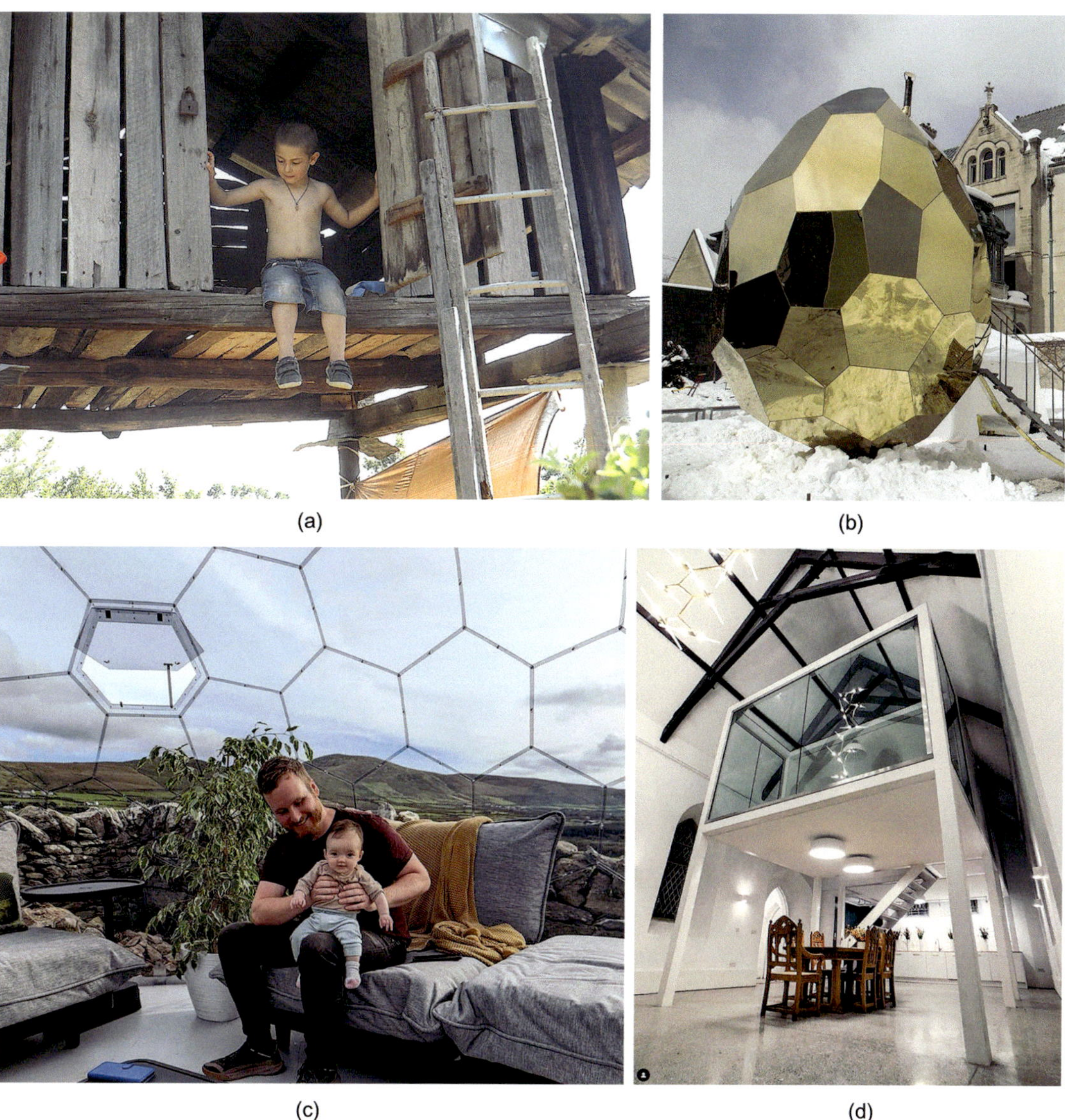

(a) (b) (c) (d)

5.8
Thin Place Sanctuary Space Strategies
a) Treehouse, b) Solar Egg Sauna, c) Dingle Sanctuary Dome, d) Dingle Home Sanctuary Space

(Sources: Wikimedia Commons, Oisin Havery, and Triona Butler Havery)

sustainability, aesthetics, and access to wellness goods, services, and health-care facilities.

Acre and Wyckmans cite four determinants in their definition of spatial quality. The first is views and the quality includes visibility, visual openness, composition, access to daylight, safety, and privacy. The second is internal spatial arrangements that include entrances and thresholds, through-circulation, internal space definitions, zoning and interconnectedness, and spatial generosity, function or activity. The third is spatial transitions that include clear boundaries, control and flow of public and private spaces, indoor and outdoor relationships, and spatial domain materiality. The fourth is spatial density which is spatial complexity, porosity, degree of enclosure, type of use, and people-to-space density.[39]

The Charles Jencks postmodern house in London has incredible spatial variety with rooms designed for the seasons, rooms for solar observation, rooms with views of the moon, and rooms for playfulness, Figure 5.9a. Room names include Spring, Summer, Autumn, Winter, the Cosmic Loo, Sundial Arcade, Solar Stair (with 52 steps), and Moonwell. The house is a re-working of the original 1840s late-Georgian building and was designed upon symbolic and elemental themes. This interior space has complexity, openness, diversity of use, and discrete zoning as well as connectedness, symbolism, and spatial generosity. As discussed in Chapter 6, Charles Jencks' wife Margaret Keswick Jencks was the inspiration for the Maggie Centres found throughout Europe for the treatment of cancer.[40]

The High Gothic Chartres Cathedral exists today almost as it was some 700 years ago. Known for the housing of the tunic or veil of the Virgin Mary, reportedly worn during the Annunciation and for the Miracle of Chartres after the great fire in 1194, the cathedral has been an important pilgrimage site. It was feared that the veil was lost in the fire, but on the third day after the fire, it was found safe. The quality of space in the Cathedral is extraordinary with the labyrinth, vertical space 120 feet (37 m) tall, exquisite stained-glass windows (176 windows), and grand colonnades. According to John James, Chartres is an architecture that enhances structure over form to create spaces held together in dynamic equilibrium.[41] The incredible uplifting spatiality of the nave and the beautiful west rose window are contrasted with the grounded labyrinth that was often navigated on pilgrims' knees, Figure 5.9b.

As wellness strategies, spatial variety accommodates multiple and changing personal and cultural needs, and spatial quality is influenced by basic elements of design and their connections to natural elements, quality of materials, and authenticity. In healthcare settings, spatial quality can contribute to self-healing through the use of sensory gardens, access to indoor air quality, and natural light. The wellness benefits to spatial variety and quality include

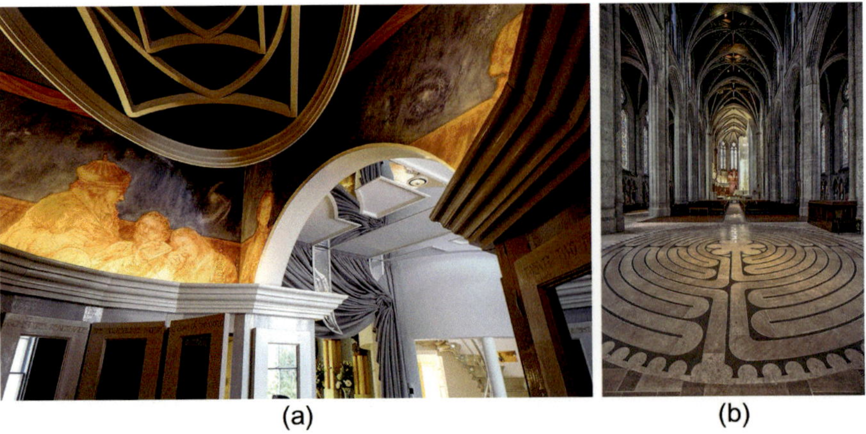

5.9 Spatial Variety and Quality a) Charles Jencks Residence Interior, b) Chartres Cathedral Interior Space

(Sources: Alamy Stock and Wikimedia Commons)

responses to a variety of physical, cognitive, emotional, and social needs. In this regard, architectural space not only contributes to physical health through spatial quality but also affects emotional and spiritual well-being. These benefits are defined further by the experience of awe and wonder resulting in possible stress and depression reduction, improvement of moods, increased generosity, and pro-social behaviors. Spatial quality can extend to interior attractiveness, public image, and users' well-being. Positive spatial experiences lead to what Aaron Antonovsky calls salutogenic designs responding empathetically and coherently to physical, cognitive, social, and spiritual pillars of wellness.[42] Spatial quality refers to one's ability to experience the space in comprehensible, manageable, and meaningful ways. And in the context of this work, in wellness ways.

Interior scale summary

The interior design scale offers opportunities for specific design strategies to incorporate health and wellness benefits that range from the aesthetic quality and reduction of contaminating materials and finishes to promoting natural light, natural ventilation, and direct access to nature. It addresses the materials, colors, and spaces in which we most intimately come in contact. This scale offers the opportunity to create a more seamless connection between inside (safe haven and refuge) and outside (prospect and access to nature). Due to the smaller impact of the interior scale, wellness design strategies and opportunities can easily be addressed with both existing and new construction. They can be focused on the interior of a single room or an entire building. However, they may be applied to outdoor "*urban rooms*" such as plazas, courtyards, and streetscapes. The outcomes at this scale contribute to pro-individual benefits through intimate and everyday wellness strategies, contribute to pro-social benefits through fostering community and family and friends' gatherings, as well as pro-environmental benefits through protection from negative climatic effects and positive interactions with nature. It must be noted here that implementation of these wellness design strategies does not guarantee positive health outcomes but it can provide greater opportunities for them to occur. Table 5.1 was originally developed by Gove Depuy and Phillip Tabb.

INTERIOR SCALE STRATEGIES

1. Incorporating nature within.
2. Daylighting strategies.
3. Natural ventilation strategies.
4. Prospect and refuge.
5. Wellness-oriented materiality.
6. Living color.
7. Workspace wellness strategies.
8. Thin places sanctuary spaces.
9. Spatial variety and quality.

STRATEGY	DESIGN INTENTIONS	WELLNESS STRATEGIES	WELLNESS OUTCOMES	REFERENCES
Nature Within	Designs for introducing nature within buildings with either living examples or abstract representations, providing indoor views to outdoor natural settings and events like changes of the seasons, and incorporating biophilic attributes indoors.	Incorporating living plants, flowers and images of the natural world , incorporating outdoor spaces or rooms such as conservatories, green rooms, greenhouses and living walls, and providing abstract biospheric design elements within the interior like tile, screen, wall covering patterns and artwork.	Can be therapeutic, encourages physical activity, reduces obesity, improves mood, can trigger a calming effect, improves air quality, reduces stress, sharpens attention, may boost productivity, can promote longevity, helps support biospheric values, and improve outlook on life.	https://www.healthline.com/health/healthy-home-guide/benefits-of-indoor-plant+H33 https://www.terrapinbrightgreen.com/reports/14-patterns/
Daylighting	Reduce negative effects of artificial lighting, increase natural light, provide varying kinds of daylight (direct, filtered, diffused), reduce lighting energy costs, and to stimulate internal clock.	Careful building orientation and placement of windows and other apertures, reduce heat gain and glare and provide sun control and modulation to adjust light levels and quality, incorporate skylights, clerestories and skyspaces, and provide opportunities for shared daylight and zone coupling.	Improves mood, less fatigue, reduced eyestrain, improves alertness, greater job satisfaction, more effective learning, reduces Seasonal Affective Disorder, improves sleep, and provides energy savings and reduction of greenhouse gasses, and helps regulate cycle of sleep.	https://www.velux.com/what-we-do/research-and-knowledge/deic-basic-book/daylight/benefits-of-daylight https://www.lheschong.com/visual-delight
Natural Ventilation	To provide direct access to the outdoors, provide air quality and thermal comfort, provide effective and economical ventilation methods, to reduce noise of conventional HVAC systems, and to control airborne infections.	Incorporate operable windows, patio doors, and walls with careful placement, stacking effect, movable skylights, wind catchers, encourage cross ventilation, orient for natural breezes, interior zone coupling, and open space planning.	Reduction of respiratory illness, increase productivity and concentration levels, high user satisfaction, fast refurbishment, improves air quality, provide thermal comfort, creates dynamic stimulation, and reduction to communicable viruses.	https://www.govinfo.gov/content/pkg/GOVPUB-C13-4bfff386c2f003c32b2ebdb2fc1eabc6/pdf/GOVPUB-C13-4bfff386c2f003c32b2ebdb2fc1eabc6.pdf https://www.ncbi.nlm.nih.gov/books/NBK143274/

Prospect and Refuge	To provide ample views outward to perceived threats as well as to the beauty of nature. To provide safe interior spaces for shelter in place and internal thin place experiences.	Site buildings for advantageous views to streets, entries and approaches to the dwelling. Provide quiet sanctuary spaces. Design for passive survivability.	Improves physical safety, moods, stress reduction, provides critical resources during disasters or extreme weather events.	https://www.resilientdesign.org/tag/passive-survivability/ https://cgscholar.com/bookstore/works/prospect-and-refuge-theory
Wellness Materials	Reduce/eliminate indoor air pollution, material outgassing, provide the warmth of natural materials, enhance biophilic effect, provide materials that are durable and aesthetic pleasing.	Where appropriate use of natural materials (timber, bamboo, stone, clay, earth, wool, cotton and natural pigments), use of recycled materials, and design for healthy ergonomics, and avoiding Red List materials, biospheric, acoustic and appealing.	Reduced inborne and outgassed toxic air, exposure to biophilic effect, supports semantic associative processes, positive emotional response and mood, cancer prevention, protects vital organs, reduce inflammation, slows down aging, and reduced respiratory illness.	https://living-future.org/red-list/ https://www.amazon.com/Cradle-Remaking-Way-Make-Things/dp/0865475873
Living Color	Incorporate color that is curative, stimulating, calming and restorative, colors that are reflective of nature, and aid in wayfinding and user experience creating positive effects.	Utilize natural pigments, color temperatures, color combinations, naturally recognized color symbols (safety, means of egress, visual language, and information), and color with light to accentuate form.	Improves cognitive and emotional health, increases alertness, forms differing mood responses depending on color (stimulating to calming), and provides symbolic meaning and personal preferences.	https://foyr.com/learn/color-theory-in-interior-design/ https://blog.bluebeam.com/color-in-architecture/
Workplace Wellness Strategies	To create healthy and productive workplaces that support physical, mental, emotional, social and financial benefits.	Indoor-outdoor connections, spatial quality, colorful and creative interiors, introducing nature inside and a variety of social and meeting places.	Stress and anxiety reduction, encourages social interaction, promotes creativity and teamwork, and achieves economic efficiency.	https://workplaceinnovation.eu/what-is-workplace-innovation/#:~:text=%27Workplace%20Innovation%27%20defines%20evidence%2D,%2C%20engagement%20and%20well%2Dbeing

Thin Place and Sanctuary Spaces	To provide spaces and interior opportunities for safe sanctuary experiences, "calm corners," places of spiritual renewal, refuge transformation, and emotional escape.	Applicable to most building types provide spaces and rooms that are safe, free of distraction, accessible and calm, usually intimate and comfortable with connections to nature, and capable of being completely isolated.	Stress reduction, reduced anxiety, improved mood, promotion mental wellbeing, lower blood pressure, reduction of temporal density, awe and serene experiences, and sanctuary from infectious disease.	https://www.taylorfrancis.com/books/mono/10.4324/9781003354888/thin-place-design-phillip-james-tabb https://www.sassysisterstuff.com/ideas-calm-corner-emotional-escape-room/
Spatial Variety & Quality	The immaterial essence of interior space to elicit transcendent an healing experiences through choices, variety and quality.	To provide functionality, dimensional quality, nobility, soulfulness, awe and serenity in spatial experiences.	Reductions of stress, depression and anxiety, enrichment of cognitive, emotional, social and spiritual benefits. Creating comprehensible, manageable and meaningful experiences.	https://www.archdaily.com/498519/the-story-of-maggie-s-centres-how-17-architects-came-to-tackle-cancer-care

Table 5.1
Interior Scale Strategies

NOTES

1. Environmental Protection Agency, (Accessed March 30, 2020), https://snowbrains.com/brain-post-much-time-average-american-spend-outdoors/
2. *The Power of Pets*, Department of Health and Human Services, (Accessed March 20, 2023), https://newsinhealth.nih.gov/2018/02/power-pets
3. Lobell, John, *Between Silence and Light: Spirit in the Architecture of Louis I. Kahn* (Boulder, CO: Shambala Publications, Inc., 1979).
4. Stern, M. et al., Blue Light Exposure Decreases Systolic Blood Pressure, Arterial Stiffness, and Improves Endothelial Function in Humans. *European Journal of Preventive Cardiology*, 2018.
5. Heschong, Lisa, *Visual Delight in Architecture: Daylight, Vision, and View* (London, UK: Routledge, 2021).
6. EnviroAtlas Benefit Category: Clean Air, (Accessed October 29, 2023), https://www.epa.gov/enviroatlas/enviroatlas-benefit-category-clean-air
7. Alexander, Christopher, et al., *A Pattern Language: Towns, Buildings, Construction* (New York, NY: Oxford University Press, 1977).
8. Tabb, Phillip, *Solar Energy Planning: A Guide to Residential Development* (New York, NY: McGraw Hill Book Company, 1984).
9. Appleton, Jay, *The Experience of Landscape* (New York, NY: John Wiley & Son, Inc., 1975).
10. Lorenz, Konrad, *King Solomon's Ring* (London, UK: Methuen, 1964).
11. Buss, David M., *The Evolution of Happiness*, (Accessed August 25, 2023), https://labs.la.utexas.edu/buss/files/2015/09/TheEvolutionofHappiness.pdf
12. Wilson, Alex, (Accessed January 12, 2020), https://www.buildinggreen.com/feature/passive-survivability-new-design-criterion-buildings

13. Kellert, Stephen R., Judith H. Heerwagen, & Martin Mador, *Biophilic Design: The Theory, Science, and Practice of Bringing Building to Life* (New York, NY: John Wiley & Sons, Inc., 2008).
14. Buss, David M., *The Evolution of Happiness*, (Accessed August 25, 2023), https://labs.la.utexas.edu/buss/files/2015/09/TheEvolutionofHappiness.pdf
15. Kellert, Stephen R., Judith H. Heerwagen, & Martin Mador, *Biophilic Design: The Theory, Science, and Practice of Bringing Building to Life* (New York, NY: John Wiley & Sons, Inc., 2008).
16. Ikei, Haumi, Chorong Song, & Yoshifumi Miyazaki, *Physiological Effects of Wood on Humans: A Review*, https://jwoodscience.springeropen.com/track/pdf/10.1007/s10086-016-1597–9 (on-line publication: September 10, 2022).
17. Miyazaki Y., Y. Motohashi, & S. Kobayashi, (1992), *Changes in Mood by Inhalation of Essential Oils in Humans II. Effect of Essential Oils on Blood Pressure, Heart Rate, R–R Intervals, Performance, Sensory Evaluation and POMS* (in Japanese).
18. Kopec, Dac, *Person-Centered Health Care Design* (New York, NY: Routledge, 2021), p. 110.
19. EPA, *Indoor Air Quality: What are the Trends in Indoor Air Quality and their Effects on Human Health?* (Accessed January 20, 2024), https://www.epa.gov/report-environment/indoor-air-quality
20. *Red List Index*, (Accessed October 23, 2023), https://www.iucnredlist.org/assessment/red-list-index
21. EPA, *Ten Things You Should Know about Mold*, (Accessed January 20, 2024), https://www.epa.gov/mold/ten-things-you-should-know-about-mold
22. *13 Ways Less Toxic Living Will Benefit You*, (Accessed March 20, 2023), https://www.nontoxicforhealth.com/less-toxic-living.html
23. *The Nature of Wood: An Exploration of the Science on Biophilic Responses to Wood, Terrapin Bright Green*, (Accessed March 15, 2023), http://www.terrapinbrightgreen.com/wp-content/uploads/2022/01/The-Nature-of-Wood_Terrapin_2022-01.pdf
24. Whitehead, Jennifer, *Ways Biophilic Design Promotes Human Health and Well-being* (Accessed November 14, 2023), https://uca.edu/art/2021/03/30/ways-biophilic-design-promotes-human-health-and-well-being/
25. *Italian Curiosities: Why are Burano's Houses for Colorful?* (Accessed November 14, 2023), https://italoamericano.org/why-are-buranos-houses-so-colorful/#:~:text=Legends%20say%20that%2C%20because%20of,them%20more%20visible%20and%20recognizable.
26. Coates, Gary, *Erik Asmussen, Architect* (Stockholm, Sweden: Byggforlaget, 1997), p. 129.
27. Food Studio, *Vidar Clinic: A Place to Nurture and Heal*, (Accessed February 20, 2023), https://foodstudio.no/blog/column/the-vidar-clinic-a-place-to-nurture-and-heal-your-whole-being/
28. Mazur, Caitlin, *What is the Average Work Hours in the US? (2023*), (Accessed October 9, 2023), https://www.zippia.com/advice/average-work-hours-per-week/
29. (Accessed October 8, 2023), https://www.pewresearch.org/social-trends/2020/12/09/how-the-coronavirus-outbreak-has-and-hasnt-changed-the-way-americans-work/
30. Workplace Innovation Europe, (Accessed October 8, 2023), https://workplaceinnovation.eu/what-is-workplace-innovation/#:~:text=%27Workplace%20Innovation%27%20defines%20evidence%2D,%2C%20engagement%20and%20well%2Dbeing.
31. Food Studio, *Vidar Clinic: A Place to Nurture and Heal*, (Accessed February 20, 2023), https://foodstudio.no/blog/column/the-vidar-clinic-a-place-to-nurture-and-heal-your-whole-being/
32. Wells, Rachel, (Accessed October 9, 2023), https://www.forbes.com/sites/rachelwells/2023/10/08/6-ai-wellbeing-tools-for-work-you-should-try-this-mental-health-month/?sh=3525defc38f8
33. Keltner, Dasher, *Awe: The New Science of Everyday Wonder and It Can Transform Your Life* (New York, NY: Penguin Press, 2023).

34. Roberts, Kay & Cheryl Aspy, *Development of the Serenity Scale* (PubMed: *Journal of Nursing Measurement*, 1993), pp. 155–156.
35. Xi, Juan & Matthew Lee, *Inner Peace as a Contribution to Human Flourishing: A New Scale Developed from Ancient Wisdom*, (Accessed October 20, 2022), https://academic.oup.com/book/39523/chapter/339352679
36. Tabb, Phillip James, *Biophilic Urbanism: Designing Resilient Communities for the Future* (New York City, NY: Routledge, 2019).
37. Tabb, Phillip James, *Biophilic Urbanism: Designing Resilient Communities for the Future* (New York City, NY: Routledge, 2019).
38. Qi, Zhen, Qiong Huang, & Qi Zhang, *Contribution of Space Factors to Decision on Comfort and Healthy Building Design*, (Accessed December 12, 2023), https://www.researchgate.net/figure/Building-space-factors-related-to-comfort_tbl1_336443324
39. Acre, Fernanda & Annemie Wyckmans, *Dwelling Renovation and Spatial Quality: The Impact of the Dwelling Renovation on Spatial Quality Measurements*, (Accessed December 14, 2023), https://www.sciencedirect.com/science/article/pii/S2212609015000023
40. Medina, Samuel, *The Storey of Maggie's Centres: How 17 Architects Came to Tackle Cancer Care,* (Accessed December 15, 2023), https://www.archdaily.com/498519/the-story-of-maggie-s-centres-how-17-architects-came-to-tackle-cancer-care
41. James, John, *The Master Masons of Chartres* (Woodbridge, Suffolk, UK: Boydell & Brewer, 1982), p. 5.
42. Mittelmark, Maurice & Georg Bauer, *Chapter 2, The Meanings of Salutogenesis,* (Accessed December 14, 2023), https://www.ncbi.nlm.nih.gov/books/NBK435854/

6 WELLNESS LANDSCAPE STRATEGIES

LANDSCAPE SCALE STRATEGIES

Health and wellness strategies at the landscape scale involve measures for connections to landscape environments and urban outdoor spaces. This can happen through creation and inclusions of parks and greenways, public plazas and courtyards, designs for edible gardens and tiny urban forests, healing gardens and wells, forest bathing, and contemplative landscapes at the smaller scale, as well as responses to agriculture, forest reformation and reforestation efforts. The experience of a good landscape can affect personal, social, and environmental health. According to Catherine Ward Thompson, "the importance of the landscape appears to be as relevant as ever in the context of modern urban lives."[1] Ward Thompson further connects landscapes and health as early as the Persians and Ancient Greeks, and later in Mediaeval landscapes including paradisal and health-oriented environments. Landscape strategies benefit in particular ways with physical, psychological, mental, social, economic, environmental, and spiritual outcomes.

The landscape scale strategies in this section include access to greenspaces in the forms of parks, public greens, open spaces, farms, and water and waterways as well as other natural areas, the design for edible landscapes and urban agriculture, salutogenic environments, and the design for healing gardens and contemplative landscapes that possess energetic qualities and historic or symbolic significance. There are certain landscape patterns, like biophilic attributes, that contribute to contemplative and wellness experiences. According to Agnieszka Olszewska-Guizzo, these landscape models include landscape layers, landforms, biodiversity, color and light, physical and visual connections, archetypal terrestrial elements, and character and sense of solitude.[2]

The landscape benefits stimulate positive awareness of ourselves, enhance our connections with nature, culture and people, are safe and do us no physical harm, provide meaningful stimuli, encourage times of relaxation and physical exercise, allow for productive interactions, contain a balance between familiarity and wonder, and are beautiful.[3] Health and wellness benefits from the strategies at this landscape scale range from improved mood and respiratory function to stress reduction and improved mental health. There are many pathways linking natural environments and landscapes, and health and well-being.

DOI: 10.4324/9781003472902-6

1. **Green spaces and parks**

Creating a healthy balance between built and natural environments is important, which means maintaining healthy edges to settlements, responding to ecological flows through urban and suburban land, integrating agriculture and made landscapes in the forms of parks, greens, playgrounds, and greenways, and creating landscaped streetscapes. Since the majority of Americans describe themselves as living in urban areas (27%) and in suburban areas (52%), this represents nearly 80% of the population who live further from rural and natural areas (21%).[4] And as much as 87% of Americans spend time inside buildings and 6% inside automobiles, so it is no surprise that we are an "*indoor culture*" susceptible to "*nature deficit disorder*," especially among children.[5] Tree canopies in urban areas have been shown to have health benefits by promoting lower obesity levels, better social cohesion, lower blood pressure, alleviation of heat stress, noise pollution reduction, reduction of street-level air pollution, and the economic benefit of an increase of property values.[6]

Biophilia is an emerging planning and design concept that supports greater access and connections to nature. It is the confluence of fields of natural and social sciences, philosophy, anthropology, public health, evolutionary psychology, environmental engineering, planning, urban design, landscape architecture, architecture, and interior design. Biophilia is defined as the love of life. Biophilia's epistemology derives from the two Greek terms *bio* meaning "life," and *philia* meaning "affection or friendly feeling toward." It is the inborn affinity human beings have for other life forms. According to Kaplan and Kaplan, landscapes today that resemble savannas or are parklike are preferred.[7] Biophilic environments can reduce anxiety, anger and fear, are known to lower pulse-rate and blood pressure, improve the immune system, and boost the length and quality of sleep. Planning and design with biophilic principles is an effective wellness strategy.

Singapore is possibly the most biophilic city worldwide. Biophilic planning, architecture, and landscape architecture play important roles in Singapore's efforts to become greener. The biophilic patterns that are most present in Singapore are human-nature connections focusing on abundant connections to and direct experiences of the natural environment, with manifestations of plants, animals, water features, geography, and responses to seasonal changes. As mentioned in Chapter 3, Singapore has envisioned itself as a garden city, which initially took the form of a tree-planting initiative and national parks system. Later the vision of a garden city changed from a "*garden in the city*" to a "*city in a garden*," bringing gardens, natural green spaces, and biodiversity to every resident. With this conceptual shift, the Singapore Park Connector Network was created and today is an innovative "*green matrix.*" The Park Connector Network ties together six loops with a network of jogging, cycling, skating, and walking pathways.

As mentioned in Chapter 3, James Oglethorpe established Savannah, Georgia in 1733, which has long been an excellent example of early American planning. In the USA, Savannah, Georgia is most recognized for its original development around 24 nature-filled squares located evenly throughout the town fabric. Typically, the squares are surrounded by four residential and four civic blocks, and together each square is known as a ward. Two of the squares were demolished leaving 22 active squares today. All of the squares measure approximately 200 feet (61 meters) from east to west, but they vary north to south from approximately 100 to 300 feet (30–91 meters). Buildings located along the east-west sides of the squares typically house civic functions, while north-south blocks are residential (*tythings*), refer to Figure 6.1b. The wellness strategies provide access to nature, integrated mixes of use, and places of casual encounters providing pro-individual, pro-social, and pro-environmental benefits.

Similar to the distributed parks of Savannah is the concept of "*tiny forests*," which are small biodiverse urban forests. Typically, no larger than basketball or tennis courts they are made of native plants and are based on what is called the Miyawaki method of planting.[8] Originally developed by ecologist Akira Miyawaki in the 1970s, the Miyawaki method is an afforestation technique for cultivating four fast-growing species near one another. The purpose is to foster layers of the tiny natural forest as the plants compete for sunlight. Benefits include carbon sequestering, mitigating heat and flooding, and providing shade. Although not in an urban context, Figure 6.1c shows a tiny forest surrounding a Shinto shrine in Sasayama City, Japan. Tiny forests have been planted in Japan, across Europe, in Africa, throughout Asia, and in North and South America, Russia, and the Middle East. They provide distributed access to nature (due to their small size), bird habitats and soundscapes, butterflies and other colorful insects, carbon sequestering and clean air, and help reduce the heat island effect.

Strategies are simply to provide ample green space with easy access, especially in the initial planning stages of development in both cities and suburban environments. Tradeoffs can be made with the densification of urban development and the land use provision of green open spaces. Further, rethinking the role of the automobile and the institution of more pedestrianization will provide opportunities for increased greenspaces. Green space multifunctionality is also important emphasizing recreation, social interactions, cultural heritage, foodscapes, aesthetics, and ecological functions. Benefits include access to nature, CO_2 sequestering, noise reduction, stress reduction, and pro-environmental behaviors. Developed by Stephen and Rachel Kaplan experiences of nature result in attention restoration which provides improved focus, increased ability to concentrate, and recovery from mental fatigue.[9] This includes the concept of increasing "soft fascination" or our attention held by less stimulation and activity. And finally, tiny forests are an effective strategy for creating carbon sequestering and relief from urban concrete jungles.

6.1
Nature and Greenspaces
a) Singapore Garden Networks,
b) Parks of Savannah, Georgia,
c) Tiny Forest

(*Sources: Shutterstock and Wikimedia Commons*)

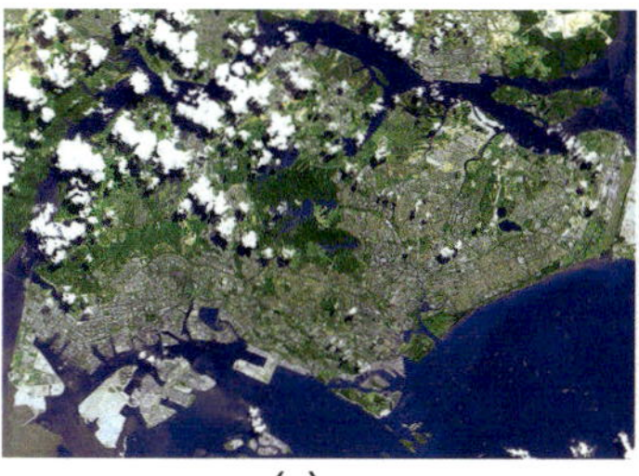

(a)

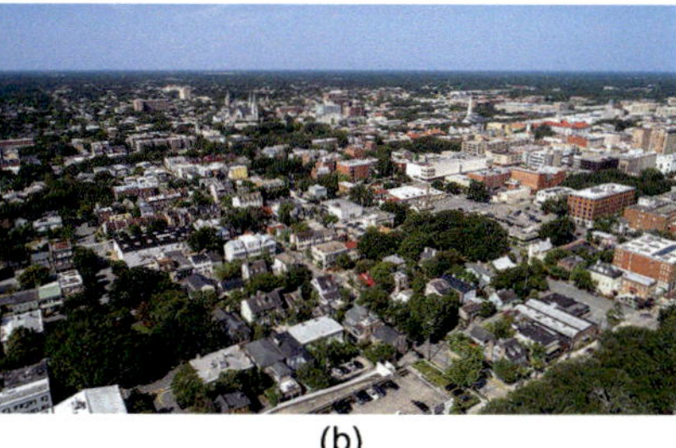

(b)

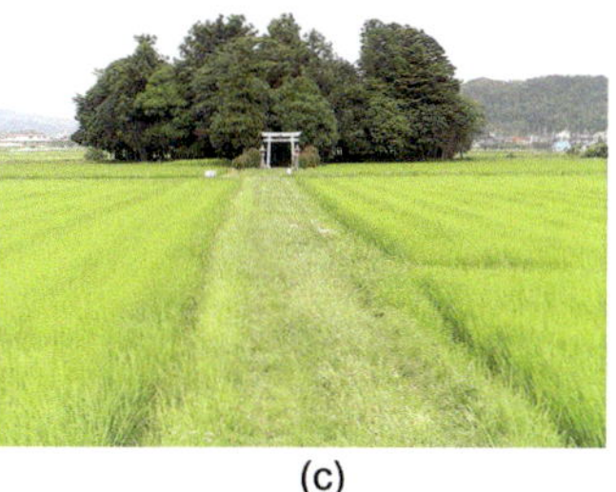

(c)

2. **Blue spaces**

Blue spaces as defined by the European Commission are outdoor environments that prominently feature water either directly (in, on, or near water) or visually (ability to hear, see, or sense water). Blue spaces and aquatic environments include coastlines, rivers, lakes, canals, waterfalls, fountains, and other water features. Waterway restoration is aimed at a variety of rivers, estuaries, and streams in restoring natural conditions, functioning and habitat, improving biodiversity, regeneration, and recreation. Blue spaces also include urban open spaces designed to sequester greenhouse gasses and absorb heat, reducing the urban "*heat island effect*." Sailing, rafting, surfing, swimming, ice skating, skiing, or even walking in the rain allow for direct contact with the natural forces of the motion of wind and water. These immersive experiences contribute to blue space wellness outcomes, including improvements in physical and mental well-being. And according to Mathew White, proximity to water is associated with at least a 10% premium in house prices.[10]

The prime substance of a blue space is water. In planning and landscape architecture it is associated with waterbodies and waterways. Because of the hydrologic cycle, water is constantly moving and transforming. Rivers, lakes, reservoirs, and wetlands supply us with fresh water for drinking, growing food, and producing energy. In addition, water elicits numinous experiences because of its mysterious underworld nature, emotional energy, and healing qualities. Clean water hydrates, flushes out toxins within the body, prevents water-borne illnesses, and raises sanitation levels.

Hot springs and natural geothermal springs occur worldwide. Hot springs are known to possess remarkable healing powers. Holy wells are found throughout the world on six of the seven cotenants. Holy wells in different forms occur in a wide variety of cultures, religious environments, and historical periods. In Ireland alone, there are nearly 3,000 wells. Wells are unchanging and are life-giving, homes of spirits, and sources of wisdom, renewal, prophesy, and wellness. Today, however, wells do not serve a necessary function unless in remote areas where public utilities are not available. They are not in everyday use anymore; however, they do still serve as sacred place destinations and places of renewal.

Good examples are the Glastonbury Chalice Well and its cascading pools which are considered one of the most spiritual places in England, and the Salk Institute's infinity pool. Glastonbury Tor in Somerset, England is a hill with the Chalice Well near its summit, with its small stone surround and movable wood and iron opening. Down slope from the Well are gardens and two overlapping pools formed by Vesica Pisces geometry (two overlapping circles). The Salk Institute for Biological Studies in La Jolla, California was designed by Louis I. Kahn and opened in 1965. Located between two of the laboratory blocks is a large plaza with a single infinity pool directed to the Pacific Ocean, Figure 6.2b. For Kahn, at sunset the infinity pool combined the Empedoclean terrestrial elements (fire, water, earth, and air) into a transformative silent space.

Seas, lakes, reservoirs, rivers, streams, and tributaries have become polluted and are cause for waterborne diseases such as cholera, dysentery, and

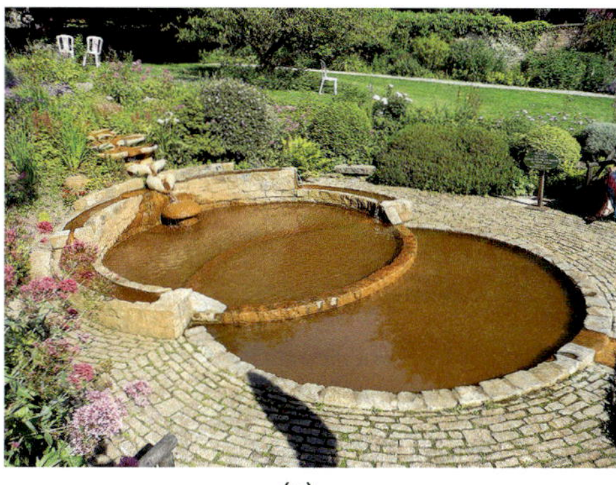
(a)

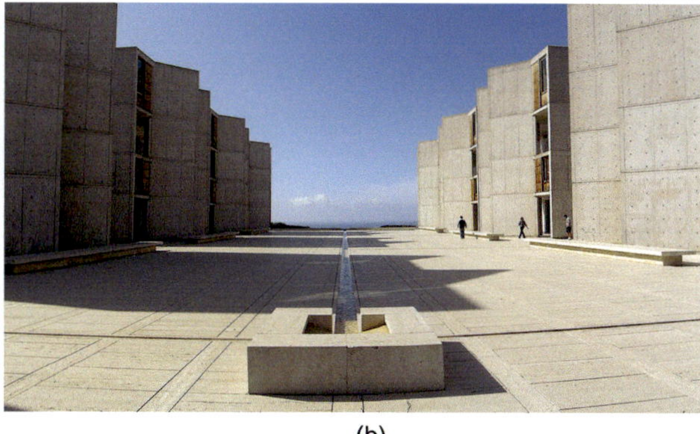
(b)

6.2
Blue Spaces
a) Glastonbury Vesica Pools, UK,
b) Salk Institute Blue Space
(*Source: Wikimedia Commons*)

hepatitis. In addition, long-term exposure to contaminated water can lead to cancer and reproductive issues. Living closer to blue space is associated with statistically significantly higher physical activity levels, and larger amounts of blue space are also associated with higher levels of activity.[11] So, it is important to restore and maintain these essential resources serving our wellness as well as planetary health. Blue spaces stimulate healing, promote calmness and better sleep, and encourage physical activity. According to Glasgow Caledonian University, blue spaces lower risks of stress, anxiety, obesity, cardiovascular disease, mental health, and premature death.[12] Blue spaces occur almost everywhere, even in the rain. According to Jantra Jacobs, walking in the rain exposes one to cleaner air, promotes exercise, can prevent overheating, can help shift perspective, and the scent of rain, sometimes called "*petrichor*," is calming.[13]

Urban waterways are common in most cities across the world. Throughout history, cities and towns have often been established along the banks of rivers, because these waterways provided a source of drinking water, and power, followed by connecting roads, and transport links to other communities. In the United States, 40% of the population lives near the coast, and about 15% live near the Great Lakes. Urban infrastructure within these areas impacts 60% of all freshwater fish, mussel, and crayfish species in North America, over 1,200 species altogether. It has contributed to local extinctions of 260 species, sometimes at great distances from city boundaries. Therefore, waterway restoration is an important wellness strategy not only for the environment, but for human health as well.

3. Waterway restorations

The San Antonio Riverwalk is a 15-mile restoration and flood management project and is considered the largest urban ecosystem in the United States providing a serene and pleasant way to navigate the city. It is filled with mixes of use including restaurants, cafés, shops, the Alamo, historic districts, and vital nightlife all with pedestrian access. It represents both an individual and city-wide wellness intervention with a host of benefits, refer to Figure 6.3a. The Los Angeles River Master Plan recognizes the Los Angeles River as a body of resources of regional importance and recognizes that those resources must be rendered less dangerous yet protected and enhanced as a blue space. Since the mid-1980s there has been a renewed interest in the river as a valuable natural asset for the entire Los Angeles basin. As a multi-use resource, the river can serve both ecological as well as human needs in a much broader sense than it does today. Along its banks, many new, job-producing facilities could be developed, and new recreation sites can be provided for people living in the basin.

Residents of Los Angeles have been stuck in a concrete landscape, especially along the Los Angeles River. The new Greenway of Los Angeles is an example of serene network urbanism, and will connect our neighborhoods, ease our commutes, build healthier space, invest in the communities, and restore the river's natural beauty. However, the Greenway is more than just a pathway for transportation—it will be a destination in itself, charting new possibilities from bike-in movies to yoga classes. The Greenway is a new way of living for Los Angeles, connecting beautiful neighborhoods, connecting natural landscapes, and connecting to one another. Instead of crowded streets and honking horns on your morning commute, imagine chirping birds, flowing water, and numerous coffee shops along the way to work. Families have longed for more open space for recreation. The Greenway creates healthier spaces where families can ride bikes, play in parks, and breathe fresh air along the water. It lowers the risk of flooding and death due to drowning. The LA River acted as a flood control channel until January 1st of 2014, and now is getting a new use as a navigable waterway. New public events along the river have already begun, like bike-in movie nights, Figure 6.3b.

The wellness strategies that include blue space and waterway resources of regional importance recognize that those resources must be rendered less dangerous yet protected and enhanced as wellness places providing not only needed greenspace to inner cities, but also a more vital network of connectivity for both people, increasing their recreational possibilities, as well as providing for better animal habitats. While some water bodies bring risks to humans, the benefits of blue spaces include improved water quality, improvements to the natural environment, increased accessibility for human activity (instoration), reduced obesity, increased cognitive restoration, increased positive mood and happiness, increased respiratory health, and enhanced pro-social and pro-environmental behaviors.

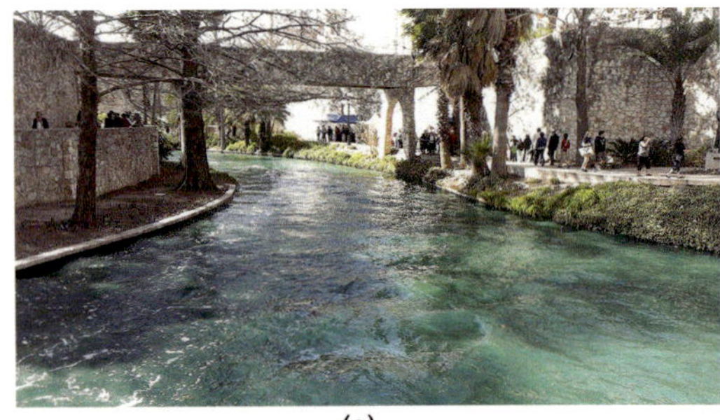

(a)

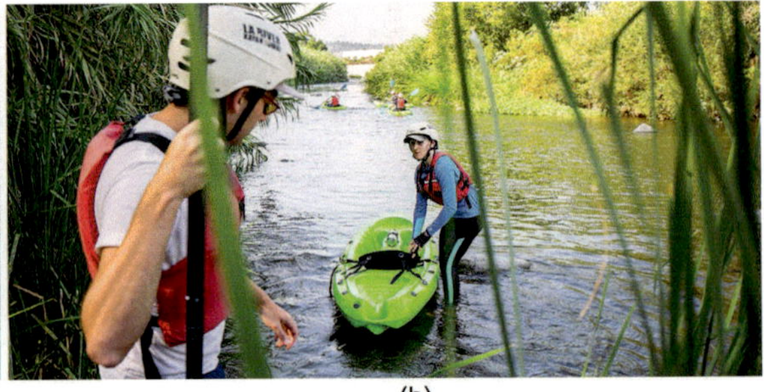

(b)

6.3 Waterway Restoration a) San Antonio, Texas Riverwalk, b) Los Angeles River Revitalization

(Source: Wikimedia Commons)

4. **Edible landscapes and foodscapes**

While many homeowners spend weekends maintaining traditional lawns and landscapes, there is an opportunity to have life-giving and food-producing landscapes with positive benefits. Edible gardens can take several forms from gardens, to orchards, streetscapes, and micro farms. Edible gardens provide healthy food and great accessibility. Typical among these gardens are fruit trees, culinary herbs and vegetables. In addition to producing food, there is a positive social aspect to creating edible landscapes. Edible landscapes double as food-producing gardens, and *foodscapes*, as well as ornamentals full of color and seasonal change. Edible ornamentals can provide beauty, shade, and food production, in addition to helping conserve water, reduce pollution, and provide habitat for wildlife.

Foodscaping (landscaping with food) is the practice of integrating edible plants into landscapes.[14] Plants include baby greens, kale, lettuces, tomatoes, beans, peppers, berries (strawberries, cherries, black raspberries), and culinary herbs (rosemary, sage, parsley, dill, and basil). In addition, they should also be pollinator-friendly. Foodscapes encourage interdependence among people, food, and place. Foodscapes are geographical and spatial and vary accordingly (including soil types and climatic conditions) with biophysical food products combined with food management processes (including crop type, water management, and agronomic inputs) on local levels. Foodways are the cultural, social, and economic practices enabling foodscaping. Edible gardens and foodscaping provide convenience and accessibility, reduce transport energy, promote food security, and are carbon sequestering.

Edible streetscapes and verge gardens typically parallel streets, sidewalks, and footpaths. They typically use native plants, are relatively maintenance-free, and are water-wise. They should be able to accommodate rainwater surge and runoff. Often verge gardens are shrubbery-laden, textured, succulent, colorful, sometimes rock or stone-centric, and non-toxic. Verge gardens should not interfere with underground services such as water, gas, and sewage pipes or block easy access to and from the street. Benefits are air filtration, shade, slowing rainfall runoff, carbon sequestering, and reducing the heat island effect.

The wellness strategies include development planning for domestic gardens and small-scale greenhouses, provision for neighborhood community gardens, foodscape gardens for commercial restaurants' farm-to-table, and creating streetscapes with edible plants. The wellness strategies associated with edible gardens include allocating ample space for either public or private gardens, preparing the soil, growing vertically as much as possible, succession planting, and extending the growing season. Effective physical barriers should be considered to keep out deer, vermin, and other troublesome visitors. Insects can be addressed with intercropping, planting pest-repelling herbs, and encouraging beneficial insects. Having both visible and physical access to the garden is important for both surveillance and enjoyment. The benefits include engaging in physical activity, relaxation and lowering stress levels and blood pressure, providing healthy nutrition, increasing vitamin D levels by being outdoors, promoting social interactions, boosting mood, enhancing the biophilic effect, and creating

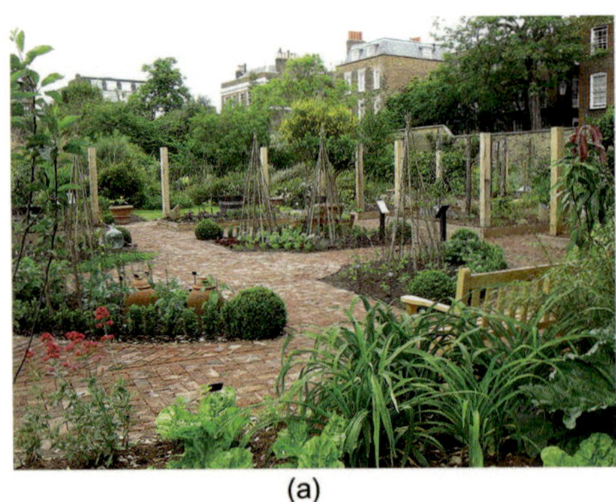
(a)

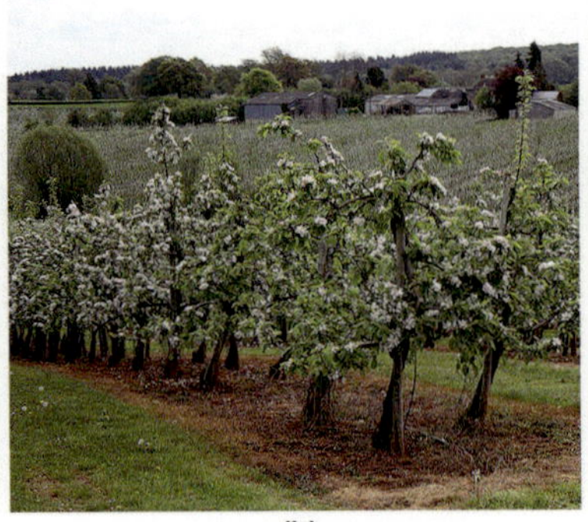
(b)

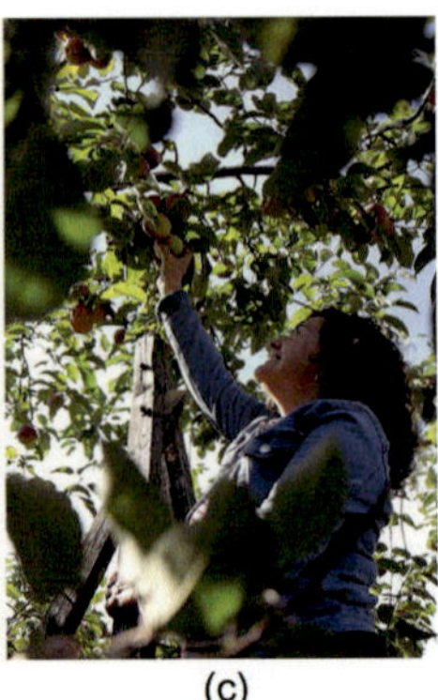
(c)

6.4
Edible Landscapes
a) Edible Gardens,
b) Apple Orchards,
c) Picking Apples
(*Source: Wikimedia Commons*)

enjoyment. Gardening has also been associated with building self-esteem. The benefits of orchards include providing vital greenspace, sequestering greenhouse emissions, increasing physical activity through harvesting, and contributing to food security. Benefits also include agroecology regeneration.

5. **Healing gardens**

While most gardens possess an intrinsic appeal and benefit to humans, healing gardens suggest improved health and wellness outcomes and therefore are considered therapeutic landscapes. Therapeutic environments or sanctuaries are considered safe spaces specifically designed for physical, mental, social, psychological, and spiritual healing. They are generally plant-dominated environments purposefully designed to facilitate interaction with the healing elements of nature. Water in the garden also serves as a healing elicitor. Interactions can be passive or active depending on the garden design and health and wellness needs. And, most recently, were seen as beneficial during the COVID-19 pandemic. They serve as places of recovery, and restoration of the mind, body, and soul. Healing gardens have a long history most likely beginning with ancient Egyptian, Persian, and Greek cultures with landscapes of medicinal plants. In the Middle Ages, monastic compounds provided enclosed and protected gardens for herbal remedies and dietary prescriptions.

With the world's population now having greater percentages living in urban areas, it is not surprising that there are negative consequences. Living in cities is associated with developing higher risks of mood and anxiety disorders, as well as mental health disorders, than living in a rural environment.[15] Living in rural areas is not without risk due to higher percentage of older adults, higher rates of obesity, and many rural communities are isolated with less access to healthcare. However, places with rich views and access to nature reduce stress and increase concentration with wellness benefits. In this regard, places supporting healing and contemplative environments are restorative with their natural geometries, biodiverse qualities, and experiential vitality. Today, contemplative landscapes possess certain spatial characteristics that contribute to their effectiveness that include landscape layering and perspectives, sensuous landforms, rich biodiversity, vibrant color and light, physical and visual access, and awe-inspiring, soulful, and contemplative qualities.

Healing gardens are used to produce medicinal plants while others may be grown for ornamental plants and their serenity healing. They are often a part of hospitals, healthcare, and aging-in-place settings. Healing gardens have appeared worldwide and, according to Roger Ulrich, healing gardens help reduce pain, improve sleep, reduce stress and anxiety for patients and their families, lower infection occurrence, and improve patient satisfaction.[16] Therapeutic gardens often engage in the active and deliberate needs of particular populations. Where healing gardens, on the other hand, generally aim for a more passive involvement and are designed to provide benefits to a diverse population with many differing needs.

Maggie Centres in the United Kingdom incorporate healing gardens as an integral part of their health and wellness activities for cancer patients. The first Maggie Centre opened in Edinburgh in 1996 and expanded in the United Kingdom and Hong Kong. The intention was to provide buildings that uplifted and supported healing. There was also the desire to create an environment that was inviting and domestic – a kind of "home away from home." This extended to healing gardens as well. The Manchester Maggie's was opened in 2016 and the building was designed by Foster and Partners and the garden was designed by the Dan Pearson Studio, refer to Figure 6.5a. It was conceived as a home away from home and a place of refuge. The garden and greenhouse were integral parts of the design, and provided a place for gathering, working together, and enjoying the therapeutic qualities of touching the earth. The garden has year-round color and gives a calming transition away from the hospital and becomes an extension of the kitchen table with people sitting out and meeting each other in the beautiful surroundings. Benefits occur to patients in healthcare facilities, their families and friends who visit, and to those who work in the gardens as a therapeutic process.

Several kinds of healing gardens support healing, enabling, meditation, rehabilitation, and restoration. Healing gardens can occur in a variety of contexts both indoors and outdoors. Healing is focused on physical, mental, emotional, and spiritual health. Enabling meditation, gardens focus on physical recovery and active participatory engagement. Meditative gardens encourage serenity and calm and are stress-relieving. Rehabilitation gardens not only affect human health, but also the land, soil, and surrounding natural environment. Restorative gardens are sanctuaries that respond to relieving stress and traumatic events and supporting spiritual renewal. Beyond the nutritional values of healing gardens, they provide an intimate and biological relationship with nature, a context for contemplation, psychological comfort, and decreased temporal density.

The wellness strategies for healing gardens include the creation of private and safe gardens with places to walk, sit and gather with others, places of social support, places with a sense of control, places that encourage physical activity, and places with beauty and serenity. Benefits include the creation of places that are serene places, fostering lowered blood pressure, increased respiratory function, cardiovascular and pulmonary fitness, and greater endurance. There can be increased social skills, positive moods, and overall sense

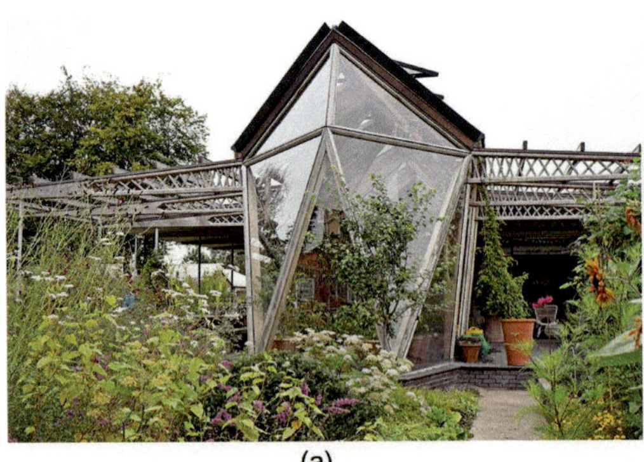

(a)

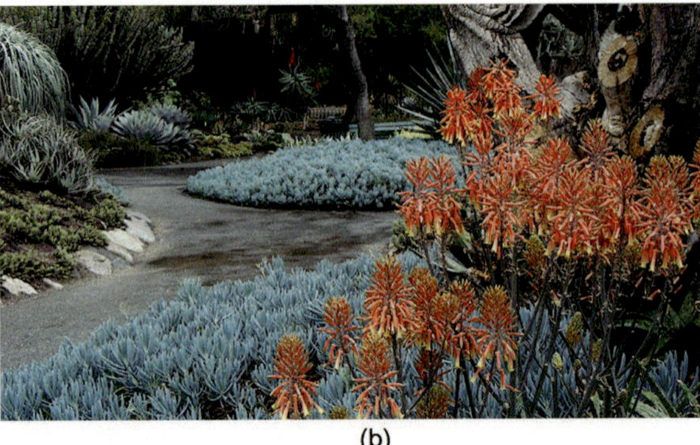

(b)

6.5
Healing Gardens
a) Maggie Centre, Manchester, UK,
b) Desert Healing Garden in San Marion, California

(Sources: Shutterstock and Wikimedia Commons)

of well-being and hopefulness, increased safety, boosting of the immune function, and cultural, social and spiritual connections to place. These promote pro-social, pro-spiritual, and pro-environmental behaviors.

6. Forest bathing

Our ancient ancestors were hunter-gatherers whose lives were intertwined with the wilderness, endless grasslands, dense forests, and vast stretches of green landscapes. Deep inside us is an instinctual connection with an understanding that much health and wellness can be sourced from nature. Forests and trees in particular are appealing as they provide oxygen, shelter, food, building materials, safety, windbreaks, and in some cases water. On a spiritual level, trees reflect connections with things greater than ourselves and they ground the earth with heaven. Forests were the source of myths and mystery, and were often seen as being enchanted. They were home to certain gods and spirits. Often certain trees were seen as holy and considered worthy of spiritual respect. Trees can also serve to create a sense of place and place identity. While forests often elicit a sense of mystery, enchantment, and wonder, they also express vitality, strength, protection, and transformation. Forests are places of contrast as in ground and sky, dark and light, and changes of the seasons. It is no wonder that there are a multitude of wellness benefits from experiences of trees and forests.

Although not a new concept, forest bathing emerged in Japan in the early 1980s by the Japanese Ministry of Agriculture, Forestry and Fisheries as *shinrin-yoku* literally meaning "taking in nature" where taking in the qualities of the forest, its atmosphere, or in a broader sense experiencing all of nature, is a wellness immersion process. In addition to *shinrin-yoku*, forest bathing is a central exponent of biophilia with the love of and affiliation with nature. Long-term benefits derive from the combination of the physical activity of slowly walking and becoming increasingly more present with the surrounding nature, breathing in oxygen-rich air, and exposure to the presence of phytoncides or natural oils of the forest. Forest bathing significantly improves physical and psychological health. Other benefits are stress reduction, encouragement of physical activity, creation of positive moods, improving sleep patterns, strengthening the immune system, lowering blood pressure, lowering of concentrations of cortisol, lowering pulse rate, enhancing the biophilic effect, reversing the "*nature deficit disorder*,"[17] and encouraging pro-environmental behaviors. Forest bathing exposes us to lower levels of salivary cortisol concentrations and higher levels of tree-produced phytoncides which in turn help human immune systems with increased levels of white blood cells with NK (natural killer)-cell activity.

Forest bathing is recommended for a minimum of 20 minutes a day, while for the full forest bathing experience, a two-hour period is recommended in order to gain the full benefit. Walking quietly, opening the senses, periodic pauses, and finding a thin place or special spot to stop and attune to the place can elicit the best results. Two experiences often occur. The first is a serene, calming, or relaxing experience, safe from negative aspects of nature and filled with sensual experiences. The second is an introspective, inspiring, or insightful experience evoking peaceful states of mind and mindfulness. Forest bathing can be awakening, instinctual, and evoking a sense of aliveness and awe. It can also be amplified with therapeutic guided tours and retreats. With forest bathing caution should be expressed in certain situations, including dehydration and exposure to predatory animals, venomous snakes, ticks, and other insects.

According to Agnieszka Olszewska-Guizzo, darker, more dense elements of nature could be non-beneficial to health and even dangerous.[18] However, the experience of what is called an "*awe walk*" and a "*wild awe*" are both safe and exhilarating and can be positive for health and wellness. According to Diane E. Bowler, et al., a meta-analysis provided some evidence of the positive benefits of a walk or run in a natural environment in comparison to a synthetic environment.[19] And recent studies show that people who move to greener urban areas benefit from sustained improvements in their mental health.[20] Benefits also include stress and tension reduction, improved respiratory system, lowered blood pressure, increased mental activity and powers of concentration, improved mental health, improved memory, improved mood, endocrine and immune system activity. Furthermore, moving to greener spaces, encourages social interaction, which in turn contributes to a spirit of place, and supports pro-social and pro-environmental behaviors. Health and wellness benefits can also be derived from desert, meadow, and glacial bathing.

6.6 Forest Bathing a) Walking in the Forest (Active Experience), b) Placebound Forest Bathing (Passive Experience)

(*Sources: Wikimedia Commons and Shutterstock*)

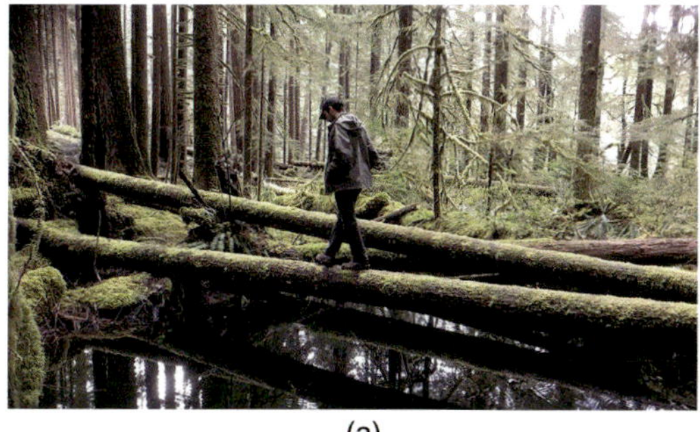

(a)

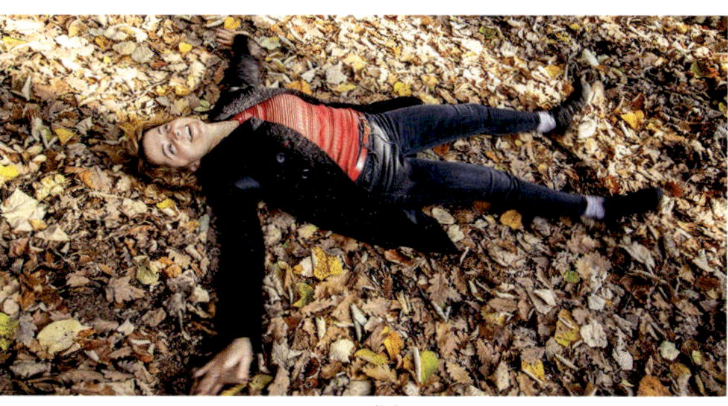

(b)

7. Reforestation, afforestation, and carbon sequestering

Globally we are deforesting, and forest loss accounts for around 25 million acres (10 million ha) of forests each year. This is mainly due to expanding cities and towns, mineral extraction, transportation and infrastructure projects, and the need for more ranches and farmland. Most deforestation occurs in areas of mature rainforests that are especially important for biodiversity, carbon storage, and regulating regional and local climate effects. At present, there are three global deforestation hotspots – the Brazilian Amazon, Congo Basin, and the Bolivian Amazon. This process affects climate (global warming), biodiversity, and human well-being.

Reforestation is a natural or intentional way of replenishing existing woodlands but could also suggest the nurturing of other ecological landscapes. The principal benefits are maintaining healthy ecosystems, oxygen production, CO_2 sequestering, climate change mitigation, improving biodiversity and wildlife habitats, increasing soil fertility, and enhancing and encouraging pro-environmental behaviors. And of course, there are economic benefits from reforestation. In the United States, there are about 766 million acres of forestland, which absorbs approximately 16% of carbon dioxide each year.[21] The process of absorption transforms the carbon dioxide out of the air, binds it up in sugar through photosynthesis, releases the oxygen, and use the sugar in their branches and roots. Evergreens, pine, cedar, spruce, and conifers have the greatest health benefits.

Worldwide, forests comprise approximately 31% of the total habitable land area. Forest loss is primarily due to population increase with expanding metropolitan areas, the need for more land-intensive agriculture, and increasing consumption. While deforestation is not a new phenomenon, half of the loss, the size of the United States, has occurred over the past century Figure 6.7a. Curbing forest loss is a combination of improvement in crop yields, improvement in agricultural production technology, improving diet with less red meat, consuming less wood products (paper, packaging), and planting of more trees.

Reforestation strategies include investment in new forests, and afforestation, which are nature-based assets. The Heathland New Forest located in Hampshire in the south of England is the largest pasture and forestland in the south of England, and the beautiful forest of Estonia is shown in Figure 6.7b. It was

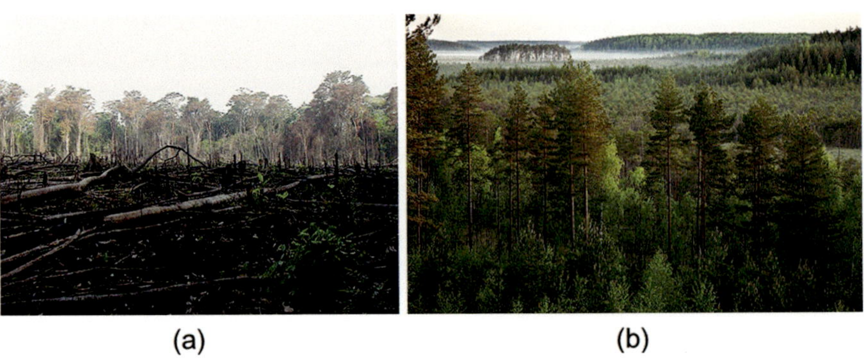

(a) (b)

6.7
Reforestation
a) Deforestation in Lacanja, Mexico,
b) Forest in Estonia,

(Source: Wikimedia Commons)

established in 1079 as a Royal Forest. The benefits are not only for carbon-dioxide absorption, but for the nurturing of abundant wildlife and biodiversity. Carbon is released back into the atmosphere as carbon dioxide and is absorbed by the soil and vegetation, including trees. According to an *Earthday* publication, forests are home to an estimated 80% of the world's terrestrial species.[22]

Urban forestation, simply put refers to trees we live with daily, from yards, streets, parks, school yards, along waterways and flood plains, and suburban forests. It is defined as the planting, maintenance, care, and protection of tree populations in urban settings. Urban reforestation is an attractive strategy addressing carbon sequestering, the heat island effect, and shaded human outdoor spaces and streetscapes. With more than half of the world's population living in urban areas, the combination of heat released by human activity, hard surfaces like streets, pavements, parking lots, and absorptive building materials, rooftops, and unobstructed solar radiation is cause for the heat island effect. Vegetation can reduce this effect, but caution should be given to locations with water shortages as urban trees and vegetation can compete with other critical water needs.

Another strategy along the lines of nature's restoration is *rewilding*, a progressive approach to conservation biology, ecological processes, biodiversity, as well as wildlife habitat preservation. It posits a reduced human intervention, and the creation of natural, resilient, and self-regulating ecosystems. Introduced by Michael Soule and Reed Noss, rewilding included the role of large carnivores. Not without controversy, the concept can bring risks to existing ecosystems thereby harming biodiversity. The biggest issues with rewilding are the level of uncertainty associated with the practice of reintroducing species to an area, and the possible dangers to people and livestock. However, there generally is support for rewilding practices. Some rewilding efforts may still employ human land management approaches, such as hunting, farming, forestry, and fisheries, leading to conflict. However, rewilding and restoring ecosystems can protect against climate change, and provide health and well-being benefits through access to vital natural environments.

Strategies include the creation and maintenance of parks, forests, and other green areas. It is important to preserve forested areas, where possible, with close daily accessibility. It is the immersion into surrounding forest environments where the felt senses, touch, hearing, smell, sight, and sometimes taste can be experienced. Afforestation within urban areas is limited by the availability of land otherwise taken by human land uses for transportation, infrastructure, buildings, and public spaces. Trees not only reflect environmental health, but human wellness as well.[23] Both natural and urban forestation will aid in mitigating climate change, help reduce the heat island effect, and provide pleasant places within which to recreate, forest bathe, facilitate wellness benefits, or simply enjoy.

8. Incorporating land art installations

Experiencing art in any form engages the senses, stimulates thoughts, and elicits emotions. Art in the landscape, also known as land art, environmental art, or earthworks, was developed in Great Britain and the United States in the 1960s and is a particularly engaging form. Rather than indoors or in galleries, works of art are created outdoors typically within monumental landscapes, often in remote locations. The artwork is most often made with local natural materials, wood, stone, sand, and trees depending upon what is available at the site. While the initial impetus of the movement was a reaction to the commercialization of urban indoor art and an intention to connect and inspire social and ecological change. Often the movement espoused utopian and spiritual connections to the landscape and to Planet Earth. Land art goes beyond the viewing of an object in a site but includes the experience beyond the object or work of art emphasizing the landscape context within which it exists.[24] Notable artists include Robert Smithson, Agnes Denes, Nancy Holt, Maya Lin, Christo and Jeanne-Claude, Donald Judd, Andy Goldsworthy, and Mary Miss.

Earth or land art was a movement using the natural landscape as a palette for environmental artistic expressions. They generally were a reaction to the commercialization and commoditization of modern art, especially gallery art. Materials, such as wood, branches, stone, sand, gravel, and soil, are extracted directly from nature. Often the works were fashioned to elicit an enhanced awareness of a place or natural phenomena. They tended to honor or amplify the site from which they were derived. This art form also centered around astronomical and celestial phenomena. Earth or land art provides a grounding, and clarity about the environment, and an immersive experience. Benefits include reduction of depression and anxiety, stress relief, and reinforced emotional bonds with the earth and others.

Burning Man is a participatory-focused event held annually in the Black Rock Desert near Rock City, Nevada. Beginning in 1991, and as the name suggests, there is a ceremonial culmination to a week-long event with a symbolic burning of a large wooden effigy. Also included throughout the week's event are the creations of experimental sculptures, unusual buildings, art cars, and performances. The principal benefits include physical activity, creativity, social cohesion, promotion of a strong sense of community and sense of place, and encouraging the process of giving and decommodification. Moreover, the event has positive economic benefits to local businesses along the route to Black Rock City.

Robert Smithson's "Spiral Jetty" built in 1970 is a 1,500-foot (457 meter) spiral arrangement of rocks at the edge of the Great Salt Lake, Utah. It was inspired by Smithson's visit to the Pre-Columbian Serpent Mound constructed in south-central Ohio east of Cincinnati. Spiral Jetty is entirely constructed of local mud, basalt rocks, and salt crystals. Due to the changing water levels of the Great Salt Lake, the sculpture is both visible and submerged. The geometry utilizes a counterclockwise spiral emerging out from the shore. Visitors are welcome to walk along the jetty and experience the pink color of the saltwater algae and the oolitic sand. The benefits include physical activity, connections to nature, contemplative moments like those when experiencing a labyrinth, and stress reduction. The site was chosen because of its vast surroundings and the Golden Spike monument marking the 1869 completion of the transcontinental railway.

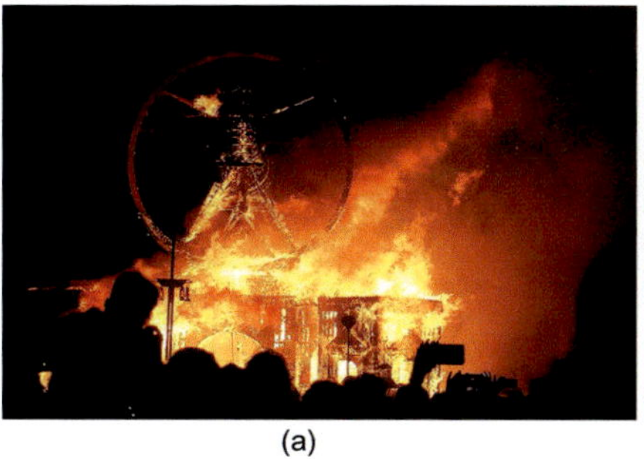
(a)

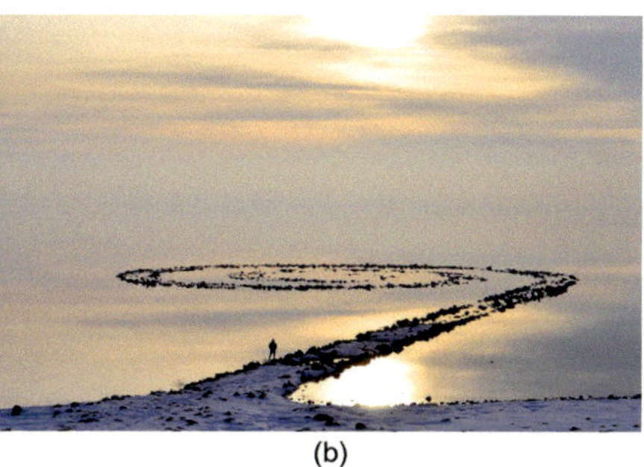
(b)

6.8
Land Art Experiences
a) Burning Man, Nevada b) Spiral Jetty, Utah
(*Source: Wikimedia Commons*)

Strategies for land-art wellness include encouraging works by local artists who can connect to site-specific and culturally relevant works of art. They create places that inspire either awe or serenity emotions, and reinforce connections to nature through the juxtaposition of the art piece and natural context or features of the site. They often amplify or bring attention to important natural features of a site, and invite engagement. Further, it is important to invite participation with these works of art and the communities at large. Participation is central to the Burning Man events in Nevada, Figure 6.8a, and nature is inseparable with the Spiral Jetty in Utah, Figure 6.8b. The benefits of land art projects include mindfulness of natural conditions, appreciation of the good in nature, experience of beauty, stress release, promoting healthy thinking and creativity, evoking biophilic effects, cognitive stimulation through direct engagement, promoting physical activity, and supporting pro-social and pro-environmental behaviors.

9. Soundscapes

Noise is unwanted or harmful outdoor sounds created by human activities that are typically caused by air and automobile traffic, railroads, loud construction and industrial sounds, sirens, street repairs, and even recreational activities. With increased urbanization and development comes increased anthrophony or human-made noise. People exposed to sudden loud or prolonged noises can damage the auditory nerve. Hearing loss, according to the CDC, is the third most common chronic health condition in the United States. The negative effects include sleeplessness, raised blood pressure, increased heart rate, hearing loss, nonauditory physiological effects, increased occurrence of hypertension, cardiovascular disease, negative moods, depression, cognitive fatigue, increased stress, and high levels of annoyance.[25] Soundscapes are an antecedent environmental noise and can be either natural or human-generated. The term, "*soundscape*," currently is credited to Michael Southworth in 1969 who studied the sonic environment in cities. Natural sounds can be generated by biospheric sources, such as wind, stream water, ocean waves, singing birds, grazing sheep, and wind chimes. Soundscapes can also be caused by human conversations, music, and sounds of children playing. The association between positive soundscape perception (e.g., happiness, serenity, calmness, etc.) and positive health effects (e.g., increased recovery rates, reduced stress-induced mechanisms, etc.) is one of the key interests in soundscape research.[26]

Acoustic ecology or ecoacoustics is a movement started in the late 1960s by musician R. Murray Schafer that promoted mediated sound among animals, humans, and nature. His work also included the idea of *soundwalks*, with a focus on tuning into and listening to the environment. Strategies to create natural and human-made soundscape settings can contribute to the wellness effects of forest bathing, blue spaces, healing gardens, and meditation and sanctuary spaces.[27]

Research has shown that noise pollution (unwanted or unpleasant sound) in the built environment not only drives hearing loss, tinnitus, and hypersensitivity to sound, but can cause or exacerbate cardiovascular disease, type 2 diabetes, sleep disturbances, stress, and mental health and cognition problems, such as memory impairment and attention deficits.[28] Noise is associated with negative human and ecological values, especially when it is derived from anthropogenic sound sources. The major causes of urban noise pollution are airplanes, ground transportation, traffic, industrialization, construction activities, and social events. Some natural noises can be unwanted as well, including thunderstorms, lightning, crashing waves, and high winds. Sound perception enables most species, including all known vertebrates, to surveil their surroundings, and for humans this includes from wild to urban environments.

Soundscapes can offer acoustic environments generally consisting of natural sounds (geophony) and animal vocalizations (biophony). They also include pleasant sounds produced by human activity (anthropophony). The wellness benefits include stress and anxiety reduction, relaxation, improved sleep, and calming heart and breathing rates. Sound therapists and mental health professionals incorporate nature sounds and white noise as a part of therapeutic interventions, particularly for conditions like anxiety, insomnia, and PTSD. Research has found that natural soundscapes produce decreased stress annoyance and improved health outcomes (decreased pain, lower stress, improved mood, and enhanced cognitive performance).[29] They can improve concentration boosting productivity, improve communication with higher-quality interactions, and provide privacy. Soundscapes with environmental triggers are considered restorative with reductions in arousal. Since people spend most of their time inside, nature-based interior soundscapes help mask unwanted noise (AC systems, construction, traffic, copy machines, and distractive speech), and can produce wellness effects including improved breathing, heart rate, and reduced muscle tension.[30]

Running through the heart of the city of Idaho Falls, Idaho is the Snake River and a series of waterfalls, Figure 6.9a. The waterfalls were originally a series of rough rapids and later were modified to accommodate surge water from upstream. Friendship Park, also known as Pedersen Sportsman's Park, is an urban oasis overlooking the waterfalls where the sounds of the falling water are hypnotic and restorative. Within the park are water features, rocks for crossing ponds, and shaded areas where you can just sit and enjoy the view. Refer to Figure 6.9a. Natural sound sources comprise ocean surf, waterfalls, rain, gentle tree breezes, wind-blown grasses, and animal vocalizations and calling behaviors such as certain insect chirps, grazing sheep, songs of humpback whales, and cooing and birdcalls as might be imagined by robins in Figure 6.9b. More

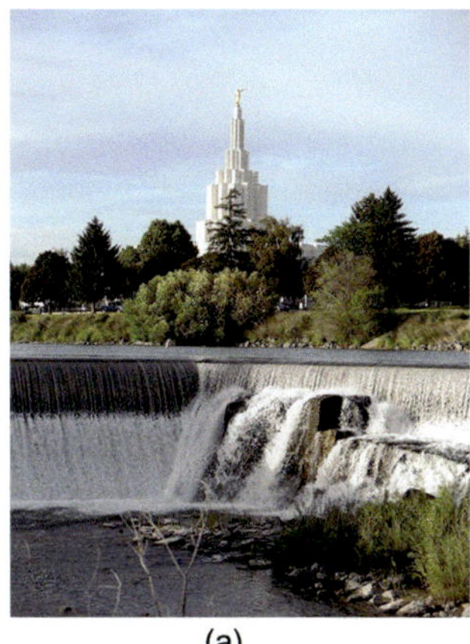

(a)

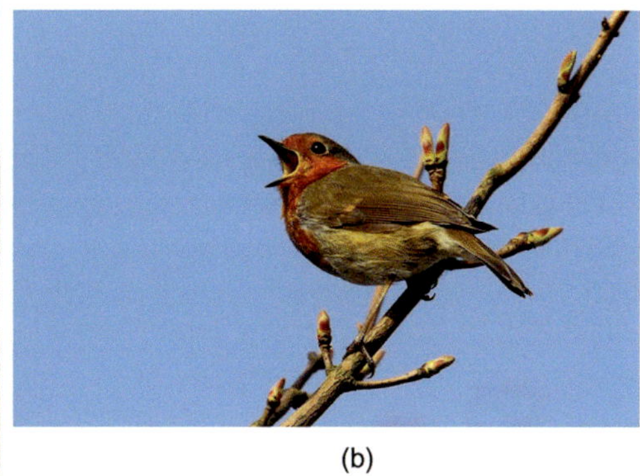

(b)

6.9 Soundscape Environments a) Idaho Falls, Idaho Sounds of Waterfalls, b) Robin Singing

(*Source: Wikimedia Commons*)

than single animal vocalizations are wholistic models of soundscape ecology that introduce an entire chorus or spectrum of life.[31]

Landscape scale summary

The landscape design offers opportunities at varying scales and for specific design strategies to incorporate health and wellness benefits. They range from the aesthetic and wellness qualities of experiencing the natural environment to engagement with healing gardens and land art installments. This includes forest bathing, incorporation of foodscapes, and purpose-built healing gardens. Landscape wellness occurs at an important scale because it is accessible and most often surrounds or is within the cities, neighborhoods, campuses, and buildings within which we live. This scale can impact each of the other scales (planning, architecture, and interiors) with their interactions with nature and green spaces. The wellness outcomes at this scale contribute to pro-individual benefits through intimate and everyday experiences of the various forms of nature. They contribute to pro-social benefits by fostering community and family and friends' gatherings, with casual encounters, and through gardening and forest bathing. They contribute through pro-environmental benefits with protection from negative climatic effects, reforestation, and positive interactions with nature. Reimaging our responses to population growth, urban development, transportation modes, consumption patterns, agricultural practices, and renewable and hybrid energy sources will help protect and revitalize our natural and urban landscapes for future generations.

The strategies are intended to positively influence a project's intentions and goals, site selection, conceptual design processes, and design details. They represent a pathway to achieving wellness design. Further, they are intended to suggest solutions for healthy people, healthy places, and a healthy planet. To Wilbert Gesler, "*healing and place are inseparable*."[32] This also would include wellness. Note that the strategies were not meant to be exhaustive, but rather a broader set of health and wellness indicators spreading across the planning, architecture, interior, and landscape design scales informing wellness best practices. What is important is access to the wellness strategies in terms of frequency (*how often*), duration of exposure (*how long*), and intensity (*how much and the quality*) of the interaction.

The resulting individual, social, and environmental outcomes are interactive and mutually supportive of one another and designed to influence the planning and design processes at varying scales. The wellness strategies are intended to be concrete examples resulting in positive additions and changes within the built environment. It must be noted that implementation of these wellness design strategies does not guarantee positive health outcomes, but it can provide greater opportunities for them to occur. Following is a listing of the strategies presented in this paper. Table 6.1 was originally developed by Gove Depuy and Phillip Tabb.[33]

LANDSCAPE SCALE STRATEGIES

1. Green spaces and parks.
2. Blue spaces.
3. Waterway restorations.
4. Edible landscapes and foodscapes.
5. Healing gardens.
6. Forest bathing.
7. Restoration and sequestering.
8. Land art installations.
9. Soundscapes.

STRATEGY	DESIGN INTENTIONS	WELLNESS STRATEGIES	WELLNESS OUTCOMES	REFERENCES
Parks & Green Spaces	To protect and provide parks, plazas, pockets and green spaces that are accessible, regenerative and climate responsive, and safe. Provide the greening of streetscapes as appropriate to climatic context and urban ecology.	Connect parks and greenways to existing ecological flows, connect circulation through greenspaces to existing urban fabric, provide a variety of activities, allow for natural or "wildspaces," consider seasonal changes. Add tiny urban forests.	Stress reduction, increase activity and strengthen muscles, increase calming, improves mood, oxygenated air, decrease cortisol levels, supports biospheric values, and promotes pro-social and pro-environmental stewardship and behaviors.	https://www.cdc.gov/healthyplaces/healthtopics/parks.htm https://montgomeryplanningboard.org/wp-content/uploads/2019/01/Attachment_A_EPS_Design_Guidelines_Working_Draft.pdf
Blue Spaces	Preserve existing rivers, lakes, waterways, and incorporate fountains, wells and water features in planning and design. Encourage aquatic activities.	Create blue spaces that are accessible, safe, with spatial variety and low negative environmental impact, easily manageable, sustainable, and create an elicitor of a sense of place.	Stress reduction, increase activity, increase calming, improves mood and mental wellbeing, increases sensory experiences and emotional arousal, and increase pro-environmental behaviors.	https://www.healthline.com/health-news/spending-time-in-blue-spaces-linked-to-better-mental-health https://www.sciencedirect.com/science/article/pii/S1618866719304625

Waterway Restorations	To preserve biodiversity, animal habitats, and provide healthy recreation.	Maintain constant natural connection among the biological communities, eliminate pollutants entering watershed, and integrate human activity.	Improvements to the natural environment, increase human activity, reduced obesity, increase cognitive function, increase positive mood and happiness, increase respiratory health.	https://www.anthropocenemagazine.org/2017/08/urban-effects-on-rivers-have-long-reach/
Edible Landscapes and Foodscapes	Provide ample and accessible urban agriculture, community gardens, allotments, and individual kitchen gardens to provide organic nutritious food integrated to ornamental landscapes.	Design public and private foodscapes, that are sustainable, regenerative, and accessible, provide edible edges, design for extended growing seasons, provide protection from vermin and pest, and consider sustainable water sources.	Providing access to nature and natural processes, increase of urban biodiversity, healthy nutritious food, reduced "harvest-to-table," advancing equity in nutrition, plant-based diet, and promotes pro-social and pro-environmental behaviors.	https://www.nature.org/en-us/what-we-do/our-priorities/provide-food-and-water-sustainably/food-and-water-stories/regenerative-food-systems/
Healing Gardens	Protect and provide outdoor healing spaces and plant-populated landscapes, that function as places of refuge and recuperation. Design for accessibility and ease of navigation.	Create safe, protected, identifiable and accessible places of refuge and prospect, design for privacy and spatial variety for diverse physical therapies and emotional settings, minimize intrusions, include water, and provide ease of circulation and clear sense of entry.	Stress reduction, fresh air, increase activity, improved mental wellbeing, increase of positive emotions and mood, increases "presence," supports decrease of cortisol levels, and promotes pro-social and pro-environmental behaviors.	https://journals.sagepub.com/doi/10.1177/1937586715606926 https://journals.sagepub.com/doi/10.1177/1937586715606926
Forest Bathing	Health connections such as forest bathing. Trail systems to be safe and interesting with a variety of spatial experiences. Protecting thin places.	Provide sensory-rich circulation network and contemplation "sit-spots," include historic, geologic topologic and water features, paths should be safe with optimum gradients.	Direct access to nature, increase sensory experience, sense of presence, and physical activity, increase mindfulness, stress reduction, and decrease in blood pressure.	https://www.nationalgeographic.com/travel/article/forest-bathing-nature-walk-health

Reforestation Afforestation and Carbon Sequestering	Preserve existing forests, encourage reforestation, encourage urban afforestation, and limit horizontal low density urban growth.	Protect existing forests and biodiverse lands, encourage new forests and urban afforestation, and limit urban growth with focus on infill, densification, streetscape and limit urban hard surfaces.	Direct access to nature, supports decrease of cortisol levels, biospheric values, pro-social and pro-environmental behaviors.	https://www.livescience.com/forest-bathing https://www.mdpi.com/1660-4601/18/4/2067
Land Art Installations	Preserve natural and historic land and earth art works. Purpose to raise awareness of social or environmental issues, and to augment rather than disrupt environment.	Provides places for interaction and gives voice to and highlights spiritual, environmental and social issues, and can connect and focus attention to beneficial healing qualities of nature.	Stress reduction, improve mood, improve thinking, empathy and life satisfaction, can form social cohesion and cultural identity, and promotes pro-social and pro-environmental behaviors.	https://www.americansforthearts.org/2018/08/30/five-reasons-why-public-art-matters
Soundscapes	To provide noise masking and access to soothing and restorative natural, animal and human-made sounds.	Reduce or limit unwanted noise, reserve healthy ecosystems, provide positive sound-producing features like fountains, trees, and rain roofs.	Stress and anxiety reduction, improve cognitive performance, moods, and concentration and increase productivity, an improve sleep.	https://www.ted.com/talks/bernie_krause_the_voice_of_the_natural_world/transcript

Table 6.1
Wellness Landscape Scale Strategies

NOTES

1. Thompson, Catherine, (Accessed October 10, 2023), https://www.sciencedirect.com/science/article/abs/pii/S0169204610002860
2. Olszewska-Guizzo, Agnieszka, *Neuroscience for Designing Green Spaces: Contemplative Landscapes* (New York, NY: Routledge, 2023).
3. Landscape Institute, *Public Health and Landscape: Creating Healthy Places*, (Accessed March 25, 2023), https://landscapewpstorage01.blob.core.windows.net/www-landscapeinstitute-org/migrated-legacy/PublicHealthandLandscape_CreatingHealthy-Places_FINAL.pdf
4. Bucholtz, Shawn, *Urban. Suburban. Rural. How do Households Describe Where They Live?* (Accessed November 6, 2023), https://www.huduser.gov/portal/pdredge/pdr-edge-frm-asst-sec-080320.html
5. Louv, Richard, *Last Child in the Woods: Saving our Children from Nature-Deficit Disorder* (Chapel Hill, NC: Algonquin Books, 2008).

6. Urban Canopy, *Trees are Essential to Healthy Communities*, (Accessed April 25, 2023), https://www.urbancanopyworks.com/services-of-urban-trees.html
7. Kaplan, R. & S. Kaplan, *The Experience of Nature: A Psychological Perspective* (Cambridge, MA: Cambridge University Press, 1989), p. 48.
8. Collis, Leo, *These 'Tiny Forests" are Popping Up in Cities Around the Country – And They're Having a Shocking Effect on Communities*, (Accessed January 8, 2024), https://apple.news/ARwhwqrJHT36s3tbehHAOIA
9. Ackerman, Cortney, *What is Kaplan's Attention Restoration Theory (ART)?* (Accessed April 24, 2023), https://positivepsychology.com/attention-restoration-theory/
10. European Science-Media Hub, *A Scientist's Opinion: Interview with Dr Mathew White about the Role of Aquatic Environments on the Health of Urban Populations,* (Accessed October 10, 2023), https://sciencemediahub.eu/2020/04/14/a-scientists-opinion-intervie w-with-dr-mathew-white-about-the-role-of-aquatic-environments-on-the-health-of-urban-populations/
11. National Ocean Service, (Accessed October 8, 2023), https://oceanservice.noaa.gov/facts/population.html
12. *Living Near a Blue Space can Reduce Mental Health Conditions,* (Accessed October 10, 2023), https://www.gcu.ac.uk/aboutgcu/universitynews/living-near-a-blue-space-can-reduce-mental-health-conditions#:~:text=Living%20near%20a%20blue%20space%20can%20reduce%20the,of%20the%20most%20deprived%20areas%20in%20North%20Glasgow.
13. Jacobs, Jantra, *5 Reasons why Walking in the Rain is Good for Your Heal*th, (Accessed November 16, 2023), https://www.pacificprime.co.uk/blog/5-reasons-why-walking-in-the-rain-is-good-for-your-health/
14. *A Landscaping Just as Good as Beautiful*, (Accessed October 10, 2023), https://garden-culturemagazine.com/foodscaping-a-new-way-to-create-a-garden/
15. Olszewska-Guizzo, Agnieszka, *Neuroscience for Designing Green Spaces: Contemplative Landscapes* (London, UK: Routledge, 2023).
16. *Natural Design for Better Health: An Interview with Dr. Roger Ulrich*, (Accessed October 12, 2023), https://naturesacred.org/natural-design-for-better-health-an-interview-with-dr-roger-ulrich/
17. Louv, Richard, *Last Child in the Woods: Saving our Children from Nature-Deficit Disorder* (Chapel Hill, NC: Algonquin Books, 2008).
18. Olszewska-Giozzo, Agnieszka, *Neuroscience for Designing Green Spaces* (London, UK: Routledge, 2023), p. 133.
19. Bowler, Diane E., Lisette M. Buyung-Ali, Teri M. Knight, & Andrew S. Pullin, 2010, (Accessed February 13, 2020), https://bmcpublichealth.biomedcentral.com/articles/10.1186/1471–2458-10–456?dom=prime&src=syn.
20. Alcock, Ian, Mathew White, Benedict Wheeler, Lora Fleming, & Michael Depledge, *Longitudinal Effects on Mental Health of Moving to Greener and Less Green Urban Areas,* (Accessed January 12, 2020), https://pubs.acs.org/doi/abs/10.1021/es403688w?cookieSet=1
21. Durkay, Jocelyn & Jennifer Schultz, *The Role of Forests in Carbon Sequestering and Storage*, (Accessed April 20, 2023), https://www.ncsl.org/environment-and-natural-resources/the-role-of-forests-in-carbon-sequestration-and-storage
22. *Fact Sheet: Reforestation*, (Accessed August 26, 2023), https://www.earthday.org/reforestation-fact-sheet/
23. Evans, Karen, *Why Forest Bathing is Good for Your Health,* (Accessed April 21, 2023), https://greatergood.berkeley.edu/article/item/why_forest_bathing_is_good_for_your_health
24. Cichick, Sage & Matthew Rohn, *A Report on the Value of Land Art and Biophilic Design to Draw Students into the St. Olaf College Natural Lands and Enhance an Environmental Ethos on Campus*, (Accessed April 20, 2023), https://wp.stolaf.edu/art/files/2013/10/Rohn-StOlafLandArtReport.pdf

25. Buxton, Rachel, Amber Peterson, Caludia Allou, & George Wittemyer, *A Synthesis of Health Benefits of Natural Sounds and their Distribution in National Parks*, (Accessed December 14, 2023), https://www.pnas.org/doi/10.1073/pnas.2013097118
26. Cui, Peng, Tingting Li, Zhengwei Xia, & Chunyu Dai, *Research Effects of Soundscapes on Human Psychological Health in an Old Community of a Cold Region*, (Accessed November 20, 2023), https://www.ncbi.nlm.nih.gov/pmc/articles/PMC9223413/
27. Schafer, R. Murray, *The Soundscape: The Sonic Environment and the Tuning of the World* (Rochester, VT: Destiny Books, 1993).
28. Dutchen, Stephanie, *Noise and Health*, (Accessed December 12, 2023), https://magazine.hms.harvard.edu/articles/noise-and-health
29. Buxton, Rachel, Amber Peterson, Caludia Allou, & George Wittemyer, *A Synthesis of Health Benefits of Natural Sounds and their Distribution in National Parks*, (Accessed December 14, 2023), https://www.pnas.org/doi/10.1073/pnas.2013097118
30. Benway, Evan & Fran Board, *How Natural Soundscapes Contribute to Comfort and Health in Design*, (Accessed December 18, 2023), https://designwell365.com/technology/commercial-integration/how-natural-soundscapes-contribute-to-comfort-and-health-in-design/
31. Krause, Bernie, *The Voice of the Natural World*, (Accessed December 15, 2023), https://www.ted.com/talks/bernie_krause_the_voice_of_the_natural_world/transcript
32. Gesler, Wilbert M., *Healing Places* (Lanham, MD: Roman & Littlefield, 2003), p. 1.
33. Dupuy, Gove & Phillip Tabb, "Wellness Strategies, Chapter 3," *Wellness Architecture and Design Pathways*, Self-published, 2023.

7 CASE STUDY 1 – MADO NEIGHBORHOOD

MADO WELLNESS NEIGHBORHOOD AT SERENBE, GEORGIA, USA

Health and wellness benefits and strategies across all scales are present in this award-winning development project located southwest of Atlanta, Georgia. Mado is part of a larger constellation of biophilic neighborhoods comprising the hamlet of Serenbe, Georgia. The name, *Serenbe,* combines the terms "*serene*" and "*being*," suggesting the essential connections to a vital natural environment.[1] Serenbe was initially described as a community among the trees and now is being considered one of the first truly biophilic residential developments. In 2008, Serenbe received the Inaugural Sustainability Award from the Urban Land Institute. Serenbe is considered an exemplar of land preservation, creative mix of uses, density, agrarian urbanism, connectivity, and walkability. It is also known for wellness and active living, green architecture and construction practice, and its association with biophilia. The initial goals for the project included land preservation, a sensitivity to the existing environment, community formation, integration of the arts, diversity of inhabitants, inclusion of sacred geometry, and as a 21st-century wellness model of intentional environmentally-oriented development.

SERENBE COMMUNITY

Serenbe is located in the heart of the Chattahoochee Hill Country, which occurs near the end of the Blue Ridge Mountain range. Most of the surrounding land encircling Atlanta has been developed, with the exception of a southwestern strip that includes most of South Fulton County. Chattahoochee Hills is planned for 40,000 dwellings and 65,000 people. While Serenbe shares some of the tenets of the New Urbanism, it stands apart from this movement in some important ways as it has created its own unique qualities and brand of authenticity. Serenbe is in harmony with the land, is farm-to-table, is sustainable and authentic, supports active living, attracts a diverse population, and creates a permanent, vital, and alive sense of community.

Within the city of Chattahoochee Hills, Serenbe is considered a mixed-use hamlet which is defined as a development on greater than 250 acres (101 ha), with 70% preserved openspace, offering housing, employment, and commercial opportunities (6–25% must be commercial), has limited block sizes encouraging pedestrianization, and is visually buffered from existing roads.[2] Serenbe hamlet is

DOI: 10.4324/9781003472902-7

composed of a series of connected neighborhoods where there is a similar offering of differing dwelling types, but the non-residential land uses vary with dissimilar themes or different focuses. For example, Selborne neighborhood is themed toward the arts (culinary, visual, and performing); Grange neighborhood is concerned with agriculture and equestrian activities; Mado neighborhood is oriented to health and wellness; Spela is related to family and play and has a large 400 feet by 400 feet (122 × 122 meter) park in the middle of it; and the Education Neighborhood (yet to be named) is oriented to education, schools, study-away, international studies, and continuing education. As of 2023, Serenbe has a population of more than 1,000 residents. The final buildout for Serenbe is planned for 1,800 dwelling units, a population of 3,500 residents, and 2,000 acres (809 ha) of land including the affordable neighborhood. The masterplan illustrated in Figure 7.1 was designed by Phillip Tabb, and shows the various neighborhoods with Mado in the center.

What can be seen is the multiplication of sensuous omega forms with their double-loaded spatial structure, and large areas of forest protected within the omega and surrounding the built portions. The spatial organization allows each home to front onto the omega street where social interaction largely occurs, and backs onto the forest edge with both visual and physical access. The thematic focus for the various neighborhoods contributes to land use diversity, varying identities, and vitality of each place. The concept of constellating urbanism is initiated in Serenbe and is based upon Leon Krier's concept of growth by *multiplication*

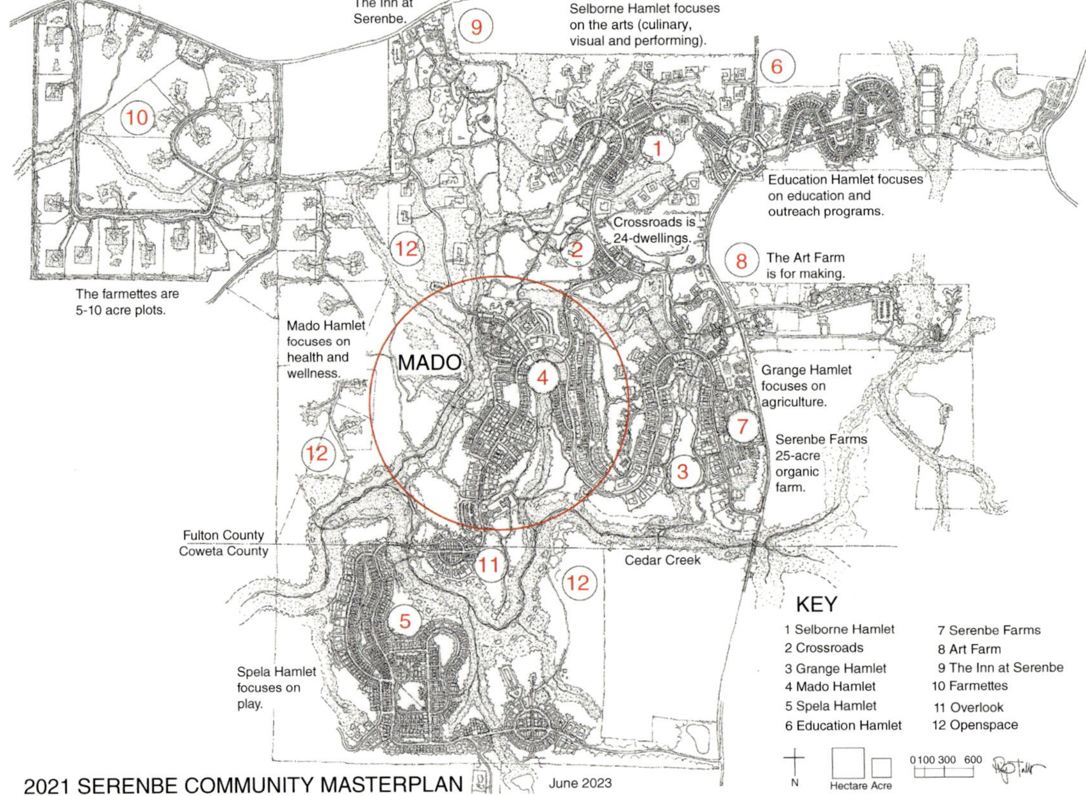

7.1
Serenbe Community Masterplan 2021
(*Source:* Phillip Tabb)

rather than sheer *addition*.[3] Systemic Constellation Theory, originally developed by psychotherapist Bert Hellinger for family dynamics, suggested that independent yet interconnected parts of a system create a combination of actions affecting the collective whole.[4] For Serenbe, this means that the interrelated neighborhoods, and the individual placemaking practices they employ, support even greater constellating, synergetic, and programmatic relationships, Figure 7.2a.

The masterplan for Serenbe supports the concept of development by multiplication. Multiplication is reinforced further through the theming of the neighborhoods apex mix of uses. The differences established by the themes create an interdependence. Each of the three neighborhood sites is positioned in a slight land-formed bowl at the interface between sloping forested portions of each of the naturally formed sites and the flat meadows or waterways below. Rather than "*gating*" or isolating each of the omega neighborhoods, there was an effort to create porous and open-ended entrances and exits with between three and four ways into the neighborhoods. A path system was created to connect the neighborhoods through the woods and floodplains. This created a sense of place and allowed for both the ridge tops and valley bottoms to be free of development.[5] The configuration of neighborhoods forms the overall community with their interrelated themes and support functions. Using the zoning mechanism of "transfer of development rights," Serenbe is able to offer varying densities and housing typologies including farmettes (approximately 1 unit per 10 acres), cottages (4 units per acre), live-work units (12 units per acre), townhomes (8 units per acre), and apartments (20 units per acre).

The omega design used in Serenbe derives from nine geometric and diagrammatic stages representing the morphology of its form. The first stage is the pure circle which represents the circularity of bounding and place-containing geometry. The second stage is creating another concentric circle within the center effectively creating a "donut" in which the center is preserved, and development occurs between the circumference of the outer circle to the inner circle. The third stage is the stretching of the circle into an elongated oval along the north-south axis. This allows the form to nestle into each site and to position residential lots adjacent to one another along the north-south axis. The fourth stage is the important opening of the south end of the oval creating a "U-shape." This allows for free movement in and out of the omega for energy, fresh air, local animal inhabitants, and people. The fifth stage is the U-shaped form slightly flaring inward, but not completing the circle and creating slightly more enclosure and a sense of place. The form then flares outward creating an inviting entrance or exit to the neighborhood and an omega-shape, "Ω." The sixth stage is the application of the Thorburn transect to the legs of the omega form. This creates a density and intensity gradient from the rural character of the site to the more urban nature of the omega apex. The seventh stage is responding to the thematic character of the neighborhood by the inclusion of the non-residential functions and services. The eighth stage is the creation or support of a central feature of the neighborhood and site. This usually is the center of the donut or inner circle and includes a water tributary (Selborne), lake (Grange), pond and wetlands (Mado), or park (Spela). The ninth stage is the creation of a unique architectural language for each neighborhood further giving them more character and identity.

For Mado the language is Scandinavian modern vernacular as developed by Erik Asmussen. The nine omega form stages are listed below:

1. Pure circle – *representing circularity, bounding, and place-containing geometry.*
2. Creating an inner circle or donut shape – *where the center is preserved and undeveloped.*
3. Formation of an oval – *stretching the circle into an elongated oval along the north-south axis.*
4. Creating a "U-shape" – *opening the southern end allowing for free movement in and out of the omega for energy, fresh air, local animal inhabitants, and people.*
5. Flaring the ends – *creating more containment and a sense of place and a welcoming sense of entry.*
6. Applying the Thorburn transect – *creating a density and intensity gradient from the rural character of the site to the more urban nature of the omega apex.*
7. Thematic land use mixes – *integrating thematic mixes of non-residential functions and services unique to each neighborhood.*
8. Creating a central feature – *including a water tributary (Selborne), farm and lake (Grange), pond and wetlands (Mado), or park (Spela).*
9. Creating a unique architectural language – *giving each neighborhood a more unique character and identity.*

Serenbe did not develop by expanding through addition creating larger and larger built elements into a single settlement plan. Rather, Serenbe has grown through a process of incremental multiplication where development has evolved in carefully controlled and sequenced parts of the plan. Beginning with the west leg of the Selborne neighborhood, pictured in yellow in Figure 7.2c, Serenbe generally expands with the most buildable legs of the omega along with some of the mixed-use at the apex. First to be developed in a neighborhood are legs occurring on flatter, more affordable and buildable land. Neighborhood legs were selected to develop first because they are double-loaded making infrastructure more affordable, and they gave a sense of the streetscape environment. As can be seen in Figure 7.2c, the development sequence moves from leg to leg and from neighborhood to neighborhood beginning with Selborne, Crossroads and Serenbe Farms, Grange, and eventually moving to Mado, Overlook, Spela, and the Education neighborhood. Hundreds of homes were not constructed in short periods with single contractors, but rather were parsed out in an incremental way over years that allowed for market adjustments. This accounted for a variety of architectural languages and styles allowing for individual expression of architecture from traditional to contemporary.

The Thorburn transect was an observation of English village entrance roads by Andrew Thorburn in 1971. It was seen as a spatial organization of varying building densities and landscape distributions in English villages.[6] Density increases as the rural road approaches the village center. The point at which the village is entered is called the "*threshold of dispersion*," often formed by a "pinch point" or tight opening between buildings or walls. In the transect, buildings are gradually placed closer to the road and closer to one another. Conversely the landscape does the reverse

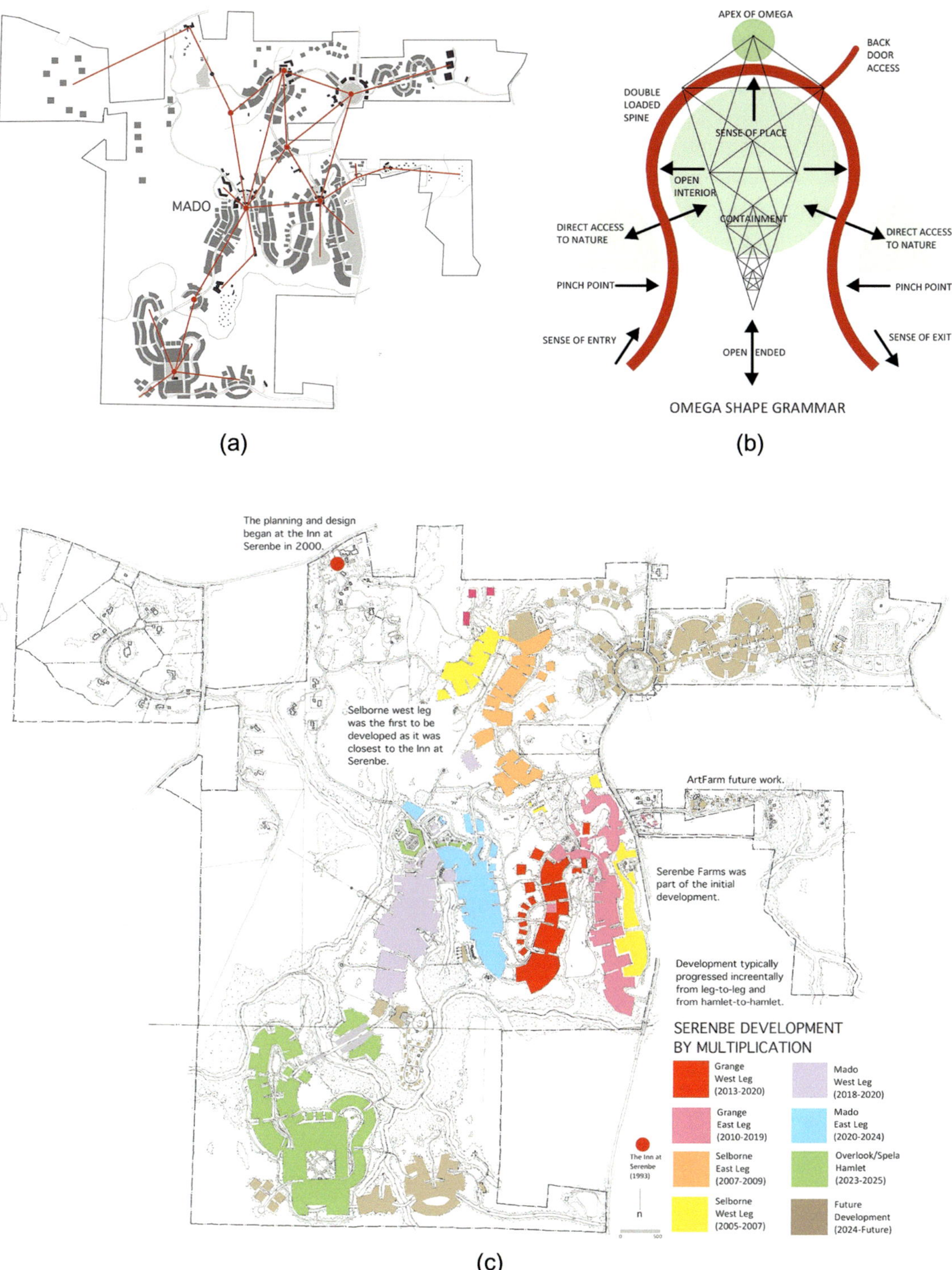

7.2
Serenbe Concept a) Constellation of Neighborhoods, b) Omega Form Language, c) Growth by Multiplication

(*Source: Phillip Tabb*)

with buffers between the road and dwellings at the perimeter. Then the dwelling positions progress to the center with mature trees along paths and walled-in gardens. This pattern was use in the Serenbe planning along the omega-shaped roads. Planned for the centers or omega apex are public "outdoor rooms" defined by attached buildings and landscapes. This transect has been applied to Selborne, Grange, Mado, and Spela neighborhoods. For Mado the transect occurs along the two north-south legs of the omega culminating at the apex where the greatest density and majority of wellness businesses and functions occur.

Planning decisions were made to reinforce the Thorburn rural-to-urban transect, with Serenbe Lane, running north and south through the neighborhood. As you enter Mado either from Grange neighborhood from the southeast, Spela and Overlook from the southwest, Crossroads from the northeast or the Inn at Serenbe from the northwest, the density grows in intensity. The character of the roads

7.3 Selborne Thorburn Transect a) Transect Diagram, b) Selborne Omega Leg (*Source: Phillip Tabb*)

(a)

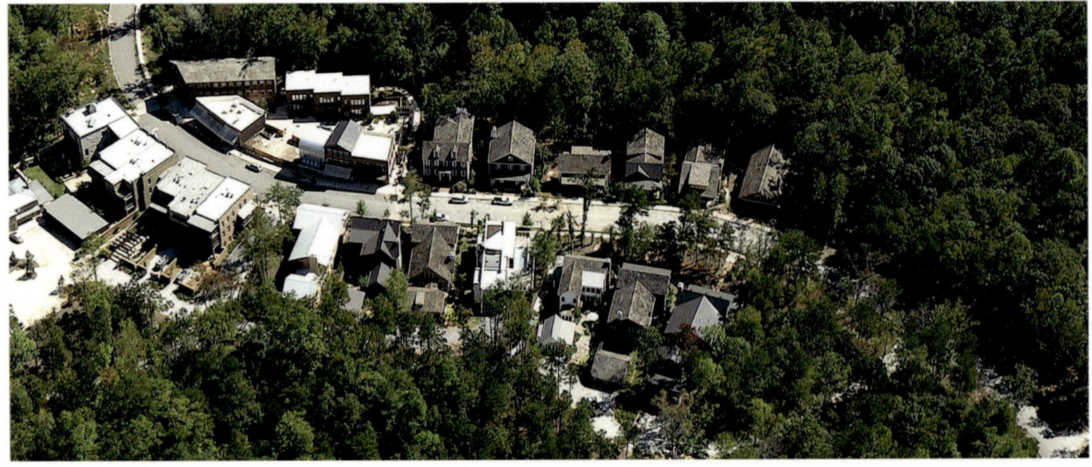

(b)

change from gravel to asphalt paving with bioswales and no curbs, and finally to paved roads with curbs and parking. Entering the neighborhood, the houses on both sides are on estate lots set back from the road with existing pines acting as natural landscape filters. Further into Mado, cobblestone and raised walkways and traffic calmer crosses the omega road indicating another transition along the transect. From this point on, the street has granite curbs and sidewalks on both sides and is treelined with cottage houses closer to one another and closer to the street. Also at these street crossings are night streetlights that indicate the points of crossing. At the beginning of the circular apex, another crosswalk appears and from this point to the center are attached buildings that align along a widened sidewalk with townhomes, live-work units, and commercial businesses on each side of the street. Outdoor dining occurs in the Halsa Restaurant at the apex, and the three-story structures indicate the center or top of the omega. Exterior building materials change along the transect from predominantly wood at the edge to brick and stucco at the center. In Mado there is a full range of exterior building colors. The diagram and omega leg illustrate the Thorburn transect for Selborne neighborhood, Figure 7.3.

NEIGHBORHOOD THEMES

The process of growth by multiplication has created neighborhoods that are organized around a series of interrelated wellness themes. There are certain land uses common to each neighborhood that include a variety of housing types from estate homes, cottages, townhomes, live-work units, and rental units. Common to each are also restaurants: The Blue-Eyed Daisy and The Hill (Selborne), The General Store (Grange), and Halsa (Mado). The Farmhouse Restaurant is in the Inn at Serenbe. Each neighborhood has a natural openspace in its center. Two omega streets connect all the neighborhoods, Selborne Lane for the northern neighborhoods and Serenbe Lane for the southern neighborhoods. Refer to the neighborhood photographs in Figure 7.4. The hamlet and neighborhood themes include the following:

- Selborne neighborhood – *is oriented toward the arts (culinary, visual, and performing), and includes the Crossroads. Selborne neighborhood is approximately 35 gross acres (14 ha) and 120 dwelling units, and Crossroads is 5 acres (2 ha) and 24 dwelling units, and two shops started in 2004. These were the first of the neighborhoods in development.*
- Grange neighborhood – *is oriented toward agriculture and is approximately 75 gross acres (30 ha) and includes Serenbe Farms, Grange Lake and Swan Ridge, and 164 dwelling units. This was the second neighborhood developed with a majority of properties now occupied.*
- Mado neighborhood – *is oriented toward health and wellness and is approximately 75 gross acres (30 ha) including the interior wetlands and 575 dwelling units. This was the third neighborhood developed with two-thirds of the properties presently occupied.*
- Spela neighborhood – *is oriented toward play and is approximately 80 gross acres (32 ha) and is planned for 380 dwelling units in the infrastructure*

construction phase. Overlook is a small cluster planned for 40 homes located in-between Mado and Spela currently in the building construction phase.

- Education neighborhood – *is oriented toward education and outreach and is approximately 50 gross acres (20 ha) planned for 500 dwelling units. This neighborhood will feature an automobile-free environment with designated central parking areas. This neighborhood is in the planning phase.*
- Affordable neighborhood – *is in the conceptual design phase and is oriented to affordable and workforce housing within easy access (walking, golfcart, or shuttle) to Serenbe and will accommodate approximately 400 dwelling units. This neighborhood will feature an automobile-free zone in the residential area, a commercial zone that interfaces with Serenbe and the larger community of Chattahoochee Hills, and surrounding forests and parklands.*

Spela and Overlook take on a different spatial order from the omega forms of the other neighborhoods, Figure 7.4d. Overlook is sited between Mado and Spela on a slightly sloping parcel of land partly surrounded by Cedar Creek. It has circular

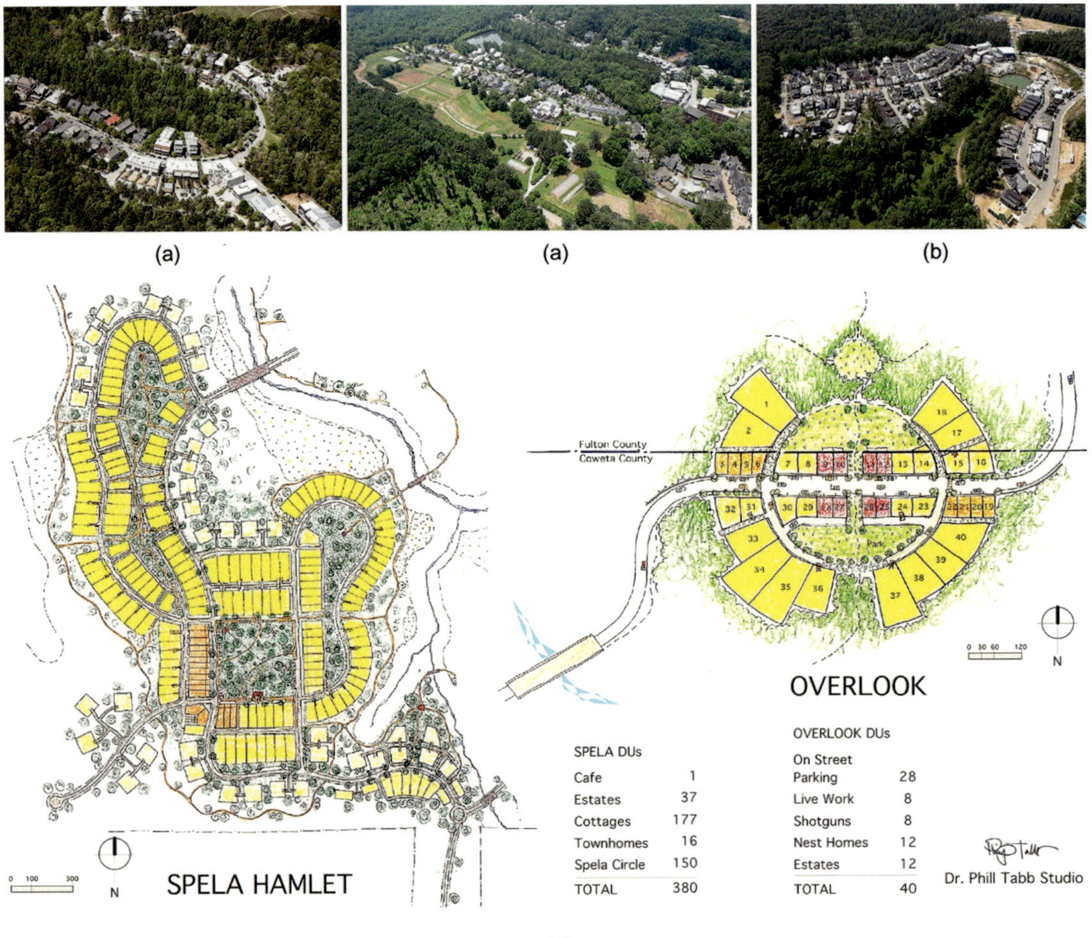

7.4 Serenbe Neighborhoods a) Selborne Neighborhood, b) Grange Neighborhood, c) Mado Neighborhood, d) Spela Neighborhood and Overlook Pocket Neighborhood (*Sources: Serenbe Development and Phillip Tabb*)

circumferential circulation connecting cottages and estate homes and a denser central street across its diameter composed of cottages and townhomes. It is similar to the Crossroads neighborhood in size and all white buildings. Over a bridge lies Spela with its curvilinear streets, internal green spaces, and the central park. The central park is a square 400 feet (122 meters) on a side and is planned as a community focus of outdoor activities including hiking, forest bathing, gardening, picnics, and a coffee bar. The park serves as a community incubator, a place of recreation and play, and a carbon sequester. It tends to provide a place of community focus, and encouragement of pro-individual, pro-social, and pro-environmental behaviors.

The neighborhoods are typically about one-half mile in diameter with green and blue spaces occupying the center and surrounded by forest land. The water features in the omega centers vary with Selborne having a small stream tributary; Grange having a tributary and lake; Mado having a tributary and wetlands; Spela having a large central park with Cedar Creek nearby, and the Education neighborhood having a sloping site down to a stream tributary. The neighborhoods have between three and four tessellations or connecting access roads into the neighborhood that pass through the threshold of dispersion or entry point into the density gradient of the built form. The threshold of dispersion is a space between agglomerated dwellings and more remote buildings not considered part of the settlement, typically more than 488 feet (150 meters). In Serenbe rural land is occupied by pastures, pasture estate lots, forestland, and farmettes. An example of a building sited outside of this threshold is the Serenbe Stables that is not part of Crossroads or Grange neighborhood as they lie approximately 500 feet away from each.

Initially home costs in Serenbe were between 400,000 and a million dollars. Today many homes in Serenbe cost between one and three million dollars, yet there have been planning strategies to generate greater choice in the context of economic diversity. Keeping in mind that all buildings need to meet EarthCraft construction standards and have geothermal systems, while using cheap materials and over-simplified housing forms were not allowed. Diversity was achieved with the planning of a large variety of housing land plots sizes from several acres per farmette site to as small as 1,000 square feet (93 m^2) for live-work units, and 1,050 square feet (98 m^2) for shotgun houses. Conversely, dwelling sizes vary from thousands of square feet for estate houses to under 1,000 square feet for the two-story shotgun homes. During the economic crisis of 2008–2009, Serenbe introduced what they called the "*nest*" homes, which were made up of smaller single-family dwellings tightly clustered together and varying in size from around 1,200 to 1,500 square feet.

In 2021, a conceptual planning effort was conducted to create an affordable and workforce neighborhood planned to coincide with the construction of new hotels in Selborne and Mado. The mix-use neighborhood was initially planned on a 132-acre site southeast of Grange for 400 dwelling units and a light commercial center, Figure 7.5a. While the plan indicates the evolving conceptual design, it is likely to change over time. The design is a dominant pedestrian plan with golf carts, emergency vehicles, and pedestrian circulation systems throughout the center of the site, Figure 7.5b. Each dwelling is planned to have emergency vehicle access. Automobile access and parking occur in remote lots adjacent to the entries, but not entering the residential part of the neighborhood. As of 2024, the conceptual design is being amended to accommodate more affordable building sites on flatter ground along the center portion of the site. The commercial area has remained the same at the southwest corner and has been designed to accommodate a small farm, grocery store, outdoor market, café, outdoor plaza, gas and electric station, and live-work units. The residential area of the neighborhood will have a denser cluster of dwellings surrounded by forested natural areas, and a linear park. The density is approximately three units per acre with 50% of the land planned as openspace. A residential block model along the main interior street was developed with three tiers of housing types including townhomes along the main interior street, shotgun homes within an intermediate space, and cottage homes at the perimeter, Figure 7.5c. At the ends of the block are road stubs for emergency vehicles. Golf cart parking occurs along the main street and dwellings are within the 300-foot (91 meter) maximum distance to nature.

In addition to the neighborhoods are several other facilities and amenities found throughout the community. These include Serenbe Farms, The Art Farm, Serenbe Stables, the Animal Village, Selborne Recreation Field, the Sculpture Park at Deer Hollow, Children's Treehouse, Trampoline Hill, and the Labyrinth. Each of these in its way, supports wellness activities. The Serenbe labyrinth has become a favorite destination for both residents and visitors to the community. It was built over a weekend in July of 2003 by family and friends of the developer. The Serenbe labyrinth is an 88-foot diameter replica of the one in the west nave or Royal Portal of the 12th century Chartres Cathedral in France. However, it is twice the size and is sited outdoors within a forested area overlooking a picturesque pond, Figure 7.6b.

A central feature of Serenbe and the second neighborhood, Grange, is the 25-acre certified seasonal organic farm located adjacent to the Grange neighborhood, Figure 7.7a. It provides farm-to-table produce to the Serenbe residents,

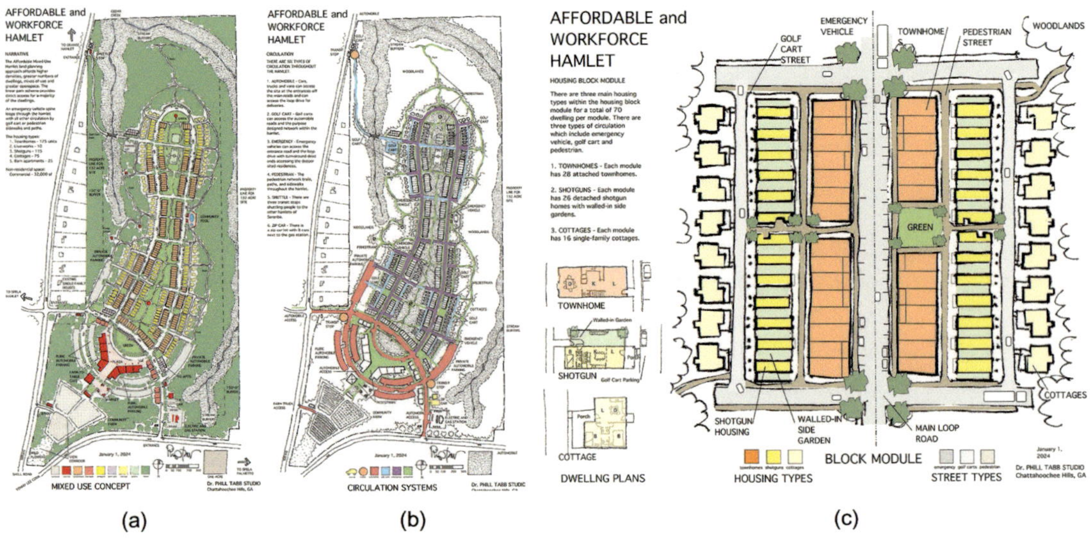

7.5
Affordable Housing Neighborhood Concept
a) Affordable Neighborhood Concept Plan,
b) Neighborhood Circulation Plan
c) Neighborhood Block Module
(*Source: Phillip Tabb*)

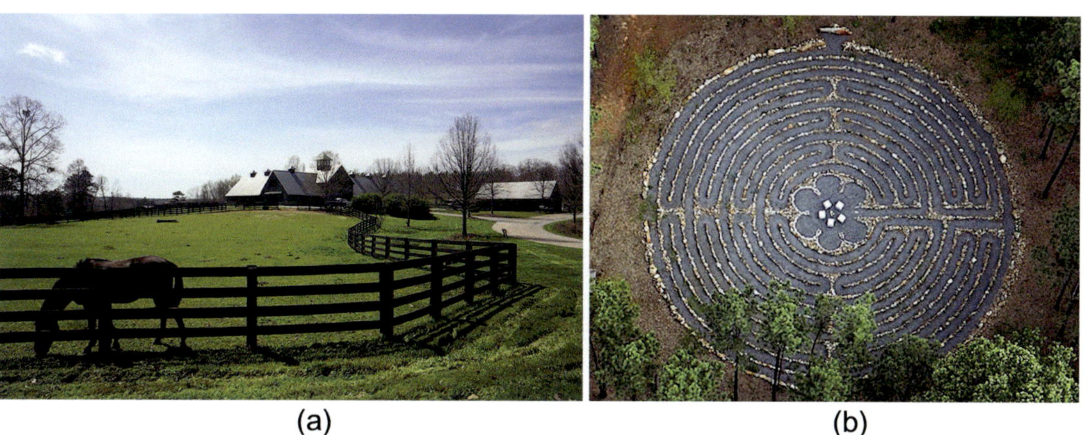

7.6
Serenbe Amenities
a) Serenbe Stables,
b) Labyrinth
(*Source: Phillip Tabb*)

restaurants, and neighboring CSA farm coops. Since 2004, the Serenbe Farms has cultivated 10 acres of farmland and is in the process of nurturing and restoring soil on an additional 15 acres. The farm has produced over 300 varieties of heirloom and hybrid vegetables, herbs, and flowers, with over 60,000 pounds of produce harvested a year. Serenbe Farms is one of the first of only 103 certified organic farms in the state of Georgia. Serenbe Farms operates within a three-part mission; to provide nourishing food for the local and greater community, to offer meaningful hands-on education for all generations, and to build community through food and farming. Both the farm in Grange and the Farmer's Market are in easy walking or golf cart distance, Figure 7.7b.

The Transfer of Development Rights (TDR) allows for the creation of density and especially nucleated neighborhood-scale developments. One of the challenges of a TDR is how to capitalize on the lower-density parcels left as a consequence of densification. Because Serenbe is interested in providing a wide range of housing choices and dwelling types, lower density development also fits into the overall scheme of things. One such way was the development of the more rural areas into five-to-ten-acre (two-to-four ha) parcels for what were called *farmettes* where buyers could construct a permanent residence, garage, shed, and either a small farm or paddocks for horses or other animals. Figure 7.7c illustrates one such farmette conceptual development plan "H" at Serenbe on a 202-acre (82 ha) site that also includes workable farms (in darker green) and home gardens (lighter green). The density averages one unit per seven and a half acres. Farm homes were clustered close to the connecting road with a small green (brighter green) to create a sense of community. Farmettes typically offer larger land plots, more privacy, and greater access to nature. Figure 7.7d is a photograph of a typical Serenbe pasture estate with an abundance of openspace surrounding the main structures, a family garden, a garage, and a swimming pool.

> *A source of local organic food, a place for nurture and nature, a place to get your hands dirty, a place of inspiration and reflection, a place to celebrate the seasons and their bounty, and a farm to create and sustain the future.*[7]

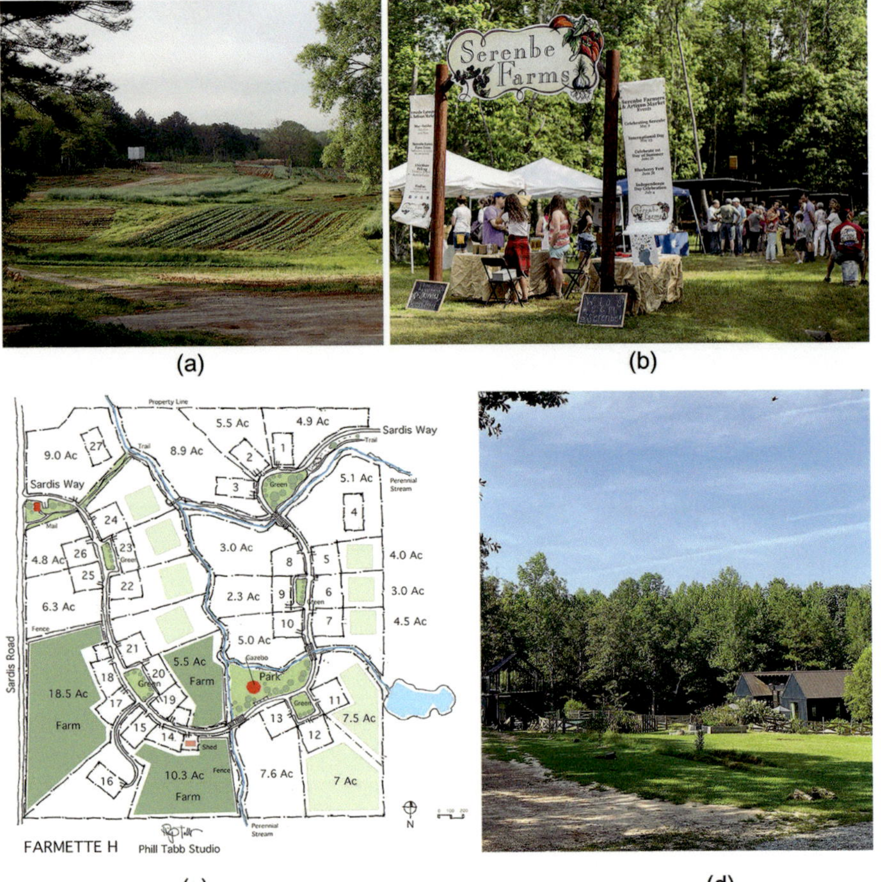

7.7
Serenbe Amenities
a) Serenbe Farms,
b) Farmer's Market
c) Farmette H Site Plan, d) Serenbe Pasture Estate

(*Sources: Phillip Tabb and Jessica Ashley*)

1. **Mado wellness neighborhood**

The Mado charrette in April of 2007, facilitated by founder and CEO of Serenbe, Steve Nygren and land planner Phillip Tabb, specifically targeted the design of the third neighborhood and its theme of the health and wellness non-residential functions. Also, it was to be the densest of the neighborhoods. Currently as of 2024, it has a population of approximately 500 residents. In the center of the neighborhood is an existing natural wetland and the 100-year flood plain, part of the Cedar Creek basin. The eastern leg of the omega is on fairly sloping forested land while the west leg is on relatively flat land, which is easier to develop. The name "Mado" comes from the Creek Nation Native Americans meaning "*things in balance*."[8] This seemed a fitting name for a focus on health and wellness. Consequently, the theme for Mado was health and wellness, so a cluster of activities was determined and dispersed throughout the fabric of the neighborhood plan. Mado is approximately 75 gross acres (30 ha) including the openspace center and wetlands, and it is 700 feet (17 meters) wide from the centerlines of each leg of the omega road. Planned for 575 dwelling units, Mado is a unique blend of residential dwelling types and health and wellness functions. It is designed for the age diversity of inhabitants, from infants to seniors.

The wellness functions, goods, and services include several buildings, clusters, and landscape features. Rather than concentrating the health and wellness activities into a single area, there was an attempt to disperse the functions throughout the neighborhood so that they were more integrated into the fabric of the place. One Mado Building is a multi-use three-story building housing many wellness-oriented businesses, offices, and services including the Halsa Restaurant, Serenbe Fitness Center, Dental Wellness, Flourish Pediatrics, Center for Positive Change, Serenbe Yoga and Body Works, Precision Performance and Physical Therapy, and the Spa at Serenbe. The adjacent live-work units provide several independently owned retail spaces on street level with residential rental units above. The Portal is a wellness retreat positioned next to the central pond offering multi-day retreats that include classes, nature walks, and healthy meals.

The Serenbe Swim Club is privately owned with membership available to the community and comprises three pools, cabanas, and eventually will have a snack bar. The Terra School Campus is located on the northwestern edge of Mado and houses preschool through 12th-grade studio classrooms. The mission at the Terra School is to inspire each child who enters its doors to find a calling that will change the world. The goal is to become a flagship school and lay the foundation for how a school design, environment, and pedagogy can support our overall mission. The Mado Aging in Place Wellness Campus is located across the street from One Mado Building, the Serenbe Swim Club and the Terra School Campus, and adjacent to the woodland openspace giving occupants views and access to the vitality of life around them. On its seven-acre campus, there will be a variety of living venues and support functions as it will support intergenerational living. The campus is modeled after Hogeweyk, the famed "dementia village" in The Netherlands. The design accounts for 40 rental apartments, 24 cottages around a courtyard, 24 individual cottages, a "wellness club," restaurant, offices, and retail.

According to landscape architect Alfie Vick, the Mado Food Forest and Medicinal Garden is a food-producing public garden that reflects the structure and diversity of the native Piedmont Forest. The garden is focused on balance and well-being; all the plants are either edible or medicinal, and many of them are both. Additionally, the garden is designed to engage residents who live adjacent to it. It is universally accessible, safe, and attractive with several spaces that encourage social interaction. Most of the vegetation is native, creating a food forest that is a microcosm of the surrounding natural ecosystems. Planning in a "V-shape" the single-story residences open to the garden and are accessible by a ramp connecting the garden to every house.

It has been an objective within Serenbe to create an architectural character that reflects diversity and individual choice while at the same time respecting a certain continuity of the overall aesthetic of the community. Like more established neighborhoods that have evolved over decades, this variable character expresses homeowners at varying stages of life, family functions, and individual tastes. The omega form is powerful enough to accommodate these differences without damaging its overall unity. For the Mado neighborhood, it

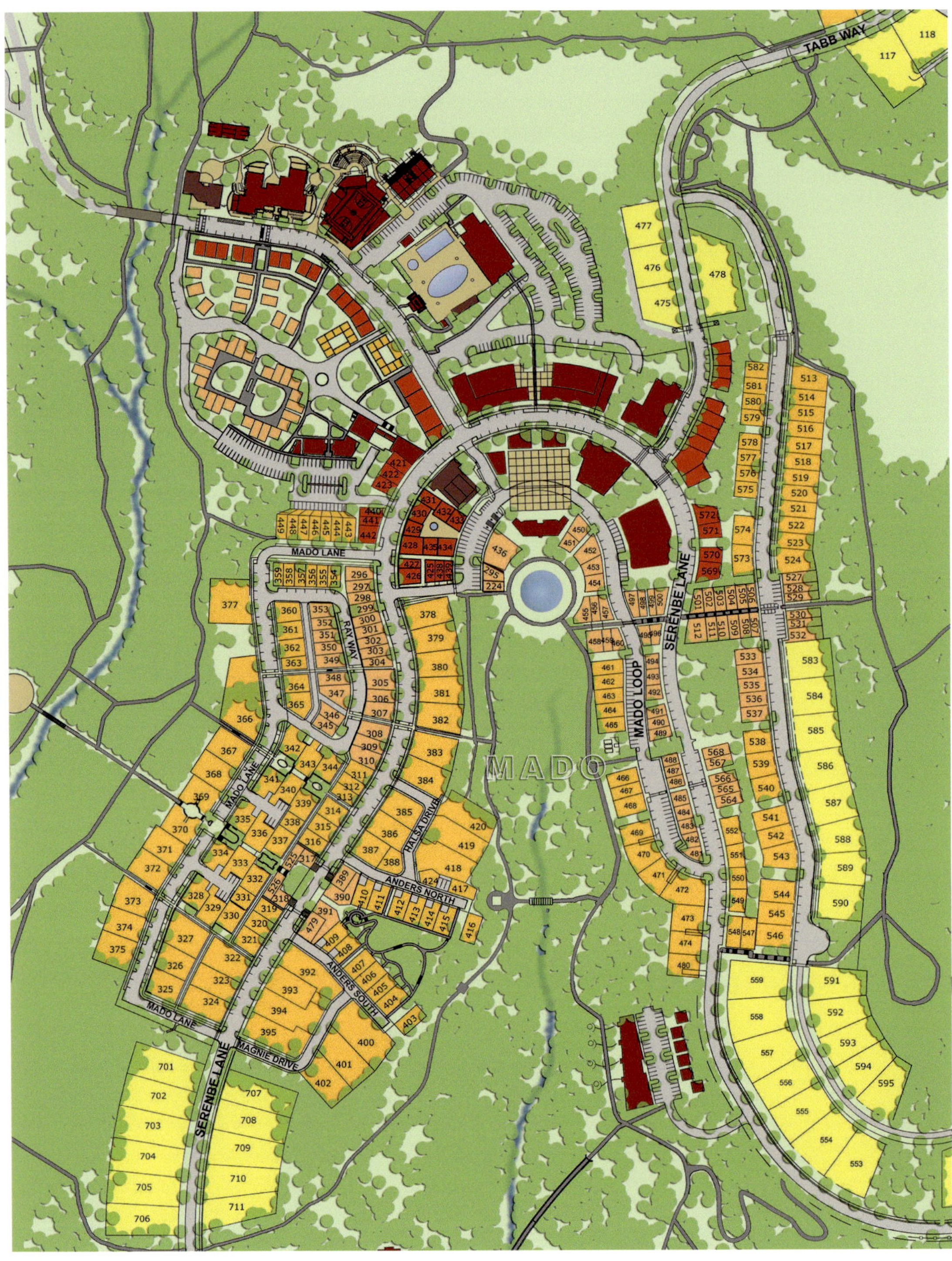

7.8
Mado Masterplan 2023
(*Source: Serenbe Development*)

was decided to reflect the wellness architecture of Erik Asmussen, a Danish architect who practiced in Sweden from the early 1960s to the end of the 1990s. While difficult to articulate in conventional terms, his work might be explained in terms like contemporary vernacular, colorful, expressive individuality with whimsical and playful moments, and as described by Gary Coates, Asmussen's architecture was "*charming and strangely attractive*."[9] Many of his ideas were influenced by Rudolf Steiner. This design language seemed appropriate for the architecture of Mado with the design strategies for wellness carefully integrated into this architectural language.

At the planning scale, Mado situates residents so they have direct connections to nature creating source experiences. This "*front door*" to nature planning approach was selected to amplify the biophilic principles demonstrating an accessible, inclusive, comprehensive, and integrated approach to residential development. The omega street is designed to provide easy access to health and wellness businesses and activities, and to nearby natural areas. Refer to the Mado site plan which shows the various building types and abundant amount of openspace, Figure 7.8.

2. Mado wellness planning and design strategies

The Mado neighborhood form and spatial structure possess certain wellness benefits. The omega design possesses certain inherent characteristics that contribute to a sense of community and wellness lifestyles. The Mado wellness design is integrated with the overall omega form and within the fabric of the neighborhood. The curvilinear neighborhood forms resemble the omega or horseshoe shapes and are characteristic of this particular typology. The neighborhood forms are not a "U" shape, but they are an "Ω" shape. This creates a slightly greater enclosure and supports greater containment, Figure 7.2b. Simultaneously, the open ends of the omega allow for natural ecological flows – solar energy, water, clean air, residents, visitors, and resident animals.[10] The omega shape slowly opens outward to create both a sense of entry and exit with connections to the neighboring neighborhoods. At the top or apex of each omega form are a collection and an intensity of mixed-use activities. They give a particular focus and identity to each neighborhood – the arts, agriculture, health and wellness, family and play, and education. The neighborhoods are connected by a serpentine road system that closely follows the contours and shapes of the natural landform omega sites.

Health and wellness were considered at the very beginning of the Mado neighborhood and carried through the omega form, integration of non-residential functions, and architectural character. Direct access to nature has been an extremely important intention for the development of the master plan and this is evident in Mado. The design nudges residents and visitors into physical activity. Serenbe preserves 70% of the land as openspace with only 30% dedicated to development. This in turn encourages physical activity, interaction with nature, and opportunities for chance encounters on a daily basis. In most instances throughout Serenbe, the serpentine omega roads are limited to singled double-loading, thereby positioning dwellings with a street frontage as well as direct forest access. With miles of trails throughout the community, residents have access to the forestland, streambeds, and other amenities located within the interstitial spaces of the neighborhood, and are connected to the adjacent neighborhoods of Selborne, Crossroads, Grange, Overlook, and Spela.

Mado is pedestrian-oriented and is situated within a one-half mile diameter circle, thereby making it an extremely walkable neighborhood. Further, there are miles of trails located on sidewalks on both sides of the streets, on cross-paths between parallel streets, within the inner omega and surrounding the neighborhood. Serenbe Lane, the primary omega street, is socially active with pedestrians walking and riding on electric golf carts to and from all the neighborhood activities. Its density also contributes to its pedestrianization. Instead of lines and lines of connected housing plots, at Serenbe the plots are periodically interrupted with paths connecting sidewalks to the openspace woodlands. Mado is the densest of the neighborhoods with approximately 75 gross acres of land and an estimated gross density of 7.7 units per acre, remembering 70% of surrounding land is openspace. The density and compactness of Mado lend to its pedestrian nature. Walking distances within the neighborhood are relatively short with the farthest homes being 1,800 feet from the apex which translates to a less than ten-minute walk at 3.5 feet per second. A majority of homes are no more than a four- or five-minute walk to the center. No home is more than 300 feet from the forest edge. Traffic calming also contributes to its pedestrianization. Mado has 13 speedbumps, narrow streets, 15-mile-an-hour speed limit, and car and golfcart parking along the streets that narrows the traffic flow-through by slowing traffic down. In addition, parking parallel on one or both sides of the streets along with perpendicular golf cart parking extends slightly into the street right-of-way.

Mado has a wide range of mixes of use, which creates greater opportunities for social interaction and reduces the need for the automobile. This includes close access to the school, healthcare facilities, healthy food, recreational activities, and immersion into the natural areas surrounding the neighborhood. The wellness businesses, facilities, and amenities are not concentrated in one single place but rather are distributed throughout the fabric of the community providing greater integration and easier access. While this theme of wellness has been developed specifically for Mado within the overall constellation of the hamlet Serenbe, it is highly connected to the other neighborhoods and the non-residential functions they house. They attract residents from the other neighborhoods and from the greater community of Chattahoochee Hills. Mado is made up of many "*sticky urban places*" that support opportunities for meeting, interacting, chance encounters, and ultimately enhancing social tolerance.

All of the neighborhoods support dark skies to reduce night pollution. Street and home lights utilize full-cutoff fixtures directing light downward. This reduces electrical energy use, provides clearer night skies, and is known for improving circadian rhythms. Each of the neighborhoods has its own unique street lighting standard giving further identity to the neighborhoods. There are several other sustainable approaches to the planning of Serenbe that include a vegetated wetland waste system, the use of geothermal heating and cooling systems, energy-efficient construction practices, and, in some instances, solar energy utilization. The biohabitats have been designed and permitted as a community wastewater collection, treatment, and reuse system. The treated water is supplied to subsurface irrigation in adjacent pastureland. Throughout Serenbe are a combination of practices including bioretention, bioswales, stream buffers, and wetland protection.

Because of the innovative planning and sustainable building practices, Serenbe won the Urban Land Institute Inaugural Sustainability Award in 2009. In Mado it is mandated that all homes incorporate ground-sourced heat pumps or geothermal systems providing space heating and cooling. Homes are encouraged to be solar-ready, meaning that there is provision of space for photovoltaic panels to be mounted to roofs. A number of the larger buildings incorporate photovoltaic systems. Explained later in the chapter, the Terra School provides 105% of its energy through its rooftop photovoltaic system. Throughout the neighborhood are stand-alone charging stations for the growing number of electric golf carts, bicycles, and automobiles. Energy efficient construction is an important part of the sustainable strategies for Serenbe. EarthCraft is a voluntary residential green building program of the Greater Atlanta Home Builders Association and Southface Energy Institute that was created in 1999. In 2004 and 2008, Serenbe was named Green Building Program of the Year by the National Association of Home Builders. Serenbe was named Development of the Year by EarthCraft, and was one of five pilot EarthCraft communities. To achieve compliance, new homes must meet both EarthCraft and ENERGY STAR certification criteria. This means achieving passing scores from diagnostic tests for air infiltration and duct leakage. The criteria include resource-efficient site planning, resource-efficient design, energy-efficient building envelope and heating and cooling systems, and use of building materials, effective waste management, indoor air quality, and water conservation. These all contribute to the overall wellness of the community.

Mado provides several places for sanctuary experiences and sacred moments both within the built portions of the neighborhood and in the surrounding openspaces. Thin places are locations or settings found in Mado that seem to possess qualitatively different energies. Thin places are often referred to as sacred places, holy places, sanctuary places, vital places, soulful places, serene places, or charged places. According to Mindie Burgoyne, *thin places* are places in which a svelte veil exists between our secular world and the sacred, where an energetic connection and nexus can more easily be made.[11] Along one of the tributaries to Cedar Creek on the west side of Mado is what locals refer to as the large waterfalls. It is considered one of the most sacred sites in Serenbe. The Blue Pyramid and Outdoor Yoga Field are considered other thin places in Mado. But most thin places are individually discovered and possess personal qualities that either elicit awe or serene emotions. (For a detailed description and discussion of thin places refer to, *Thin Place Design: Architecture of the Numinous*.)

The two Mado plans in Figure 7.9 illustrate the disposition throughout the neighborhood of wellness facilities, services, and activities (represented

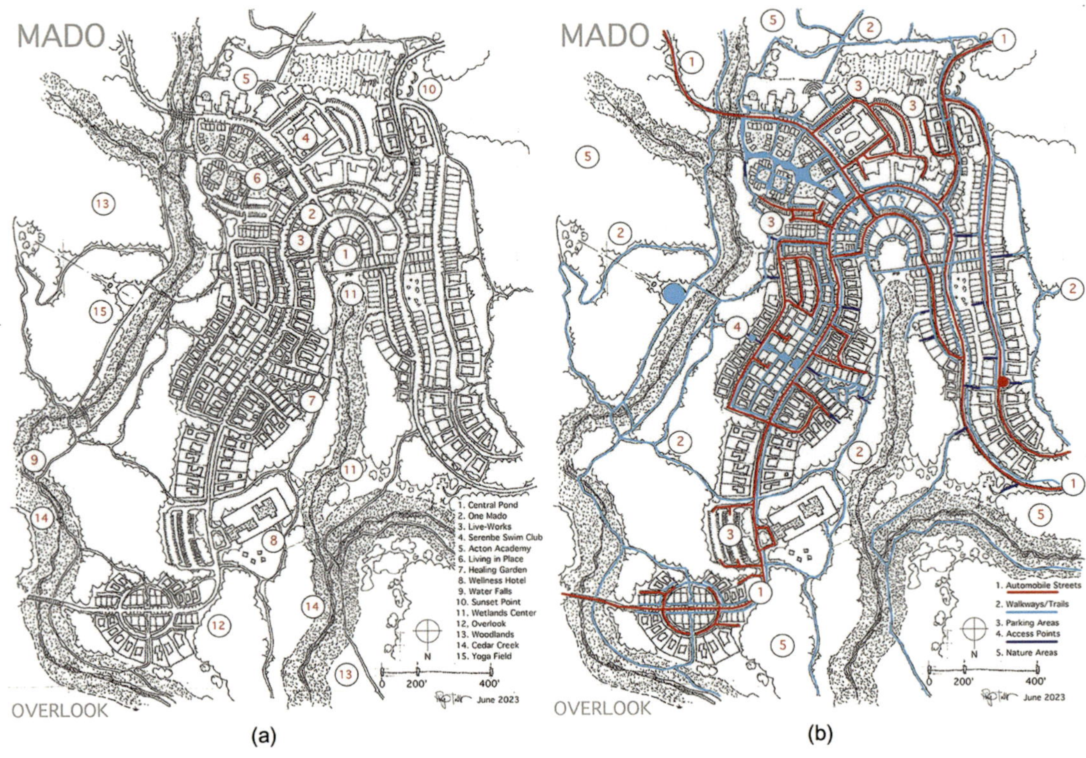

7.9
Access to Wellness Functions
a) Distribution of Wellness Functions,
b) Automobile and Pedestrian Networks
(*Source: Phillip Tabb*)

by numbers). As can be seen, there are 15 different wellness sites identified throughout the plan. These include the openspace and natural areas surrounding the center of the neighborhood. Other more personal and intimate thin places can be found in the surrounding nature and certain gathering spots within the community. The wellness functions are spread throughout the neighborhood providing multiple destination points. The wellness benefits from these physical design strategies are intended to create a strong sense of place, maximize interactions with nature, encourage pedestrianization and physical activity, increase socialization, and provide community meeting places.

In conventional suburban development, rows and rows of single-family plots are arranged along both sides of streets with little-to-no spatial variety, interruptions, or access to natural openspaces. Further, they are lined with large automobile garages and driveways, and maybe there is access to a trail or path behind the rear yards. To counteract this monotonous repetition of dwelling massing and single-use development, in Serenbe the creation of periodic breaks between the houses offers a visual and physical relief in the urban streetscape, also providing access points to the neighborhood's important natural areas, features, and amenities. The efficient automobile circulation (in red) and miles of trails (in blue) are also shown in Figure 7.9b. The pedestrian network within and surrounding the neighborhood is more than five times the length of the roads. The purple indicates points of access from the streets to natural areas and amenities. These points also provide multiple ways of

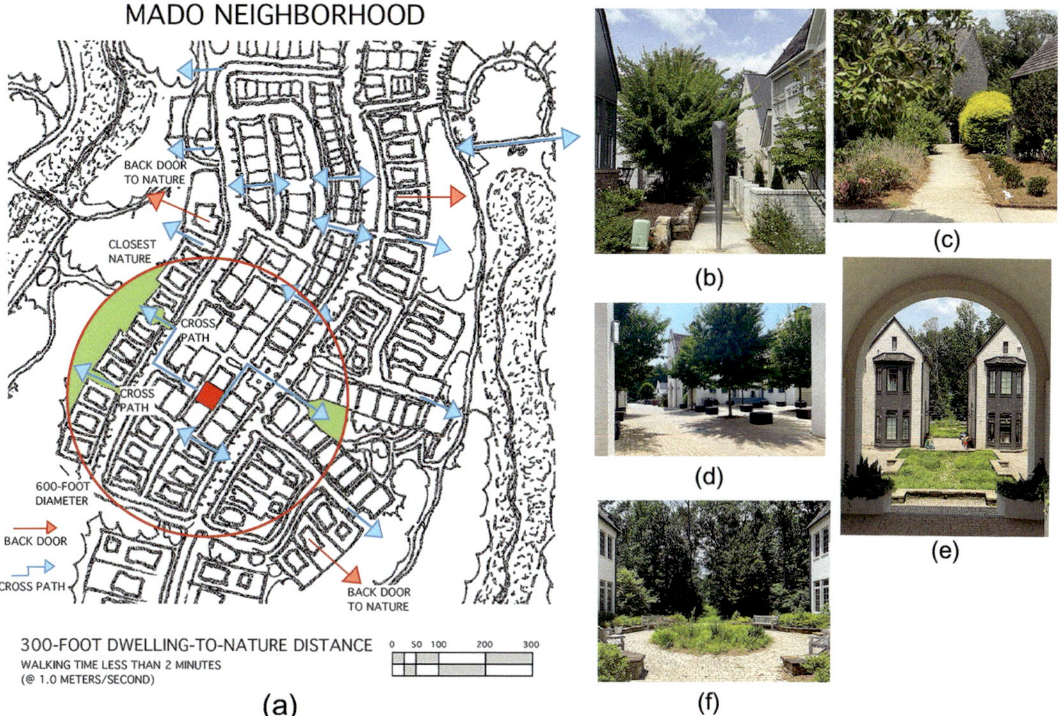

7.10
Cross Access Circulation a) Cross Path Plan b) Night Lighted Pathway, c) Between Dwellings Path, d) Anders Court at the Top of the Axis, e) Arched Axis to Yoga Field and Folly, f) Meeting Place Along the Way

(*Source: Phillip Tabb*)

accessing the homes of nearby neighbors, while others provide access points and offer long views into the site, such as Figure 7.10b and c. Figure 7.10d shows a neighborhood meeting place in the center that connects down to the forest through a series of cascading greens. In Serenbe these access points are accompanied with traffic calming street bumps, changes in pavement (usually pavers), and night lights for nighttime demarcation.

The plan indicates a good example of pedestrianization along with efficient, convenient, and emergency access to each dwelling. There is an intentional 300-foot dwelling-to-nature maximum distance to nature with most homes directly adjacent to natural areas. The wellness benefits from these physical design strategies are intended to create a strong sense of place, maximize interactions with nature, encourage pedestrianization and physical activity, increase socialization, and provide community meeting places.

A survey of Mado residents indicated the positive wellness qualities of the neighborhood, the sense of community, pedestrianization, easy access to nature, its density, and its convenience to businesses, food, and other amenities. Residents tend to frequent the fitness center, walks in the woods, and the patronage Creek Retreat (Figure 7.12e). The result – the residents stated they socialize more. A frequent complaint was the ongoing construction with its noise, nails left on the street, and increased traffic. Many who have school-aged children enjoyed the close connection to Terra School. In addition, respondents noted they made frequent visits to the woods, Halsa Restaurant, the Farm Coop, Fitness Center, the Swim Club, and the popular trampoline hill.

3. Mado wellness goods and services

As the theme for Mado is health and wellness, there are various businesses and practitioners providing goods and services and numerous outdoor opportunities for social and nature engagements. One of the first wellness facilities is the three-story One Mado Building which houses health and wellness-oriented retail and office functions, Figure 7.11a. It was designed by Lorraine Curran Locus Design. On the ground level are the Halsa restaurant, fitness center, Serenbe Real Estate, Biophilic Institute, and public restrooms. Halsa is a casual, neighborhood-oriented restaurant serving vegetable-forward healthy food. It has both indoor and outdoor seating and is a popular year-round meeting place for the community and often serves as a coworking space, an Internet café, and a place for casual business meetings, Figure 7.11c. Offices on the second and third levels include Dental Wellness, Serenbe Yoga and Body Works, the Spa at Serenbe, and Precision Performance and Physical Therapy. The fitness center or "The Gym at Serenbe" is located on the ground level, Figure 7.11b. One Mado's dramatic spiral staircase in the foreground and the partially hidden elevator in the background support the concept of nudging encouraging people to increase their physical activity by using the stairs. Circulation within the building is open connecting each of the businesses so there is constant exposure to the outdoors.

One Mado's exterior deep blue color provides uniqueness and serves as a place marker. Building exterior colors for Mado have been inspired by the architecture of Erik Asmussen with a full spectrum of colorful hues. The deep blue One Mado Building is diagonal from the pink community pool. Terra School has a combination of complementary colored buildings. The toddler building is yellow and blue, the elementary and middle schools are purple and peach, and the gymnasium when completed will be rust and moss green. Other residences throughout Mado are colorful as seen in Figure 7.17b. (As discussed in Chapter 5, different colors can trigger different emotions, for example blue's association with water and the sky suggests calmness which can lower stress levels.)

The Gym at Serenbe is a 2,000-square-foot (186 m^2) membership facility open 24 hours a day. It is outfitted with functional workout strength and mobility equipment, including cardio treadmills, ellipticals, and rowers. Indoor Peloton bikes are available for on-demand classes. Both individual and team training are available. The Gym has a membership of 300 people and an average daily use population of 90. Directly across from The Gym is the Portal, a wellness

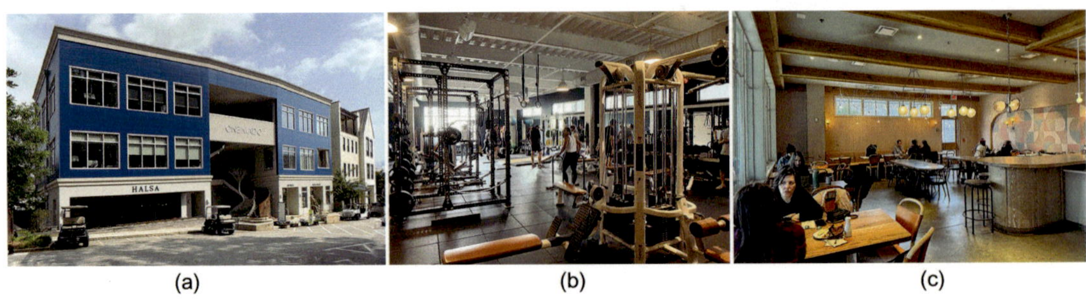

(a) (b) (c)

7.11
One Mado Building a) Street Façade, b) Serenbe Fitness Center, c) Halsa Restaurant
(*Source: Phillip Tabb*)

retreat for those who enjoy elevated curvilinear design, immersive experiences in nature, and as a complement to the eight-treatment spa. Facilities include six en-suite double bedrooms, a full chef's kitchen, living and dining rooms, and a secluded outdoor courtyard with a hot tub overlooking the Koi fishpond. They offer multi-day retreats including daily nature hikes, yoga classes, spa services, healthy meals, and access to many other wellness practices in Mado.

Other live-work units are feathered into Mado, such as The HearingSmiths, providing in-house hearing services with advanced diagnostic and hearing technology. Adjacent to One Mado Building is a cluster of three and four story live-work units. These are semi-attached and house wellness-oriented businesses that occupy the street level floors. Rental offices or apartments are located on the upper two floors. The units vary some in size averaging 3,000 square feet. Typically, the ground-level commercial spaces average about 700–1,000 square feet. The residential components on the upper two levels have two bedrooms, two full baths, living and dining spaces, and a kitchen. The residential

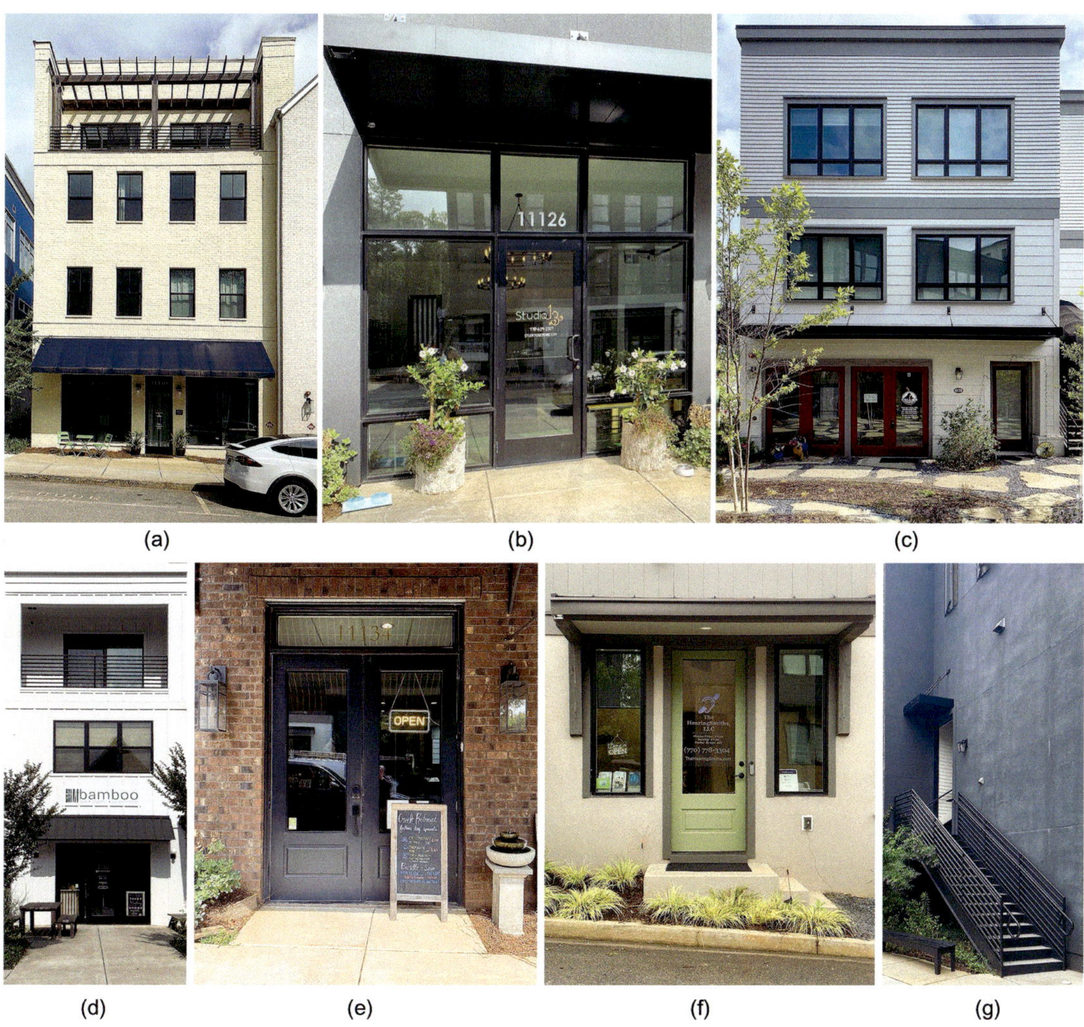

7.12
Mado Live-Work Units
a) Chai Vegan Spa,
b) Studio 13,
c) Collier Animal Hospital,
d) Bamboo,
e) Creek Retreat,
f) The HearingSmiths,
g) Residential Entrance
(*Source: Phillip Tabb*)

areas are between 1,500 and 2,000 square feet. There are private ground level entries, a foyer, and stairs with access to the upper levels from the rear or side of the units. Among the live-work units are a Vegan spa, Pilates studio, veterinary hospital, wellness retreat, hearing-aid shop, an ice cream shop, a bagel shop, and a cold pressed juice shop. The Creek Retreat accommodates chiropractic, HydraFacial, and cryotherapy wellness services. Additions to come in the near future include a pottery studio, an ice-cream shop, bagel shop, and an interior furnishings and design firm.

The Serenbe Swim Club is located next to Terra School at Serenbe, across the street from the proposed Aging in Place Wellness Hub, and close to One Mado Building. It backs onto a large horse pasture and has great southern sunlight exposure. It is designed by Curran Architects and is privately owned with membership available to community members. There is a main elliptical saltwater pool, a heated 4-lane lap pool (24 meters long), a splash pool for children (20 feet diameter), canopies and beach chairs, and restrooms and shower facilities. Soon there will be a snack bar. There are several adult and youth programs including aqua yoga, pool volleyball, infant swim classes, swim teams, and private lessons.[12] A newly constructed two-story structure has a cabana on the pool level and on the street, level below houses the Modo community mailboxes. It has a uniquely pink-colored exterior, refer to Figure 7.13.

Founded in 2010, Terra School at Serenbe is a new state-of-the-art K-12 campus with preschool, elementary, middle school, high school students.[13] Terra School is founded on Montessori philosophies and practices placing emphasis on student-centric learning. The campus plan is composed of five buildings that accommodate a toddler building with four classroom clusters, two connected elementary and middle school buildings with a total of eight classrooms, a high school, and an auditorium-theater building. The student-to-teacher ratio is 10:1. The proposed high school building has classrooms, a maker's studio, an organic farm, and a gymnasium that opens to an outdoor amphitheater. Connecting each building is a learning playground with gardens, an amphitheater, farm animals, and creative play areas. Each classroom has a covered outdoor classroom separated by large garage doors which encourage indoor-outdoor learning.

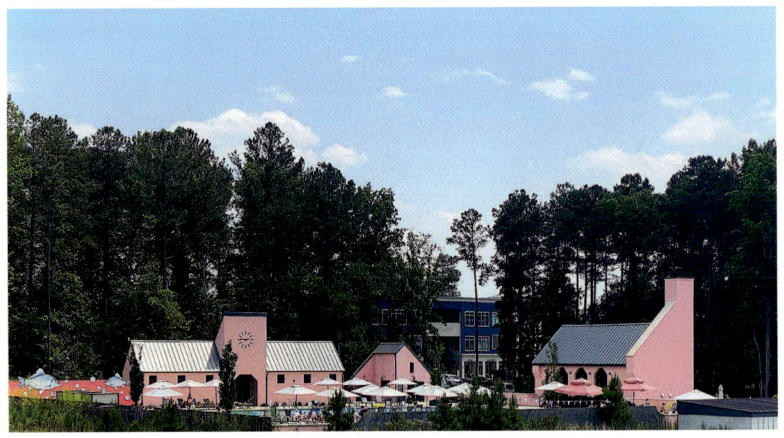

7.13
Serenbe Swim Club
(*Source: Phillip Tabb*)

The name, "*Terra School*," embodies the fostering a sense of connectedness to the land and environment of Serenbe. Environmental sustainability was at the core with geothermal system and Tesla photovoltaic roofs when complete will provide well more than 100 percent of its energy needs. Visual monitoring of the energy systems will be an integral part of the educational experience on the campus with display monitors on the wall that show a trend of power usage during the day and the water and solar generation. The original conceptual design work was done by Founder and CEO of Serenbe Steve Nygren, Land Planner Dr. Phillip Tabb, and students at Texas A&M University. Later the final architectural work was developed by local architects Jose Tavel of TaC Studio (Elementary/Middle, Highschool and Gymnasium) and Lorraine Cunanan (Toddler School). The architectural language was informed by biophilic principles and the work of Danish architect Erik Asmussen who designed the wellness community at Yarna in Sweden.[14] At the northeastern entrance to Mado is the Toddler Building that was designed with a low-profile roof and presence as if it is emerging out of the land, and it has playful tree-like columns supporting the Tesla-tiled roof. The color palette unfolds with the Elementary and Auditorium buildings expressing combinations of warm and cool complementary colors. Driving down the street adjacent to the school brings delight and joyfulness in part due to the playful forms and colors, Figure 7.14a.

The campus buildings use "*micro-school-studios*" with inside-outside architecture, views of nature, use of stimulating and calming color, integration of Asmussen-like playful biomorphic forms, and soaring roofs completely covered with Tesla photovoltaic tiles, Figure 7.14b. In the Fall of 2023, there were over 200 students, and when completed they anticipate 450 students. The Toddler Building will accommodate children from ages 6 weeks to 3 years. The Elementary School will accommodate kids from 3 years old through the eighth grade. Future phases include the High School Building and a gymnasium which also can accommodate community meetings.[15] The Montessori-based school was grown from a resident-based effort, and when complete will feature a 100% geothermal and a 105% Tesla solar shingle campus.[16] The bioinspired columns for the Toddler and Elementary schools reflect biophilic principles, refer to the two images in Figure 7.14c.

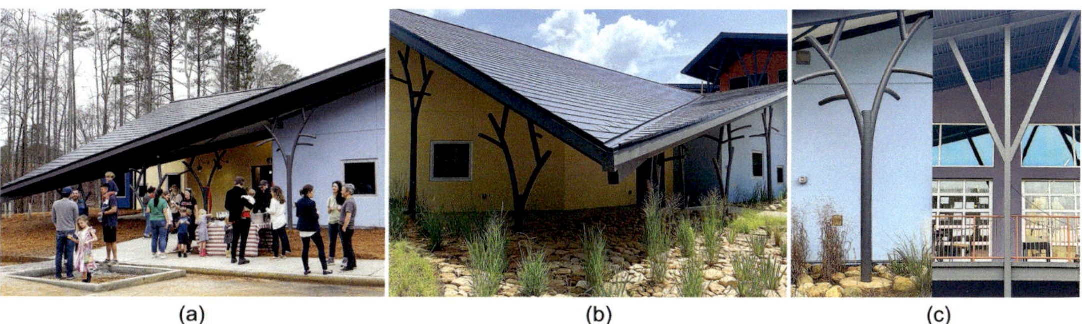
(a) (b) (c)

7.14
Acton Academy Toddler Building a) Parent Gathering at Preschool, b) Tesla Roof, c) Bioinspired Columns
(*Sources: Jessica Ashley and Phillip Tabb*)

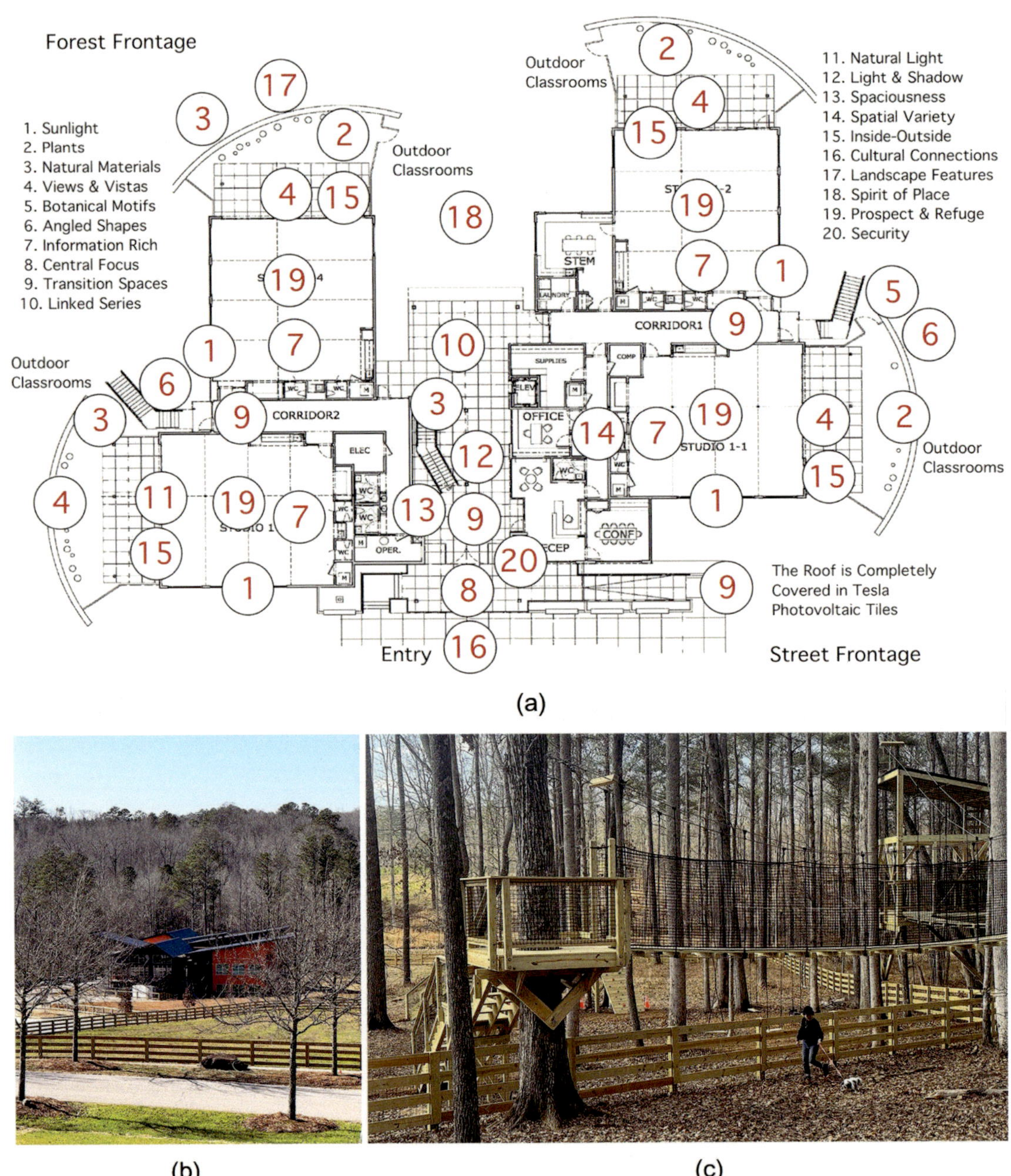

7.15 Terra School at Serenbe Elementary School
a) Elementary School Plan,
b) School Tree-houses (under construction)
(c) School Playground
(*Source: Phillip Tabb*)

The Mado Aging in Pace Wellness Hub is planned as a mixed-use campus of approximately 88,600 (8,231 m2) square feet of service-based housing, street level retail, medical offices and facilities, and a restaurant. The program is in part based on the Hogeweyk Dementia Village in the Netherlands. Hogeweyk is designed with what they call an "*innovative and disruptive*" deinstitutionalized vision with living, dementia care and well-being all mixed into a single community.[17] Similarly, the Mado Aging in Pace Wellness Hub is located in the center of Mado and across the street from the Terra School and Community

Pool to the north, One Mado Building to the east, and the forest and stream tributary to the west. Taken together these closely knit land uses are intended to support an intergenerational community. According to Serenbe Founder and CEO, Steve Nygren, *"Intergenerational interactions have always been a foundational element of life at Serenbe, and facilitated through design decisions meant to create 'accidental collisions.'"*[18]

The eldercare campus includes 24 cottages around a protected courtyard, 24 individual cottages, 40 independent living apartments, a wellness club, and a restaurant. Occupants will be served by a concierge program helping residents access the wellness services and amenities. A key concept is the use of a central pedestrian spine connecting the clusters, courtyard housing, and the main independent living building. The spine serves to interconnect the facilities within the campus, provide access to the many greenspaces, create a view corridor to the woods to the northwest, and provide emergency vehicle access to all occupied buildings in the campus. The conceptual site plan was developed by Serenbe Land Planner Dr. Phillip Tabb, and the architecture was developed by DK Levy Architecture+Design of Knoxville, Tennessee.

Mado's residential dwelling types vary from attached to detached and are sited on varying lot sizes according to the Thorburn transect. Dwelling types include shotguns, semi-attached (duplexes), townhomes, cottages, estate houses, rental apartments, nearby pasture estates, and in the Living in Place Wellness Campus are independent living cottages, courtyard housing, cohousing, and apartments. Dwelling sizes vary in size from 1,000 square foot (93 m^2) shotgun houses to well over 4,000 square foot (372 m^2) estate houses. Dwellings aligned along the streets are positioned close to the sidewalks and all have front porches intended to encourage outdoor living and social engagement with fellow residents. Most dwellings in Mado have direct access to the woodland openspace and all within the 300-foot (91 meters) dwelling-to-nature design strategy. Most of the homes in Mado are quite colorful. The variability of building typology, size, architectural language, and color contribute to particularity and identity within the urban context of the neighborhood. Mado is the densest neighborhood in Serenbe. According to one Serenbe resident:

> *The entire vision behind Serenbe is to create a biophilic community, one that connects its residents with nature. So, in your first year living in one of the hamlets or neighborhoods, you can expect to get outside often. First, Serenbe homes for sale are intentionally designed with attached porch and balcony spaces. Second, they provide residents with the chance to greet and commune with passing neighbors.*[19]

Many wellness features exist in and around the neighborhood including parks, gardens, edible landscapes, land art installations, and blue places. The Mado Food Forest and Healing Garden occurs along the east/west axis connecting the inner omega forest and the pyramid and yoga field. Designed by landscape architect Alfred Vick, ASLA the wellness landscape form connects each of the

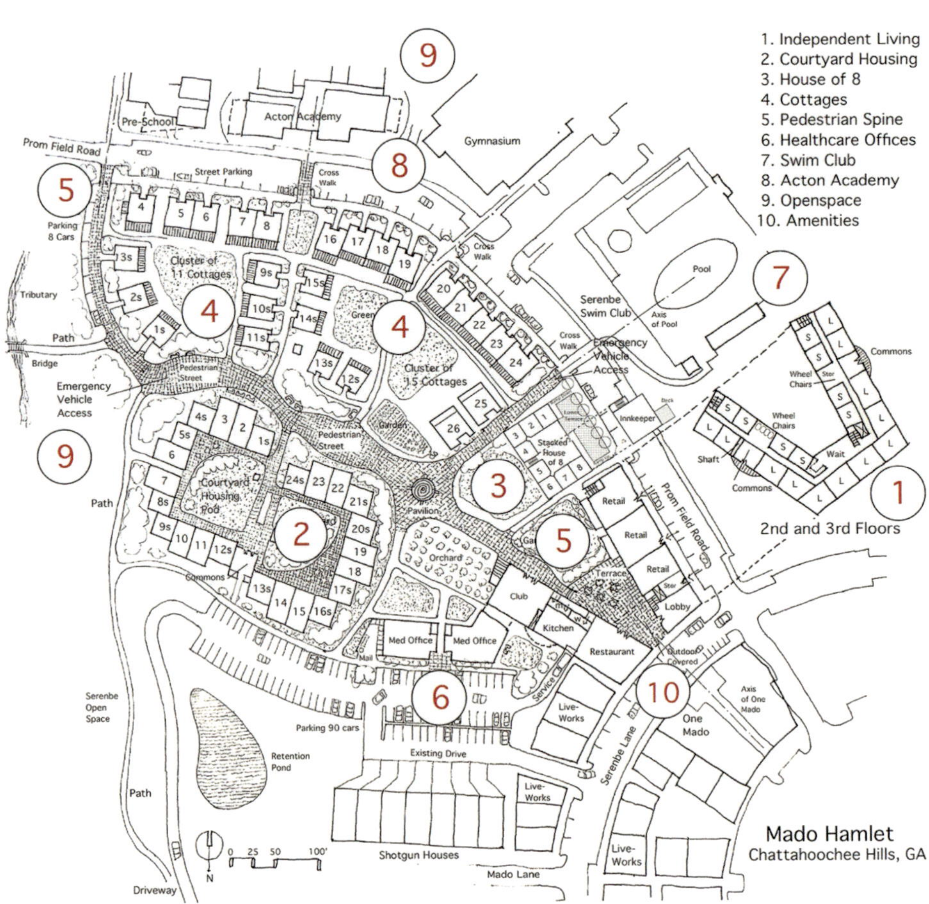

Serenbe Aging in Place Wellness Campus
Dr. Phill Tabb Studio • Revised March 18, 2022

(a)

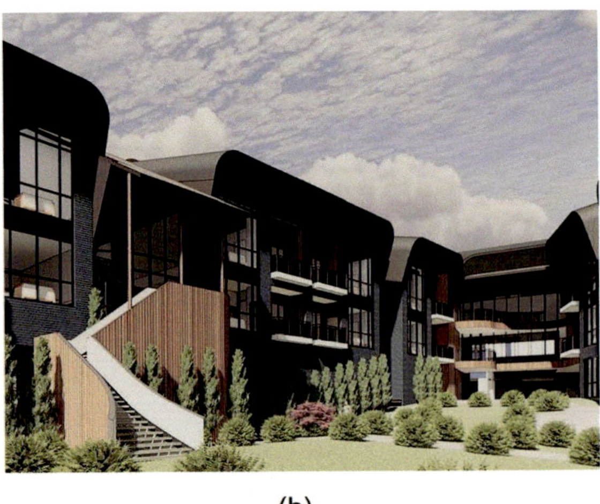

(b)

7.16
Aging-in-Place a) Serenbe Aging in Place Wellness Campus Plan b) Age Diversity

(*Sources: Phillip Tabb and Serenbe Development*)

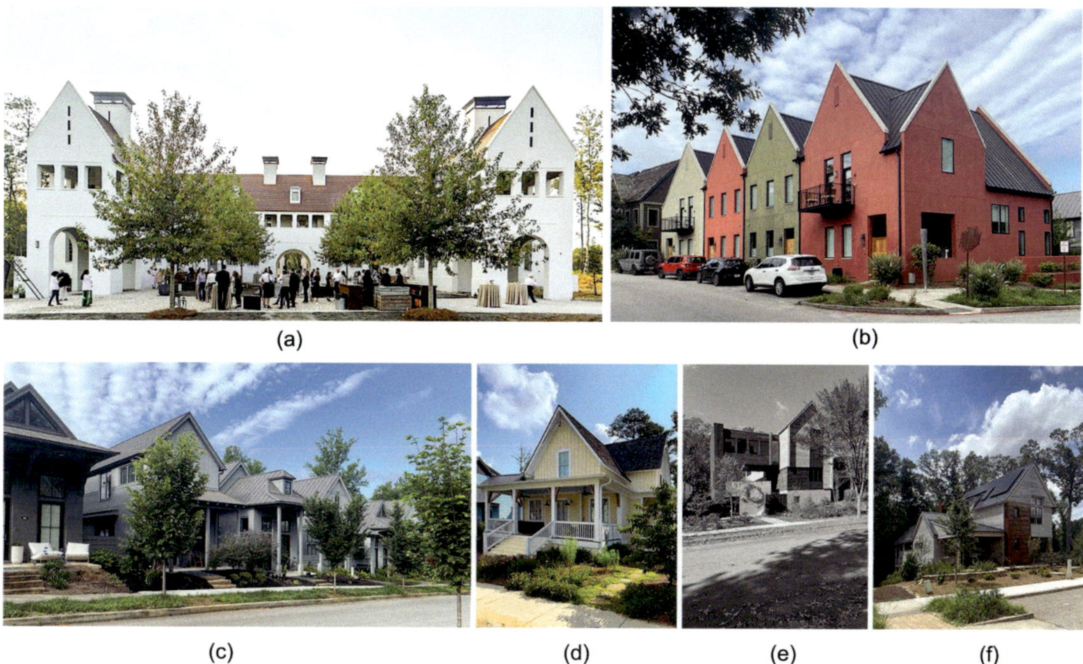

(a) (b) (c) (d) (e) (f)

7.17
Mado Residential Dwelling Types
a) Anders Court Townhomes,
b) Attached Courtyard Houses,
c) Shotgun Homes,
d) Detached Cottage,
e) Contemporary,
f) Cottage with Solar Array

(*Sources: Serenbe Development and Phillip Tabb)*

cascading homes in the "V-shaped" site with an ADA serpentine walkway with a gradient that is less than 5%.[20] The homes are single-story dwellings with direct access to the healing garden. Shared outdoor gathering spaces occur along the curvilinear walk promoting outdoor living and socialization. They function as an accessible outdoor living room and neighborhood meeting place. At the eastern end overlooking the forested omega center are a trellis and Bocce Ball court. In addition, there are 16 varieties of trees with White Oak and Shortleaf Pine being the most prevalent. There are 14 varieties of shrubs with Winged Sumac, Oakleaf Hydrangea, Sweetshrub, and Beautyberry in the greatest numbers. There are numerous herbs and grasses including Christmas Fern, Purple Coneflower, Showy Evening Primroses, Woodland Aster, and a variety of kitchen herbs, Figure 7.18. All species are native to the region, and many have documented edible or medicinal uses. Being relatively enclosed, the garden is quiet and protected from the street which allows for thin place experiences.

Each of the neighborhoods in Serenbe have neighborhood mailboxes designed to encourage interaction. Several have playgrounds associated with them for children to play while adults get their mail and socialize. In Mado there is a dog park with benches overlooking the forest. Down the center of the omega form lies a treelined tributary and wetlands leading to Cedar Creek to the south of the neighborhood. Mado Park and the Fire Pit lie at the apex of the omega center and serve both adults and children. Many of these outdoor spaces function as thin places where transcendent experiences of awe and serenity can occur.[21] A double-tiered 15-foot-high waterfall is located about a

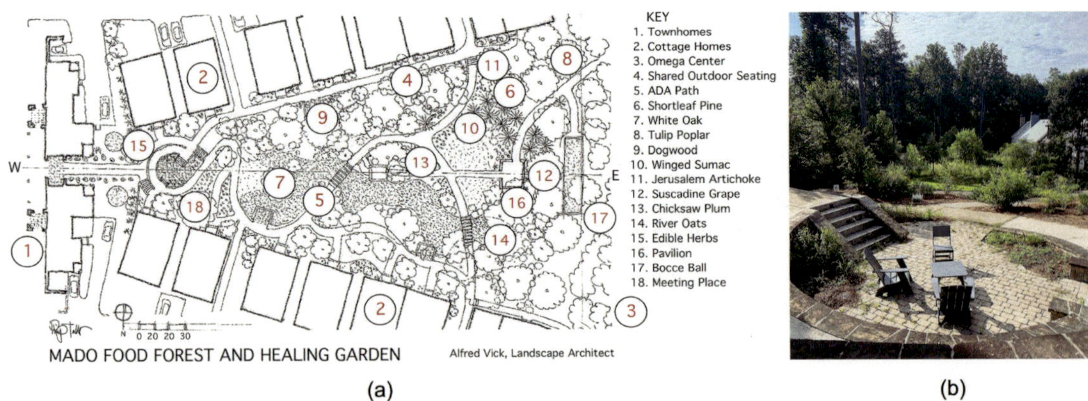

7.18 Wellness Greenspaces a) Food Forest and Healing Garden Plan, b) View from the West

(*Sources: Alfred Vick and Phillip Tabb*)

ten-minute walk from the southwest of Mado along one of the tributaries that empties into Cedar Creek. The waterfall is framed by a conifer pine tree and a deciduous beech tree. This site is considered one of the most sacred thin places in Serenbe. It is also accessible from Serenbe trail riding. Mado is connected to the 17 miles of trails found throughout the community in a series of expanding loops. In addition, annually there are 1k (for kids), 5k, and 10k races on the trails, Figure 7.19a. Due to COVID-19, it was closed. However, the tradition continues each spring and autumn now called the "*Fast Banana Trail Race*." Being only a minute or so from one's home to the woods is a real wellness benefit.

With 70% of the land at Serenbe protected and dedicated to openspace, plenty of space and many opportunities exist to engage with nature. This includes the farm, pastures, paddocks, parks, greenspaces, and woodlands all connected with miles of sidewalks and trails. Mado has openspaces surrounding the neighborhood and running through the middle of the omega form. Every resident is either directly connected to the openspaces or is just minutes away from them. Experiences through the openspaces allow for exercise, forest bathing, schoolchildren's access to the school, education, and play for Serenbe's "free-range" kids, Figure 7.20.

Children referred to by local adults as "*free-range kids*" – independently run throughout Serenbe, and walk to school. The benefits also allow for a variety of housing type choices, reduce the need for "traditional lawns," support safety and encourage the idea of free-range children, and provide a variety of supportive amenities and functions. Free-range parenting advocates argue that this approach helps children develop decision-making skills, problem-solving, resilience, and independence. Further, the trails create an intricate network connecting the neighborhoods, amenities, and natural places. Counteracting Richard Louv's "*nature deficit disorder*," is the physical contact with nature that nourishes the mind, body, and spirit.[22] Risk-aversion is meant to protect children but can impede child development in some ways with limited outdoor experiences.[23] Free-range play reduces stress, rejuvenates brain activity, and stimulates the imagination and senses. Children play independently, exploring openly, and building confidence, self-sufficiency, and skills. Benefits can occur with advanced motor skills, improved muscle strength, communication with

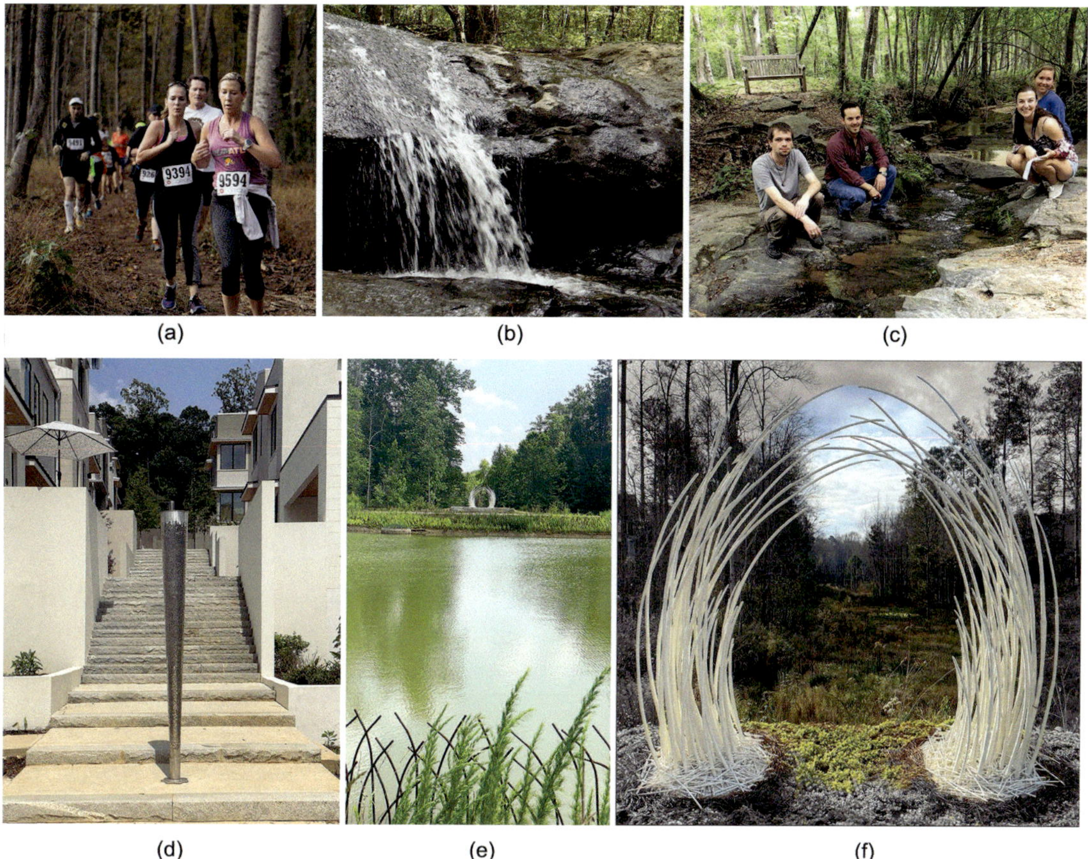

(a) (b) (c) (d) (e) (f)

7.19
Wellness Activities
a) Serenbe Trail Race, b) Large Waterfalls, c) Students at Small Waterfalls, d) Pedestrian Stairs, e) Mado Central Pond, f) Land Art in Omega Center

(*Sources: Serenbe Development, Jessica Ashley, and Phillip Tabb*)

peers, use of the five senses, fostering curiosity for new experiences, and the fostering of independence.[24] And they take risks. The full complement of planning and design strategies presents opportunities for health and wellness for individuals, families, the community, and the environment. By providing the context in which each level of wellness can interact, outdoors and more specifically, free-range activities, become more holistic and opportunistic for high-level wellness to actually be achieved, especially on an everyday basis and for people of all ages. As of the beginning of 2024, there are approximately 180 children living in Serenbe. Free-range parenting is not completely without risks depending upon the nature of the community, degree to which there is no passive surveillance, the exposure to unnecessary risks and dangers children may encounter, and the possibility that too much freedom could lead to neglect.

Within and around Mado are many meeting places and points of common interest where small groups of residents and visitors can relax and interact. Often, these interactions occur between rows of houses on or near access paths to the forested openspace, at T-junctions of roads and paths, at mail pavilions, and adjacent to parks and playgrounds. Often, they are small and intimate, and mark points of attraction like the firepit site located near the top of the omega next to a children's playground, which is frequented by parents

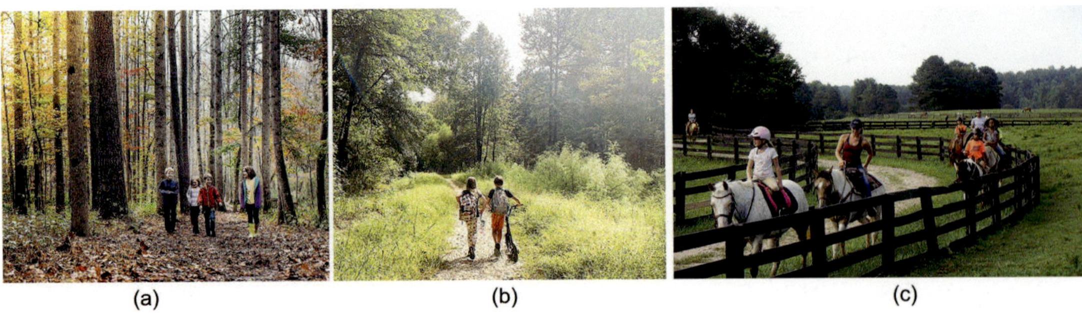

(a) (b) (c)

7.20
Free-Range Kids
a) Kids in the Woods, b) Kids Walking Along Path, c) Kids on Pony Rides
(*Sources: Serenbe Development and Phillip Tabb*)

while children play. Another place, Sunset Point, was designed to view sunsets and solar equinoxes beyond one of the horse paddocks. Hanging-out places found at entrances into the forested openspaces such as at the end of Anders Court are green. These places often do not require a great deal of space and are not expensive to create. Yet they can provide relief from single-use zoning or privately owned land uses, and can encourage social interactions. In these locations, many, if not all, of the wellness benefits are capable of being experienced by everyone. Mado is an extraordinary community experiment featuring distinct strategies such as a framework for fostering wellness outcomes. As a real living community, its benefits are experienced daily and, in time, may evolve into another Blue Zone as discussed by Dan Buettner.

At the omega apex of Mado is a geometric park designed with a community firepit to one side, Figure 7.21a. It represents another simple insertion of a site-borne amenity that supports wellness through physical activity, emotional exuberance, and playful social interactions. It serves as a place for parents to sit and converse while children play in the adjacent playground. It serves as a good example for chance encounters or a quiet moment alone. Near the entrance of Mado is a large mound of construction fill that was transformed into a trampoline hill. The trampoline that sits atop the mound is enjoyed by the young at heart of all ages, Figures 7.21b/c. Named by local children, it is now called "*Volcano Hill.*" A spiral path leads up the hill to the 15-foot diameter trampoline. As residents and visitors pass by the hill to enter Mado neighborhood or Crossroads neighborhood or walk up to the top of the mound, they see people flying mysteriously up and down. From atop Volcano Hill are great views of Serenbe Stables and horse paddocks to the east and Sunset Point, the adjacent meadows, Terra School, and Sunrise Knob to the west. Mado has many other places for shared moments and chance encounters, including Halsa, Nigel's Banana ice cream shop, Bamboo Juice, the live-work courtyard, Anders Court, the Food Forest, the mail pavilion, the landscape sculpture facing the omega center, the dog park at the end of the shotgun houses, and in the rock garden along Serenbe Lane.

4. Mado testimonials and podcasts

In testimonials and podcasts, residents offer personal views about their experiences living in Mado. Two young middle-school Serenbe residents attending

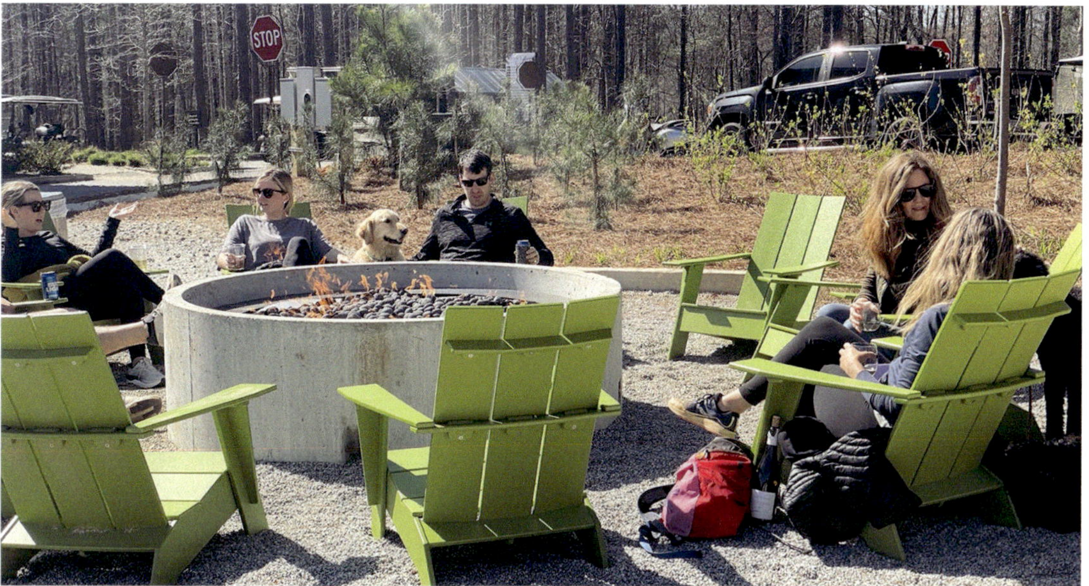

(a)

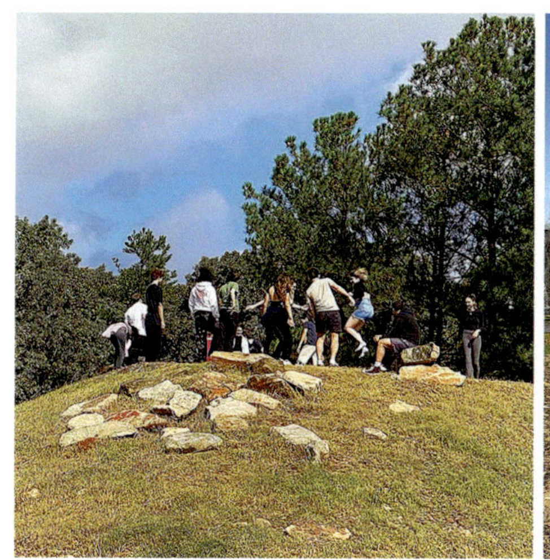

(b)

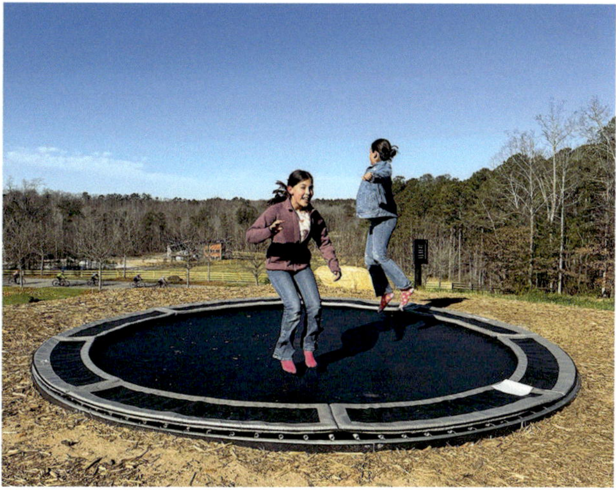

(c)

7.21
Mado Shared Moments a) Mado Park Fire Pit, b) Kids Hanging Out at Trampoline Hill, c) Jumping Children
(*Source: Phillip Tabb*)

Terra School conducted a local podcast talking about their experiences living in Serenbe and attending Terra School. One 12-year-old remarked that she found herself riding a horse around her neighborhood at age seven. Another spoke about being able to walk outside her home in Mado to the waterfalls. She, a friend, and their dogs walked along the tributaries, which they recounted, creating a wonderful adventure. Both said they liked being able to ride their bicycles to school, and they said that their brothers ages four to six can roam around freely without their parents worrying. They concluded that Serenbe is a place where you find out who you want to be when you grow up.[25] Following are testimonials and quotes from Internet respondents to Mado businesses representing a variety of positive opinions.

> *Our home is in the heart of the Mado hamlet of Serenbe. We are a short walk to the Halsa restaurant, Bamboo Juice, hiking trails, a yoga studio, a gym, and more.*[26]
>
> *Our family moved to Mado two years ago and we love the mix of people in the community and the close access to nature. We especially love taking the kids to the Foodforest and Healing Garden minutes from our house. It is so peaceful.*[27]
>
> *It [Serenbe] is a place of serenity, a place of surrender, a place of peacefulness, a place of beauty, all of those apply so that's how I originally defined Serenbe.*[28]
>
> *Be Well, Live Well, Eat Well is the overachieving vibe of this place.*
>
> *Halsa has the most inviting ambiance. The service was efficient, and the hostess was very knowledgeable of the food options.*[29]
>
> *I loved my restorative Yen yoga class! The studio was just the right size, and the owner was a great instructor. I can't wait to go again for goat yoga!!* [30]
>
> *Scandinavian-inspired eatery with delicious, fresh food. Laid back and casual atmosphere with a menu that is unique and healthy. They serve alcohol but carry a bunch of alcohol alternatives. Great place for gluten-free, vegetarian, or pescatarian diets.*[31]
>
> *I'd only been on a horse twice when I decided to ride at Serenbe, so I was a bit apprehensive. All worry was for naught, it was a small group, and the leader was a seasoned rider. We all fell in love with our horses and the trails are beautiful, along streams, open fields, lakes and you can even book a lunch ride where you can stop by the water's edge at the stream and have lunch from the local café.*[32]
>
> *Having recently moved from the incessant buzz of New York City to the tranquil hamlet of Mado in Serenbe, my family and I have experienced firsthand the profound impact that connection to nature and thoughtful design can have on well-being. We've become calmer, more balanced, and deeply connected, realizing the stark contrast between our past and present living environments.*[33]
>
> *I just got to experience riding a horse around my neighborhood at the age of seven.*[34]

The Mado neighborhood design elicits many wellness benefits both direct and indirect. Table 7.1 indicates the 43 wellness strategies related to the seven wellness benefit pillars. Highly present are the physical, emotional, social, and environmental benefits, and the intentional design strategies of community-oriented design, sense of place, aging-in-place, trails and forest bathing, pedestrianization, meeting places and socialization, wellness street design, agriculture and nutrition, abundant access to nature, healing waters, limited night pollution, and the presence of thin places. The 300-foot maximum distance to nature is afforded to every resident. At a walking speed of three-and-a-quarter-feet (one meter) per second, this translates to under two minutes. This is the length of a football field. A majority of homes are either close or directly adjacent to Mado's openspaces. Another planning strategy is to position the neighborhoods closer to one another, such as with Crossroads, Overlook, Grange, and Farmette sites which encourage social interactions, chance encounters, sharing and, to some extent, safety. The clustering of non-residential uses within each neighborhood also creates the potential for economic synergy created among the various neighborhoods.

There exist several financial benefits that are both directly and indirectly related to the wellness strategies. For example, pedestrianization and the presence of mixes of use give exposure and access to commercial activities, social meeting places, and wellness functions that economically benefit both patrons and businesses. Further, lower automobile use reduces carbon emissions, reduces energy use, fuel expenditures, and provides a safer community. Other strategies that elicit multiple benefits include the community-oriented form, the rich mixes of use, the aging-in-place campus, the miles of trails and opportunities for forest bathing, designs that encourage fluid indoor-outdoor activities, limited night light pollution. The many sacred moments found throughout the community add to wellness experiences, like Sunset Point at the entrance to Mado is on a hill overlooking a paddock to the west. At the vernal and autumnal equinoxes, the sun can be seen setting due west just over the forested ridge and Sunrise Knob beyond, Figure 7.22.

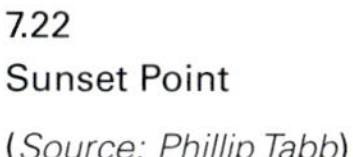

7.22
Sunset Point
(*Source: Phillip Tabb*)

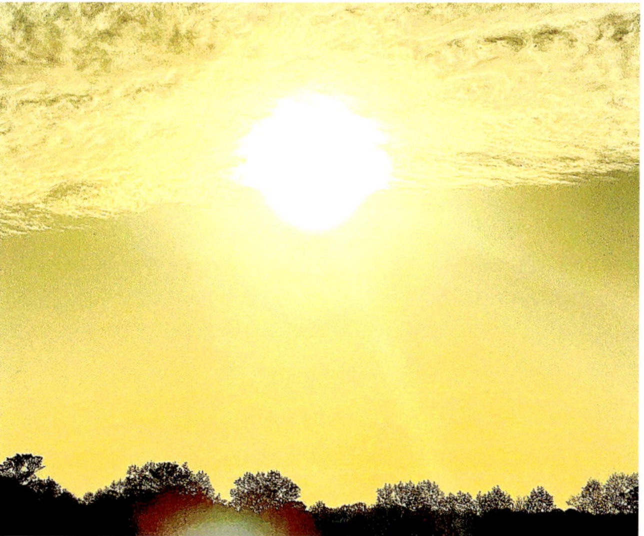

MADO SUMMARY

Mado is an exciting example of the wellness principles and design strategies applied at the neighborhood and community scale. This scale is a unique opportunity to create a multitude of strategies that interrelate, provide easy daily access, and are intergenerational. The identifiable neighborhood forms, sense of place, mixed functions and themes add to the wellness potential. Mado is the densest of the Serenbe neighborhoods and as such affords an economy of scale allowing for inclusion of so many non-residential wellness activities. This mosaic of wellness opportunities creates an explicit model and pathway for reimagining future development, especially at the neighborhood scale. Refer to Table 7.1 that follows for a listing of the wellness strategies and their relationships to the benefit pillars of physical, mental, emotional, social, financial, environmental, and spiritual wellness. The 'X' occurring in many of the cells indicates that the particular planning or design strategy may be found and informed by certain wellness pillars. This does not represent a rigorous analysis, but rather is intended to show the specific planning and design strategies relative to their impacts within the seven wellness benefit pillars.

There are a large variety of planning and design strategies for wellness in Mado. These strategies occur from the overall omega-like urban form, its incremental growth pattern, the large park within the interior of the omega and surrounding forest to numerous sidewalks, passageways and trails, access to water, and the myriad of wellness functions and facilities woven throughout the community. Following is a summary listing with brief descriptions of the wellness design strategies for Mado neighborhood:

1 Community-oriented urban form – *omega shape promotes inclusion, community building, nurturing nature, and a sense of place.*
2 Sense of place – *promotes wellness identity, groundedness, security, and spirit of place.*
3 Constellating urban growth by multiplication – *creates a network of accessible and walkable communities.*
4 300 feet to nature – *ensures that access to nature is not more than a two-minute walk away from a home.*
5 Designing with resilient infrastructure – *promotes on-site, water retention and management, renewable energy, waste recycling, and local agriculture.*
6 Mixed-use development – *provides a diversity of nutritional, social, recreational and economic opportunities and benefits, and a synergy among the wellness live-work businesses.*
7 Density gradient – *provides rural-urban transect and an increase in housing choices, and proximity to either greater access to natural areas or concentrations of non-residential amenities.*
8 Decentralized wellness activities – *promotes integrating wellness throughout the community fabric with increased access and allowing for small wellness businesses.*
9 Integrated aging-in-place campus – *provides age diversity and inclusion, easy access for seniors in daily community life, and mixing intergenerationally.*

10 Encouragement of physical activity – *provides easy access to nature and the 19 miles of trails, fitness center, trampolines, and other outdoor recreational activities.*
11 Nudge design strategies – *where planning and architectural elements, such as stairs, corridors, outdoor spaces, and connecting paths, landscape elements, lighting standards, and are encouraged through design.*
12 Miles of trails and forest bathing opportunities – *provision of 70% openspace, 17 miles of trails, and special natural places.*
13 Pedestrianization – *accessibility with urban sidewalks, rural trails, walkable streets, multiple dispersed destinations throughout the community.*
14 Traffic safety and calming – *sticky urbanism, narrow streets, street parking, speed bumps and crosswalks, common use of golf carts, high degree of pedestrian activity, and a 15-mile-an-hour automobile speed limit.*
15 Neighborhood meeting places – *provision of multiple destinations and gathering places throughout the neighborhood encouraging socialization.*
16 Clustering end uses – *creating safety and community surveillance, and possibilities for synergy, and random and planned social interactions.*
17 Chance encounters – *pauses, intersections, walks along the street, crosswalks, stairs, mailbox pavilions, treehouses, restaurant destinations, Farmer's Market, healing garden, trails, trampoline hill, and other gathering places.*
18 Neighborhood mail pavilions – *encouraging community interactions and places with adjacent playgrounds.*
19 Other shared elements – *include stairs, greenspaces, sidewalks, seating areas, land-art installations, the labyrinth, the ArtFarm performances and activities, the firepit, trampoline hill, and Sunset Point.*
20 Well-streetscapes – *native plants and trees providing shade, visual access to nature, and aesthetic value, and curving streets providing constantly changing perspectives.*
21 Sticky urbanism – *enticing street fronts, colorful façades, pedestrian activity, cars, bikes, and golf carts creating complexity, constant movement, and attraction.*
22 Encouraging indoor-outdoor spaces – *porches, balconies, terraces, courtyards, outdoor dining, greens, and recreation areas.*
23 Safety and community surveillance – *close proximity to streets, porches, clear visual access, community Facebook connections, and an active community.*
24 Agriculture and healthy nutrition – *access to nearby Serenbe Farms, gardens, Farmer's Market, and easy access to the six restaurants and cafes.*
25 Integration of edible landscapes – *occurring along neighborhood main streets, and in the Food Forest and Healing Garden.*
26 Cross pathways – *rows of housing plots interrupted by a network of passages connecting sidewalks to parallel streets, openspaces, and trails.*
27 "Front door" access to nature – *direct adjacencies to the 70% openspaces and the implementation of the 300-foot rule (two-minutes from dwelling to nature).*
28 Healing water – *access to on-site streams, lakes and ponds, day-lit stormwater, on-site water feature and fountains, and existing waterfalls.*

29 Limited night light pollution – *utilizing low wattage night lights, down lights for streets, dwellings and outdoor activities, and no lighting between the neighborhoods.*
30 Integration of living color – *with abundant nature surrounding the neighborhood, wildflower meadows, flowering gardens, and the Mado colorful buildings.*
31 Eurythmy of urban form – *rhythms of neighborhoods and massing of buildings reflect the Thorburn transect form with purely natural areas building up to a more urban density and non-residential activities at the neighborhood apexes.*
32 Energy standards – *building to EarthCraft energy standards required of all Serenbe buildings.*
33 Materialization – *encouragement and use of wood, stone, masonry, stucco, and other non-toxic materials; roofs are typically metal and wood shingles; and roads go from gravel, to paved with no curbs, to paved with granite curbs.*
34 Topography and ecology – *urban form responding to topography with minimal disruption of land and ecological flows; most development located downslope; ability to channel and hold water.*
35 Stormwater management – *primarily day-lit utilizing natural gravity, visually apparent and easily maintained, and contributes to forming retention ponds.*
36 Natural and renewable resources – *encouragement and use of solar energy for passive heating and photovoltaic electricity, mandated geothermal heating and cooling, and connections to vegetated wetland waste treatment.*
37 Economic benefits – *increases land and property values, high ROI, positive wellness branding and marketing, and efficiency and reduction of automobile uses for everyday functions.*
38 Wellness branding – *creating beautiful biophilic neighborhood, promoting sense of community, providing inviting support functions, and encouraging wellness lifestyles with abundant associations with nature.*
39 Ability to engage in free-range parenting – *access to rural areas adjacent to dwellings, strong sense of community and surveillance, safe streets, and low traffic speeds and volumes.*
40 Terra School – *neighborhood-integrated K-12 school with strong parent and community participation, and a context for life-long learning.*
41 Carbon sequestering – *through preserving adjacent forest land and meadows, integrating forests into urban form, and urban tree planting along streets.*
42 Presence of thin places – *creating natural and intentional thin places, soundscapes, blue spaces, and special markers and artforms found throughout the community.*
43 Celestial moments – *special sites, opening within forest canopy, and certain urban spaces designed for celestial observations like sunsets, moon rises, and night skies.*

As can be seen in Table 7.1, the Mado wellness strategies are cross-referenced with the benefit pillars. What becomes clear is the relatively even distributions of benefits across the 43 strategies with the physical, mental, emotional, and social benefits scoring slightly higher. Planning and urban design strategies scoring across all seven of the wellness benefits were the omega form, sense of place, 300-foot distance to nature, pedestrianization, access to nature and water, night light mitigation, carbon sequestering, on-site agriculture, the K-12 school, and thin place moments. Other strategies scoring high were aging-in-place, trails and forest bathing, meeting places and socialization, wellness street design, thin places, and celestial moments. The lowest strategies were decentralized wellness activities, topographical and ecological responses, natural renewable resources, and day-lit stormwater management. These lower rated strategies tended to be less people-centered and more environmentally-oriented. Overall, the high number of wellness strategies in this case study may be a result of the neighborhood scale, land use diversity, and the overall wellness and biophilic design of Mado. Mado neighborhood is a comprehensive and fully integrated wellness design, and possibly is one of the first intentional and contemporary urban design wellness models.

	MADO WELLNESS STRATEGIES							
1	Community-Oriented Urban Form	X	X	X	X	X	X	X
2	Sense of Place (place theming)	X	X	X	X	X	X	X
3	Growth by Multiplication	X	X			X	X	X
4	300-foot Distance to Nature	X	X	X	X	X	X	X
5	Infrastructure Resiliency	X		X		X	X	X
6	Mix Use Development	X	X	X		X	X	X
7	Density Gradient (transect)	X		X		X	X	X
8	Decentralized Wellness Activities	X				X	X	
9	Integrated Aging-in-Place	X	X	X	X	X	X	
10	Encouraging Physical Activity	X	X	X		X		
11	Nudge Designs	X			X		X	X
12	Trails and Forest Bathing	X	X	X	X	X		X
13	Pedestrianization	X	X	X	X	X	X	X
14	Traffic Safety and Calming	X	X	X		X		
15	Meeting Places and Socialization	X	X	X	X	X	X	
16	Clustering End Uses	X	X	X		X	X	X
17	Chance Encounters		X	X	X	X		
18	Mail Pavilions and Playgrounds	X	X	X		X		X
19	Other Shared Elements	X	X	X		X		X
20	Wellness Street Design	X	X	X	X	X		X
21	Sticky Urbanism	X	X	X		X	X	
22	Indoor-Outdoor Spaces	X	X	X		X		

23	Safety and Surveillance	X	X	X		X		
24	Agriculture and Healthy Nutrition	X	X	X	X	X	X	X
25	Integrated Edible Landscapes	X		X		X		X
26	Dwelling Plot Interruptions	X	X	X		X		X
27	Abundant Access to Nature	X	X	X	X	X	X	X
28	Access to Healing Waters	X	X	X	X	X	X	X
29	Limited Night Light Pollution	X	X	X	X	X	X	X
30	Integration of Living Color			X	X			
31	Eurythmy of Urban Form	X	X	X	X			X
32	Building to EarthCraft Standards	X	X				X	X
33	Use of Non-Toxic Materials	X	X	X			X	X
34	Topo and Ecological Responses	X		X			X	X
35	Daylit Storm Water Management	X					X	X
36	Natural and Renewable Resources	X		X			X	X
37	Economic Benefits (real estate)		X	X		X	X	
38	Wellness Branding		X	X	X	X	X	X
39	Free Range Parenting	X	X	X		X		X
40	K-12 Integrated School (participation)	X	X	X	X	X	X	X
41	Carbon Sequestering	X	X	X	X	X	X	X
42	Thin Places	X	X	X	X	X	X	X
43	Celestial Moments	X	X	X	X	X		X
	WELLNESS BENEFITS	Physical	Mental	Emotional	Spiritual	Social	Financial	Environmental

Table 7.1
Mado Neighborhood Wellness Design Strategies

NOTES

1. The word *Serenbe*, while initially created by co-founder Marie Nygren, is now a common or more general term used to describe the entire community at Serenbe. This includes the land, the Inn, the hamlets, the crossroads, interstitial spaces and functions, activities, and residents. Serenbe is the broader whole or constellation that comprises the larger place.
2. City of Chattahoochee Hills Comprehensive Plan Community Agenda, (Accessed May 5, 2024), https://www.dca.ga.gov/sites/default/files/chattahoochee_hills_ci_community_agenda_plan_2011.pdf.
3. Krier, Leon, Leon Krier: Houses, Palaces, Cities (*Architectural Design*, First Edition, London, UK, 1984).

4. Systemic Constellation Theory: the combination of the four hamlets and crossroads clusters evolve as proximate urban areas creating the larger development whole and sphere of influence, which is referred to as Serenbe Community. The idea of a *constellating urbanism* can have both literal and symbolic presences. Preiss, Indra Torsten, *Family Constellations Revealed: Hellinger's Family and other Constellations Revealed (The Systemic View, Volume 1)*, CreateSpace Independent Publishing, 2012.
5. Tabb, Phillip James, *Serene Urbanism: A Biophilic Theory and Practice of Sustainable Placemaking* (New York, NY: Routledge, 2017).
6. Thorburn, Andrew: *Planning Villages* (London, UK: Estates Gazette Limited, 1971).
7. Serenbe Farms website, (Accessed October 2015), http://www.serenbefarms.com/.
8. Reed, Karen – Serenbe resident naming Mado.
9. Coates, Gary, *Erik Asmussen, Architect* (Stockholm, Sweden: Byggforlaget Publishers, 1997).
10. Tabb, Phillip James, *Serene Urbanism: A Biophilic Theory and Practice of Sustainable Placemaking* (New York, NY: Routledge, 2017).
11. Burgoyne, Mindie, (Accessed November 24, 2017), http://thinplacestour.com/about-mindie-burgoyne/
12. Serenbe Swim Club, (Accessed June 22, 2023), https://www.serenbeswimclub.com
13. Acton Academy, (Accessed June 22, 2023), https://actonacademyatserenbe.com/#ourstory
14. Coates, Gary, *Erik Asmussen, Architect* (Stockholm, Sweden: Byggforlaget Publishers, 1997).
15. Serenbe Hamlet, *Cutting Edge School: New Acton Campus Taking Shape*, (Accessed June 25, 2023), https://issuu.com/serenbe1/docs/serenbehamlet-springsummer-2023_issuu/s/25140696
16. Serenbe Hamlet, *Cutting Edge School: New Acton Campus Taking Shape*, (Accessed January 29, 2024), https://issuu.com/serenbe1/docs/serenbehamlet-springsummer-2023_issuu/s/25140696
17. *The Hogeweyk: Normal Life for People Living with Severe Dementia* (Accessed January 30, 2024), https://hogeweyk.dementiavillage.com
18. Mullaney, Tim, *Pioneering Wellness Community Serenbe Plan Innovative Aging-in-Place Campus*, (Accessed January 30, 2024), https://seniorhousingnews.com/2023/07/05/pioneering-wellness-community-serenbe-plans-innovative-aging-in-place-campus/
19. Reed, Karen, *Plenty of Time Spent Outdoors*, (Accessed June 23, 2023), https://teamreed-realestate.com/blog/what-to-expect-in-your-first-year-of-living-in-serenbe
20. Green, Jared, *Serenbe's New Wellness District Features a Food Forest*, (Accessed June 23, 2023), https://dirt.asla.org/2017/04/19/serenbes-new-wellness-district-features-a-food-forest/
21. Tabb, Phillip James, *Thin Place Design: Architecture of the Numinous* (New York, NY: Routledge, 2024).
22. Louv, Richard, *Last Child in the Woods: Saving Our Children from Nature-Deficit Disorder* (Chapel Hill, NC: Algonquin Books, 2008).
23. Lothian, Tracey, *The Free Range Play Effect*, (Accessed July 8, 2023) https://www.ecoparent.ca/eco-wellness/free-range-play-effect
24. Miracle, *Why Should My Child Play Outside? Benefits of Outdoor Play for Kids*, (Accessed January 3, 2024), https://www.miracle-recreation.com/blog/why-should-my-child-play-outside-benefits-of-outdoor-play-for-kids/#physical
25. Serenbe Stories, *Serenbe Kids: Biking to School, Exploring in Nature, & Building Lifelong Friendships,* (Accessed December 4, 2023),
26. Testimonial from visitor to an Airbnb owned by Serenbe resident Brandi Kenner owner, 2023.
27. Quote from resident interview held July 25, 2023.
28. Quote from founder Marie Nygren comparing Serenbe to the children's novel, *The Secret Garden* published in 1910 by Frances Hodgson Burnett.

29. On-line review of Halsa Restaurant, July 8, 2023.
30. On-line review of Serenbe Yoga Bodyworks in Mado, July 23, 2018.
31. Halsa Restaurant review November 32, 2019.
32. Respondent review of the Serenbe Riding Trail in 2017.
33. Testimonial from Noa Hecht, Serenbe resident.
34. Quote from podcast, *Serenbe Kids: Biking to School, Exploring in Nature, & Building Lifelong Friendships*, 2023.

8 CASE STUDY 2 – FIVELEMENTS RETREAT BALI

FIVELEMENTS RETREAT BALI

Nestled on the banks of the Ayung River, Fivelements Retreat Bali is an award-winning eco-conscious wellness retreat founded in the ancient traditions of Bali. The retreat features authentic healing and wellness rituals, regenerative plant-based cuisine, and transformative sacred arts practices. Both health and wellness benefits and strategies are present across the architectural and retreat scales. Fivelements' iconic biophilic architecture promotes pedestrian movement, forest bathing, and a harmonious connection with nature and spirit. Enchanting indigenous gardens, natural-shaped pools and koi ponds, and soaring bamboo structures enhance the tropical jungle environment. A recipient of over 50 international awards, the company is recognized as an innovative leader in design, integrative wellness programs, cuisine, and hospitality. United by a shared mission to positively impact the wellness of humanity and the planet, the founders pioneered a new genre of regenerative well-being destinations, bridging the wisdom of traditional cultures with innovative healing concepts – Fivelements.

PROJECT BACKGROUND AND DESCRIPTION

Fivelements is an integrated wellness lifestyle company whose authentic destination offers an opportunity for inspiration and awareness, and progress in the 21st century. Its focus is on designing high impact wellness strategies aimed at supporting individuals, couples, and organizations through enduring life transitions and transformation, and bringing about greater health and well-being.

The founders' intention for regeneration was to revive, celebrate, and bridge ancient healing wisdom and traditions – from planning and building methods and materials to wellness programming – through authentic, immersive, and

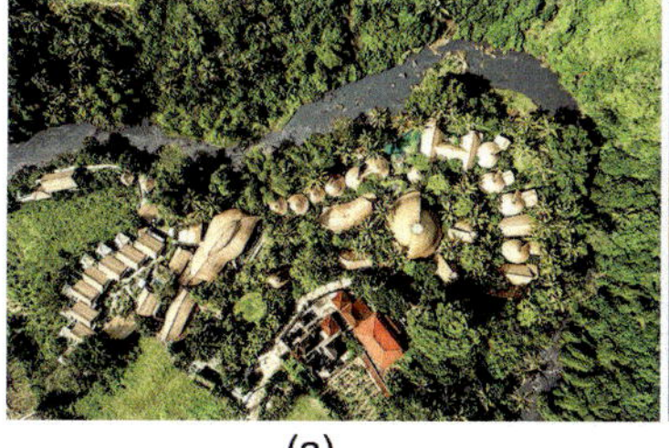

(a)

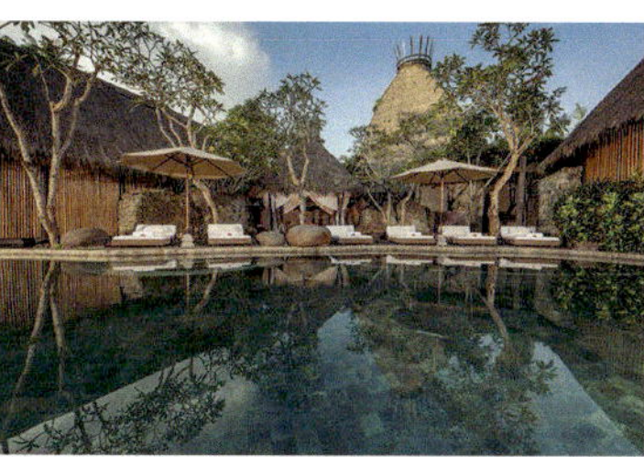

(b)

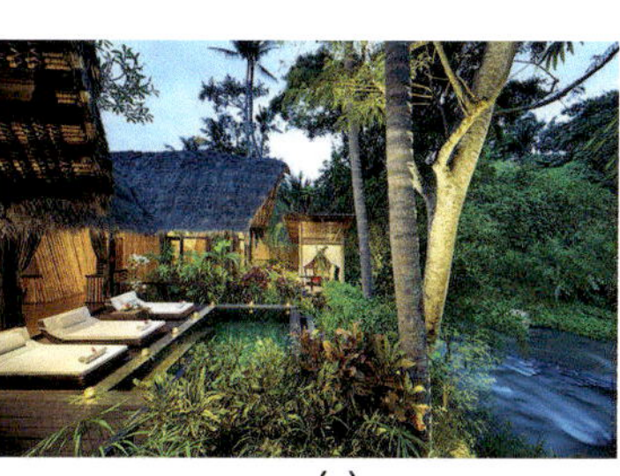

(c)

8.1 Fivelements Retreat Bali a) Site Overview, b) Pool, c) Double Suite, (*Source: Fivelements*)

DOI: 10.4324/9781003472902-8

transformational experiences aimed at self-regeneration and revitalizing social, cultural, and environmental ecosystems. A purpose-driven project, Fivelements was founded with a vision of "Learning to Love and Respect Life" and a mission, "Creating the Space for Life Transformation and Love in Action." The retreat's distinctive architecture, design, and wellness programming celebrates the philosophical, artistic, and healing dimensions of the formidable Balinese living culture.

Fivelements Retreat in Bali is located approximately 20 minutes from the cultural, artistic, and holistic center of Ubud, 45 minutes from the seaside on both the east and west coasts of the island, and about an hour-and-a-half from the international airport. An extension was later added in 2019. The area is known among local villagers for having more than 1,000 holy springs and is regarded as a sacred landscape. The retreat site has an area of 4.2 acres (1.69 ha), and the buildings' areas total 37,673 square feet (3,500 m^2). Designers for the retreat were Ketut Arthana (lead architect), Ida Pedanda Gede Kaloran (Brahman high priest and spiritual advisor), Jero Mankgu Made Wiranasapanca (high priest and spiritual advisor), Lahra Tatriele (concept and interiors), Mauro Raffellini (light and sound), Gove DePuy (sustainability), and I Wayan Kertayasa (landscape).

The masterplan illustrates an enchanting organic village-like character to the design, and it is sited adjacent to the Ayung River. The buildings and their orientation reflect indigenous planning methodologies and natural architecture from the island; however, the shapes have been redesigned and crafted to reflect the retreat's healing intention and present a new style of eco-luxury design, as well as enhance sustainability and wellness impact.

Fivelements' architecture and design approach is deeply grounded in its core healing philosophy, *Tri Hita Karana*, which, translated from Balinese Sanskrit, means living in harmony among human to God, human to human, and human to nature. For centuries, this philosophy has guided Balinese daily life as well as their architectural planning. *Tri Hita Karana*, combined with sacred geometry and biophilic design principles, have been applied to various structure formations and in the mapping of the physical *journey to wellness* with the intention to bring human, spirit, and nature together in harmony.

The masterplan and architecture were thoughtfully designed to enhance a sense of connection to self and others in the world. Both public and private spaces have been designed to hold and promote transformational healing for guests on wellness retreat stays as well as to bridge guests to a greater like-minded, conscious community and healthy lifestyle. Found throughout the design are circular, spiral geometries and mandalas incorporated to enable energy to flow in and out and to promote unity and diversity of experience. An important consideration of the design was to provide opportunities to enhance connections to nature physically, visually, and non-visually creating a sense of refuge, peace, and calm. Some examples are the intentional design of natural meandering pathways to evoke a sense of mindfulness as well as mystery as a Balinese-inspired retreat, and curating a place of peace and healing. Also important is the welcoming and nurturing dynamic airflow and diffused light with passive cooling design and orientation toward the cardinal and ordinal directions, accompanying audio playing soft mantras and kundalini yogic music along the pathways, and throughout the entire property holding the space for healing and transformation along the wellness journey. Maintaining and enhancing the presence of water with buildings facing the river and jungle waterfall, or by the design of natural ponds and fountains give blue space experiences. The use of biomorphic forms and patterns, such as the nautilus shell, the use of raw, unprocessed, and natural locally sourced materials, as well as renewable resources, such as bamboo and *alang alang* grass for thatched roofing, are among the designs which helped define and guide Fivelements' signature wellness design style. With this inspiration, great focus and attention was placed on selecting the site and designing the masterplan in harmony with spirit, human, and nature. Refer to Figure 8.2a for the Fivelements Retreat Bali original sketch plan.

PLANNING INSPIRATION FROM LOCAL WISDOM

Fivelements' master plan is based on Balinese cosmology or Balinese Vastu or *Mandala Nawa Sanga*. According to *Mandala Nawa Sanga*, the site is divided into nine squares, and each square will have its own sacred significance. Since the Balinese orient themselves to the most sacred volcano, Mount Agung and location of the most holy Balinese temple, *Pura Besakih*, the land areas, and buildings closest to Mount Agung are considered the most sacred, and the areas and buildings closest to the sea are considered less sacred. Refer to Figure 8.2a for the architect's concept sketch for the masterplan.

The Balinese guidelines for site proportions, *Asta Kosala Kosali*, were also applied to the master planning. In *Asta Kosala Kosali*, the building measurement and proportion are measured according to the measurements of the human body, and thus, the land is divided into three sections: the Head or *Utama* (considered the most sacred and important part of the land), the Body or *Madya* (the more moderate sacred part), and the Feet or *Nista* (the least sacred area on the land). Applied to the masterplan, this represents a human-oriented retreat design strategy rooted in traditional knowledge. Fivelements Retreat Bali was greatly influenced by Balinese master planning and cultural-spiritual methods, blended with modern environmental sensibilities. Following are descriptions of the major sites, buildings and activities contributing to wellness at Fivelements and in accordance with these Balinese planning methodologies.

PLANNING AND DESIGNING FOR THE HEAD OR UTAMA

The Utama is considered the most sacred and important part of the land. The Head section represents the area of the property where both spiritual and intellectual activities take place in harmony. The most important Balinese temple is placed near the northeast corner of all Balinese homes, offices, and properties. On the land of Fivelements, this temple shrine is situated accordingly, and nearby are other consecrated spaces for prayer, meditation, and contemplation. In contrast, a management and administration building, located on the opposite side of the Head section, signifies the "brain" and "leader" of the site and is in close vicinity to the main reception which acts as an important

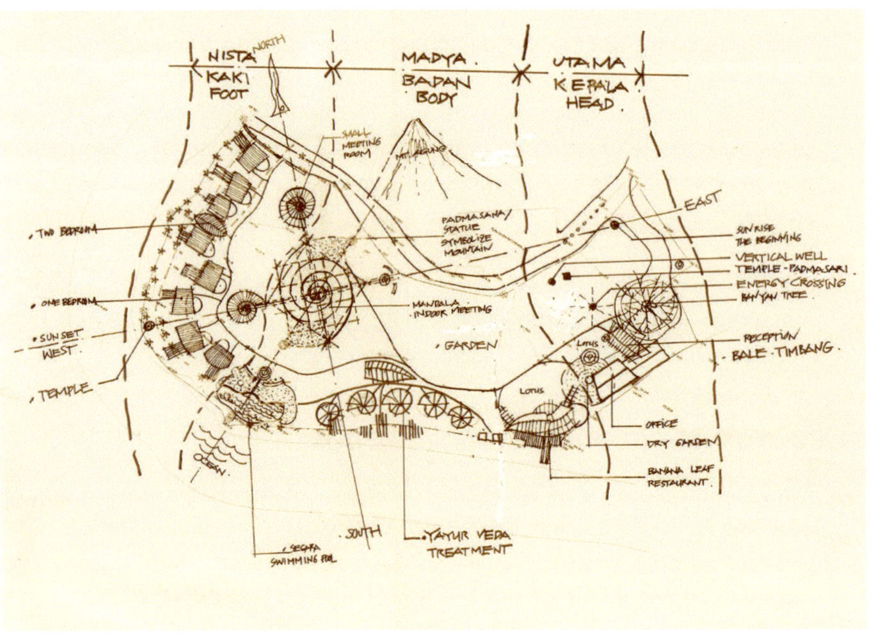

(a)

KEY

1. Banyan Tree
2. Balinese Temples
3. Sacred Space
4. Agni Hotra
5. Main Reception
6. Management & Administration
7. Multi-Purpose Buildings
8. Restaurant/Sakti Dining/Culinary
9. Healing & Wellness Reception, Boutique & Laboratory
10. Healing & Wellness village
11. Gym
12. Water Healing Pools
13. Sleeping Suites
14. Ayung Rive
15. Balinese Temple

N

FIVELEMENTS RETREAT BALI MASTERPLAN

(b)

8.2
Fivelements Retreat Bali Masterplans a) Concept Sketch Plan, b) Masterplan Drawing

(Sources: Fivelements, Ketut Arthona and Phillip Tabb)

post for the welcoming and coordination of guests' stays. At Fivelements, the Head section is intended to promote a place for inward reflection and divine connection, creativity, and abundance.

1. **The entrance and Banyan Tree meeting place – love all, serve all.**
   A small Balinese temple shrine marks the entrance to the property. A circular driveway was originally designed and constructed with round shaped river stones set by hand inside the ground and leading to a prominently positioned Banyan Tree, the symbol of a traditional meeting place, the original marketplace and welcoming point of exchange for the Balinese people. The meaning signifies a loving, inclusive welcoming to Fivelements, a place of healing intended to hold the space and gently guide guests toward a more purposeful life with newfound freedom and joy. A stone statue of Ganesha is placed nearby as a symbol of protection, blessing, and transformation, suitable for a place intended for healing. Wellness strategies for this entrance are the design of a meeting place for socialization and welcoming, combined with sacred moments. With a strong integration with nature and purpose, the wellness benefits include spiritual, social, mental, emotional, and environmental dimensions.

2. **The main reception**
   The reception is the main entrance to Fivelements and is adapted from the traditional Balinese *Bale Timbang* found in the middle of rice fields throughout rural Bali. The *Bale Timbang* is a simple structure formed by an equal number of living trees, in this case, six, supporting a thatched roof. The function of the traditional architecture serves as a place of rest in the shade and a meeting place for farmers and agriculture landowners to discuss and resolve the farming and harvesting challenges. Adapting this building as the entrance to the retreat, the intention is an expression of the retreat's mission to bridge dialogue toward self-love and resolution for a healthier and happier path forward. This reception structure is made from natural, locally sourced live materials and serves as a meeting place for guests to begin their healing journey at Fivelements. It is intentionally designed to evoke a warm welcome and a strong sense of emotional belonging.

8.3
Fivelements Retreat Bali Main Reception a) Sketch, b) Entrance Area

(*Sources: Fivelements and Ketut Arthana*)

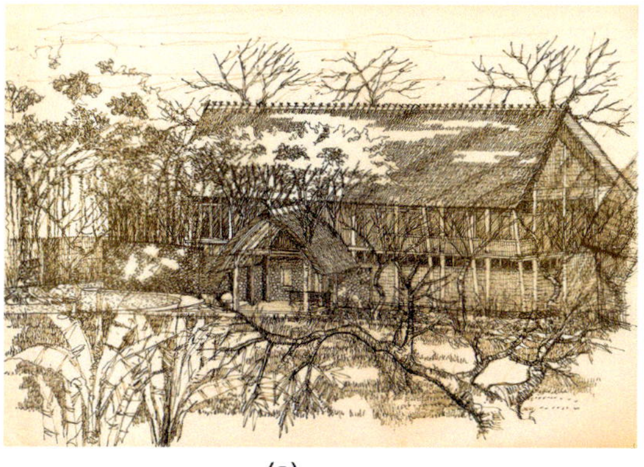

(a)

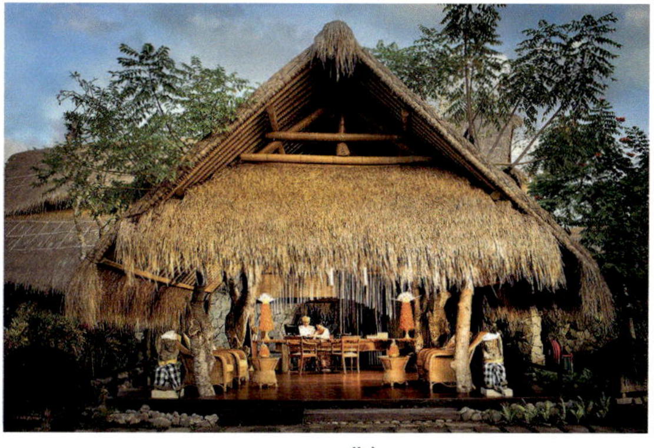

(b)

3. Balinese temples: their significance and orientation

In Balinese culture, the spiritual practice is known as "*shiva-buddha*" and is a unique blend of Hinduism (rituals and practices), Buddhism, and animism (everything with spiritual entity). In Balinese architecture and design, every space and every building has a specific orientation to God toward the mountains and nature.

To this end, there are three holy spaces that have been planned and constructed. Proceeding past the Banyan Tree in the Head or *Utama* section is the position of the most holy Balinese temple on the property, the **Padmasana** (meaning lotus throne), representing the Supreme God in Balinese Hindu belief.[1] It is built on the northeast position of the land and at the circular "vertical well" or sacred spring identified on the site by two Balinese high priests and a water dowser and land healer. Sacred springs are regarded all over the world as offering pure water, the source of life, and as places for healing. In Bali, the water from sacred springs is considered holy and is used for healing and purification ceremonies as well as other important blessing ceremonies. A natural well and water tap was constructed to access this water for these blessing purposes as well as a stream looping around the Padmasana and the Sacred Space in an infinity symbol formation or *anantha*, linked to the infinite number of cycles from creation to dissolution and recreation of the universe in Balinese and Indian Hindu philosophy.[2] It is also linked to the notion of *Pancha Mahabhuta*, the five elements, and represents continuity, balance, and the interconnectedness of all things in the macro and microcosm. The core wellness strategy and benefit is the consecration of a thin, spiritual place for prayer.

The second holy space is an energy vortex discovered on the land and designated as the **Sacred Space**. A vortex is believed to be a special spot on the earth where energy is either entering the earth or projecting out of the earth's plane in a swirling spiral form. It is also believed to connect the universe with the human body and produce a range of physical, emotional, and spiritual effects. Vortexes are thought to enhance meditation, focus, clarity, self-discovery, and spiritual growth and can be found at sacred sites throughout the world, such as Machu Picchu in Peru, the Great Pyramid in Egypt, Stonehenge, Uluru/Ayers Rock in Australia, and in numerous locations in Bali, including at Fivelements.

The discovery of an energy vortex in the Head section nearby the temple was made early in the design and planning process by the high priests and water douser and land healer. Interestingly, this was found approximately nine months after the founders of Fivelements set out to create a retreat for healing and transformational experiences. At the center of the vortex is the intersection of eight energy lines. A large, circular, mineral-rich volcanic black stone was chosen by the high priest to mark the center of the intersection signifying unity and peace, a place welcoming all beings for healing, collaboration, and positive dialogue. Eight river stones have been placed around in a circle to mark the eight lines which correlate with the cardinal and ordinal direction points of the compass. Following a sacred consecration by the high priests, the spiritual advisors of the project, the Fivelements founders designated this area as the Sacred Space for meditation and peaceful dialogue open to the management, staff, guests, and the greater Balinese community. The Sacred Space was the first area to be designed on the Fivelements land and remains the most significant part of the property for its international visitors promoting mental, emotional, and spiritual benefits. It offers guests access to a safe and tranquil meditative space and stimulates mindful, sacred moments.

Among the other sacred spaces at Fivelements Retreat is the **Agni Hotra** site used for healing fire ceremonies. *Agni Hotra* is an ancient fire ceremony originating from the sacred Vedic Hindu texts. Centuries past, the tradition of *Agni Hotra* in Bali was embraced and fused with animistic rituals; however, following a great fire, it fell out of practice more than 360 years ago. Today, there is a revival of the practice of *Agni Hotra* for its powerful healing effects not only in Bali but worldwide. Fivelements' founders brought this ritualistic building structure into their retreat for staff and visitors to participate in the spiritual ceremony and to benefit from its healing properties. There are many anecdotal stories of healing in relation to the *Agni Hotra* and even evidence of benefits to agricultural areas where *Agni Hotra* is performed.

Simplistic in design and taking on an open-walled, circular formation, the *Agni Hotra* is constructed entirely out of locally sourced, natural renewable bamboo and *alang alang* thatched roofing materials, similarly found across many of the other structures in Fivelements. The roof is designed with a passive cooling strategy in three layers consisting of the main roof structure open to the sky and two smaller roof "hats" piled on top with space between the three roofs vertically, allowing for air and smoke from the fire to escape, and keeping the main space and floor cooler. This roof concept is inspired by traditional Balinese architecture and can be seen all over Bali in rectangular shaped structures.[2]

PLANNING AND DESIGNING FOR THE BODY OR *MADYA*

The Body section represents the area of the property where the main activity takes place, such as dining, wellness treatments and sessions, swimming, and socializing. Open garden spaces and terraces, solarium, and swimming pool areas offer abundant access to the outdoors and nature as well as social gathering and event spaces. These thoughtfully designed well-being spaces offer guests an array of options to participate in traditional Balinese healing and wellness sessions, transformative water healing, or simply places of rest and contemplation.

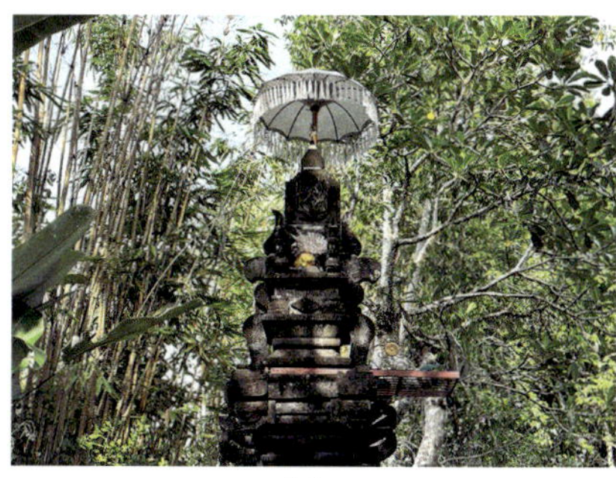
(a)

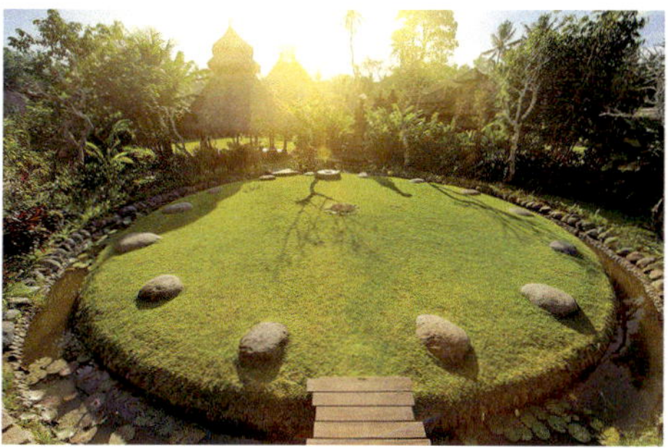
(b)

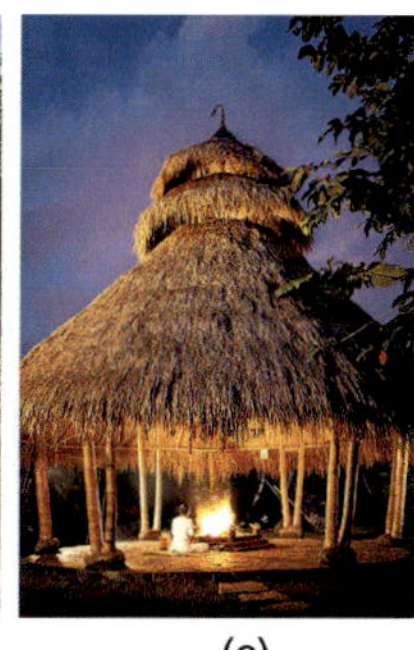
(c)

8.4
Fivelements
Balinese Temples
a) Padmasana,
b) Sacred Space,
c) Agni Hotra
(*Source: Fivelements*)

1. **Multi-purpose buildings**
   Mandala Agung, Mandala Madya, and **Mandala Alit** are three multi-purpose buildings hosting a plethora of sacred arts sessions, ranging from yoga, meditation and mindfulness, sound healing, dance, and martial arts, etc. These multi-purpose spaces and open gardens also serve as venues for special events, Masters Series, and other conferences, think tanks, or performing arts. These buildings adopted the shape of the volcanic mountains in north Bali. The largest, Mandala Agung, is positioned in the northeast direction of the Mount Agung volcano, the smaller, Mandala Madya, is positioned nearest to the swimming pool to the south and the smallest, Mandala Alit, is facing southwest, the direction of the *segara* or sea. The largest of the multi-purpose buildings, Mandala Agung, is an architectural representation of three Balinese Cultural concepts.

   The first concept is ***Rwa Bineda*** or ***Purusa Pradana*** a Balinese philosophy that describes the continuous play between opposing forces. It is a concept that gives us masculinity and femininity, creation and destruction, yin and yang, positive and negative, and the interactions between these forces. The Balinese understand this concept as integral to maintaining balance and see it in all aspects of life, even in the way they interpret the very land that they live on. It is believed that when the *Purusa* (masculine) and the *Pradana* (feminine) collaborate, the creation of something new can manifest.

   The second concept is proportion according to ***Asta Kosala Kosali***, the Balinese traditional architecture method. In the *Asta Kosala Kosali*, the building measurement and proportion is based on the human body. Every part of the building is measured based on the users' body dimension. Internationally we know that the natural proportion of the human and creature is 1:1.618… also known as PHI. One shape that also follows the PHI is the nautilus shell shape, a logarithmic spiral shape that follows the Fibonacci sequence. These Mandala multi-purpose building structures have been inspired by the nautilus and are formed in vertical spirals.

   The third concept is the ***Tumpeng***, one of the core elements of the Balinese offerings made from rice and shaped as a mountain. This type of offering is a symbol of gratitude by the Balinese for the prosperities given by nature. The shape of the *tumpeng* was adopted giving a vertical, mountain shape to the outside of the Mandela buildings and resembling the three prominent volcanoes on the island.

   Blending these three Balinese concepts, the overall shape and form of Mandala Agung was created. The structure is designed as two adjoining spirals allowing for fresh air circulation. The two spirals connect in the middle at the top representing unity and oneness. A crown was designed at the top of the building with a covered opening to the sky offering a "*channel of light*" and a connection to the divine. On the sides of the crown are ventilation holes to enhance the passive cooling design. A vacuum of air is created that sucks up the warm air into the crown and out of the holes. Further, cross ventilation is created as the structure is open air with only half slatted bamboo constructed for privacy and as a railing protection. The structure is built from 100% renewable "grass" materials of bamboo for the structure and flooring with thatched roofing. Two similar and smaller single-spiral-shaped buildings, Mandala Madya and Mandala

Alit were designed and built to host further yoga, meditation, dance, movement, and sound healing sacred arts sessions as well as special events and gatherings.

In addition to its awe-inspiring, bamboo cathedral-like architecture, further wellness strategies for this building include a eurythmy of architectural form, the use of natural renewable resources, access to a range of wellness activities, sacred geometry and biophilic design attributes. Wellness outcomes include physical movement, mental and emotional healing, social connections, environmental, and spiritual benefits.

2. Sakti Dining Room

For the Balinese, the banana leaf or *don biu* has historically been a symbol related to food. Banana leaves are used as food wrap, food plate, and even folded in a manner that can be used as a spoon. Appropriate for the retreat's signature organic, plant-based cuisine, the form and shape of the restaurant and roofline were inspired by that of the banana leaf. Blending the materials of large apus yellow and black bamboo for column and roofline structures, fibers from the coconut tree for wrapping the bamboo beams, and *alang alang* thatched roofing, the banana leaf shape was adapted and transformed for the rooftop of the open-air restaurant. Passive cooling design strategies were implemented in addition to its eurythmy of architectural form. Offering an abundance of natural light and integration with living color, the restaurant is positioned between outdoor

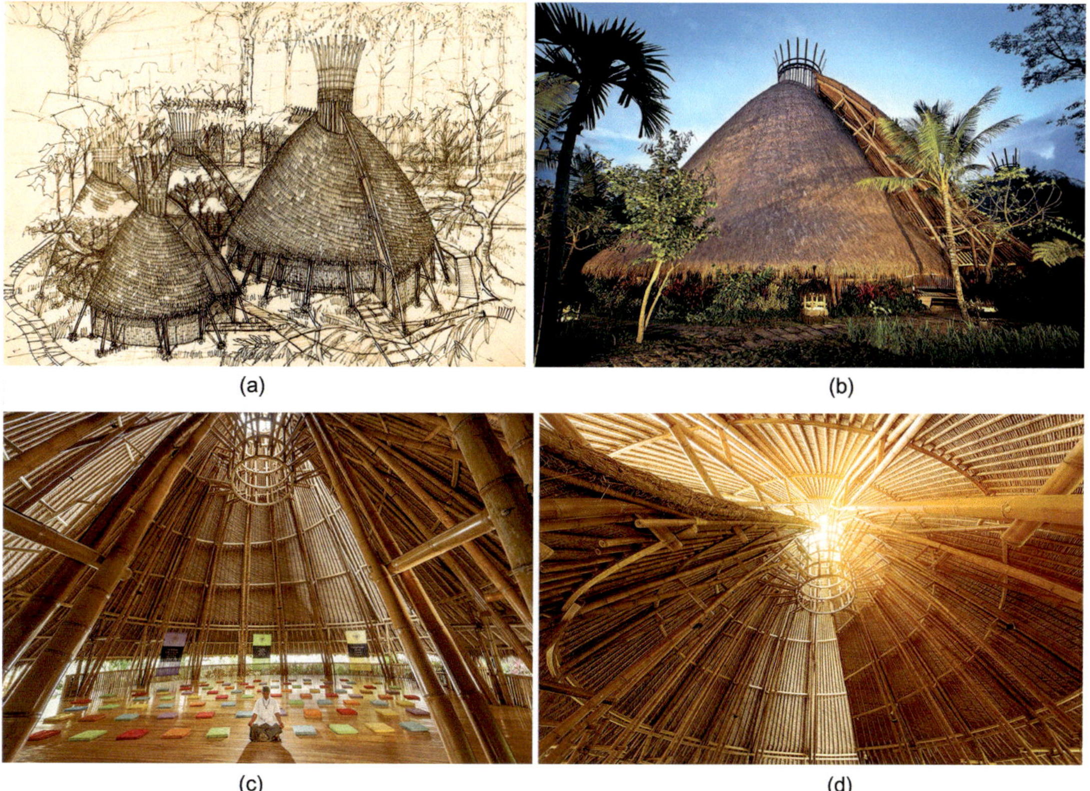

(a) (b) (c) (d)

8.5 Fivelements Multi-Purpose Building a) Mandala Sketch, b) Mandala Exterior, c) Mandala Interior, d) Bamboo Ceiling

(*Sources: Fivelements and Ketut Arthana)*

ponds and the prominent Ayung River. There is also a koi pond inside the center of the restaurant providing an abundance of access to healing elements. Cross ventilation and cooling are created by these positionings, reducing the building temperature by two to three degrees Celsius. In addition, the double story open air building and double roof system with space in between creates a natural wind vortex continuously pulling warm air up and out of the building and creating a continual flow of fresh air circulation from the ponds and river.

The award-winning Sakti Dining Room features a fine dining, eco-luxurious setting flanked between Bali's sacred Ayung River and lush tropical ponds and gardens. The prominent bamboo restaurant offers an inspiring gastronomical journey based on fresh, innovative plant-based cuisine aimed to nurture body, mind, and soul. Also offered from the restaurant and kitchen area are plant-powered nutrition and culinary training retreats and programs. The wellness benefits focus on physical (nutrient-rich cuisine), emotional (awe-inspiring design), and environmental levels (all natural materials).

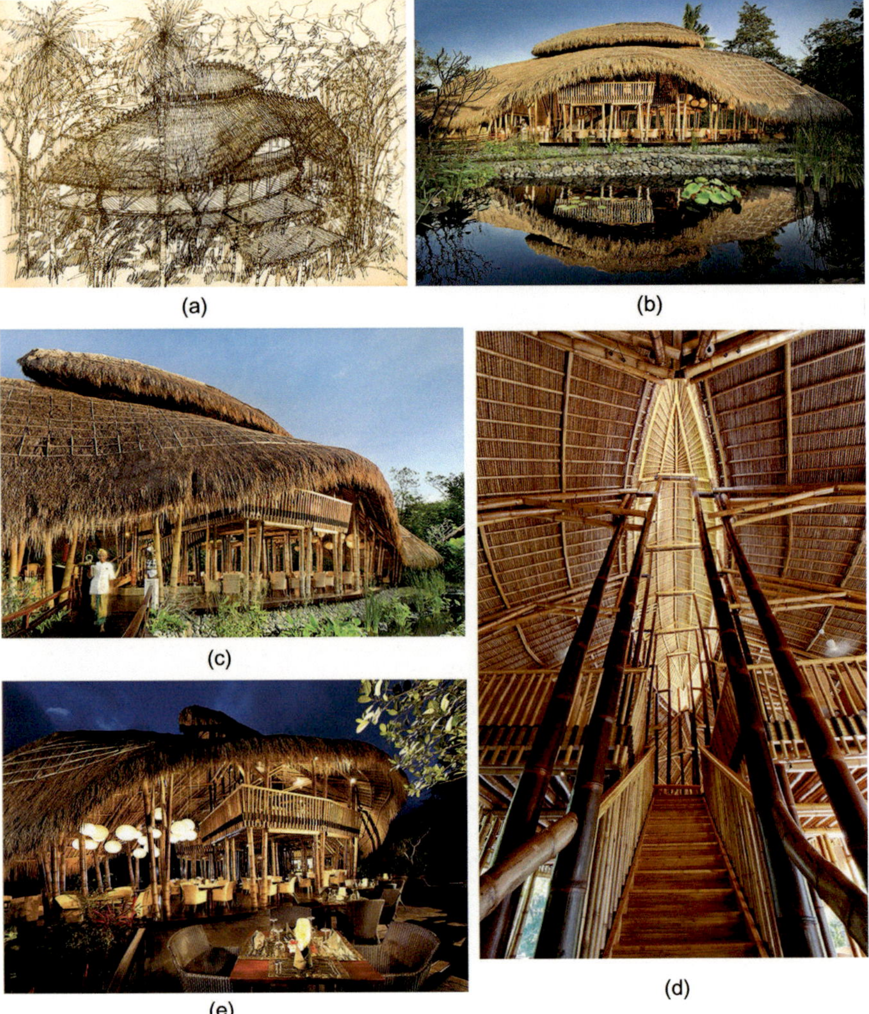

(a) (b) (c) (d) (e)

8.6 Fivelements Sakti Dining Room a) Restaurant Sketch, b) Restaurant, c) Wave, d) Black Bamboo Ceiling, e) Terrace

(*Source: Fivelements*)

3. The gymnasium

The gymnasium onsite serves as a space for fitness training, both for individuals and small group training. The building takes on an organic leaf-like shape symbolizing that we are all in a natural process and journey to well-being. One of the primary benefits is the positive impact on physical health. Exercise at the gym promotes cardiovascular fitness, muscle strength, and flexibility. It aids in weight management, reduces the risk of chronic diseases such as heart disease and diabetes, and enhances overall body function. Beyond the physical aspects, gyms play a crucial role in mental well-being. Exercise releases endorphins, commonly known as "feel-good" hormones, which can alleviate stress, anxiety, and depression. The gym environment often serves as a social hub, fostering a sense of community and connection. Interacting with like-minded individuals can provide motivation, support, and a sense of belonging. The variety of fitness classes and equipment available allows individuals to tailor their workouts to personal preferences and goals, making the gym a versatile and accommodating space for people of all fitness levels.

In addition, design elements of the space, such as incorporating glass and bamboo, further enhance the overall well-being experience. The use of glass allows for abundant natural light, creating a bright and airy atmosphere. Natural light exposure has been linked to improved mood, productivity, and sleep quality. Being surrounded by elements of nature, like wood and bamboo, even in an indoor setting, has been associated with stress reduction and increased well-being. Bamboo's inherent durability and versatility align with the sustainable and mindful ethos of wellness practices. Wellness benefits include physical, mental, and social well-being.

4. Healing Village and Wellness Sanctuary

Fivelements Healing Village (also referred to as the Wellness Sanctuary) consists of six riverfront wellness pavilions with en suite bathrooms and with bath houses featuring over-sized bathtubs, hand-carved from volcanic river stone,

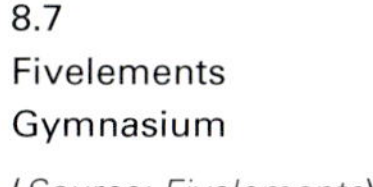

8.7
Fivelements
Gymnasium
(*Source: Fivelements*)

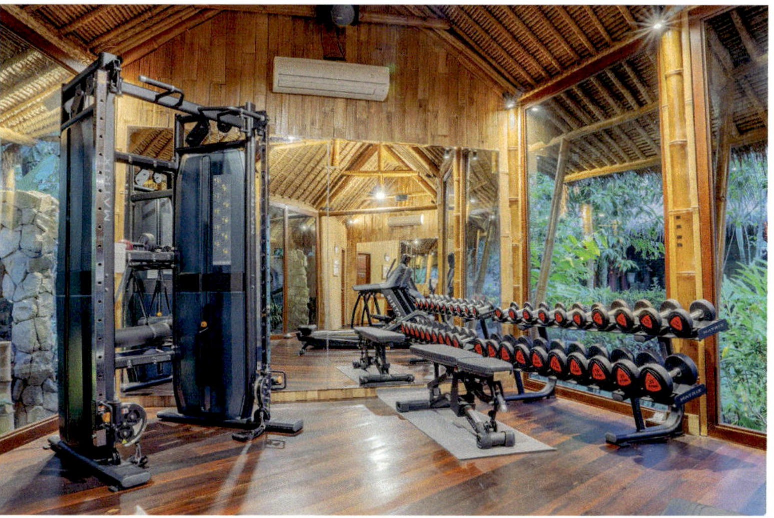

used for signature healing bath rituals. Each pavilion is in the shape of the sacred spiral and includes a terrace for pre- and post-treatment reflection by the river. Flooring is made from ironwood and structures are from bamboo with thatched alang alang grass roofs. These spaces are used for Balinese healing treatments, administered by traditional healers whose gifts in bodywork and energy healing have been passed down over generations. Guests can also enjoy more relaxing Balinese-inspired massage and body care, face care, nail and hair care rituals prepared by hand in the therapy prep laboratory along with Fivelements' signature homemade tisane and Sakti healing elixirs. Like other buildings on property, the healing and wellness reception, signature boutique, and laboratory share the same semi-enclosed building style with an organic shaped roof mimicking nature.

The wellness strategies for these buildings include abundant access to nature and natural light, forest bathing, passive cooling design, utilization of natural, non-toxic renewable materials, and recycled timbers for flooring. In addition, the integrated wellness activities include combining holistic wellness consultations, healing and beauty wellness treatments, and plant-powered nutrition as well as access to healing elements from traditional healers and village-inspired wellness rituals made fresh from the lab. The wellness benefits realized are physical and emotional through the therapeutic treatments, retreats and programs, mental and environmental through the immersive, natural riverside architecture set amongst the verdant jungle foliage, and spiritual

8.8 Fivelements Wellness Reception, Boutique & Laboratory a) Wellness Reception, b) Healing Village, c) Balinese Healer, d) Healing Bath

(*Source: Fivelements*)

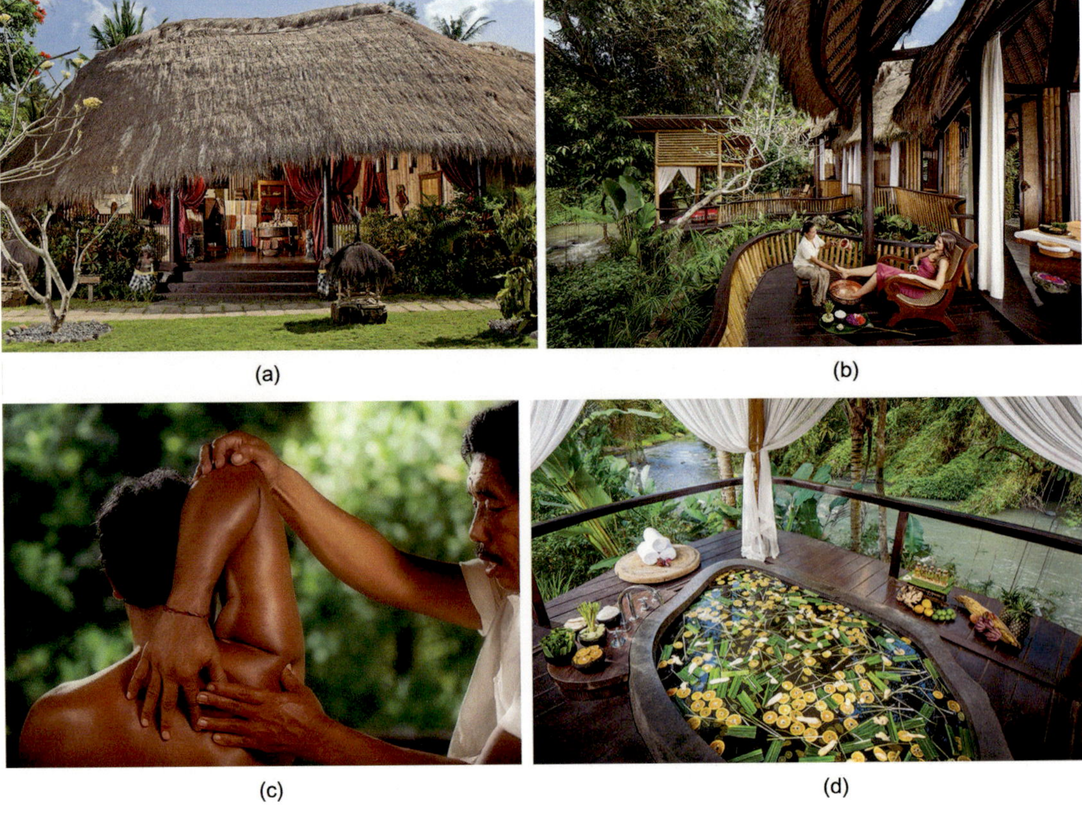

(a) (b) (c) (d)

through the engagement with devoted Balinese healers and their integrative energy healing and bodywork practices.

PLANNING AND DESIGNING FOR THE FEET OR NISTA

1. Sleeping Suites

According to *Asta Kosala Kosali*, the Feet or *Nista* section of a property signifies spaces for rest and less sacred activity. Positioned in the lower area of the property are the original Sleeping Suite villas. With riverfront views, the spacious Sleeping Suites and en suite covered, open-air bathrooms were designed in both spiral and leaf-shaped forms, offering a luxurious, immersive experience nestled in nature. Each Sleeping Suite features a private terrace with a covered *balè* housing a hand-carved volcanic stone bathtub with chromotherapy lighting for healing baths and quiet reflection by the river. Ponds connect the suites with curved bridges leading to each garden entrance. Ironwood floors ground the enclosed suites with coconut pillars for structure, split vertical bamboo grace the interior walls with *alang alang* assembled roofs. Heritage items have been carefully appointed with traditional, handwoven Balinese *songket* and *ikat* textiles made by women from the northeast mountainous areas.

Perched up on the hillside on the opposite side of the property are 11 additional Sleeping Suites built as a second stage intended to host retreat groups. Designed to feel like a meditation village, these suites are more intimately positioned with ponds connecting and traditional pitched rooflines. Each Sleeping Suite features a private plunge pool and covered terrace overlooking the expansive gardens and organic rice fields. Bamboo "*skin*" creates the exterior façade from the outside, and inside, natural furnishings with hand-woven Balinese *songket* textiles add a colorful touch of artistic tradition to the more minimalistic architecture and interior design languages.

The wellness strategies for the Sleeping Suites include access to the healing five elements, healing waters, forest bathing, large canopy roofs for shading over relaxation terraces, use of local, natural, and non-toxic materials and recycled timbers for flooring, access to abundant natural night and cross ventilation, and access to organic herb gardens. The intended wellness benefits are environmental and physical (natural architecture immersed in nature by the riverside with limited light pollution for enhancing restorative sleep and circadian rhythm balance, among others), mental, and emotional (reducing stress, improving positive outlook, and calming of the nervous system through connecting with the greater, natural ecosystem).

FIVELEMENTS TESTIMONIALS

Following are a few testimonials from industry leaders, guests, media visits, and guestbook comments for experiences of the Fivelements Retreat:

> *Fivelements Retreat Bali was decades ahead in its quest to incorporate biophilic design principles that are purposely intended to nurture the relationships between humans and nature — relationships that heal and sustain*

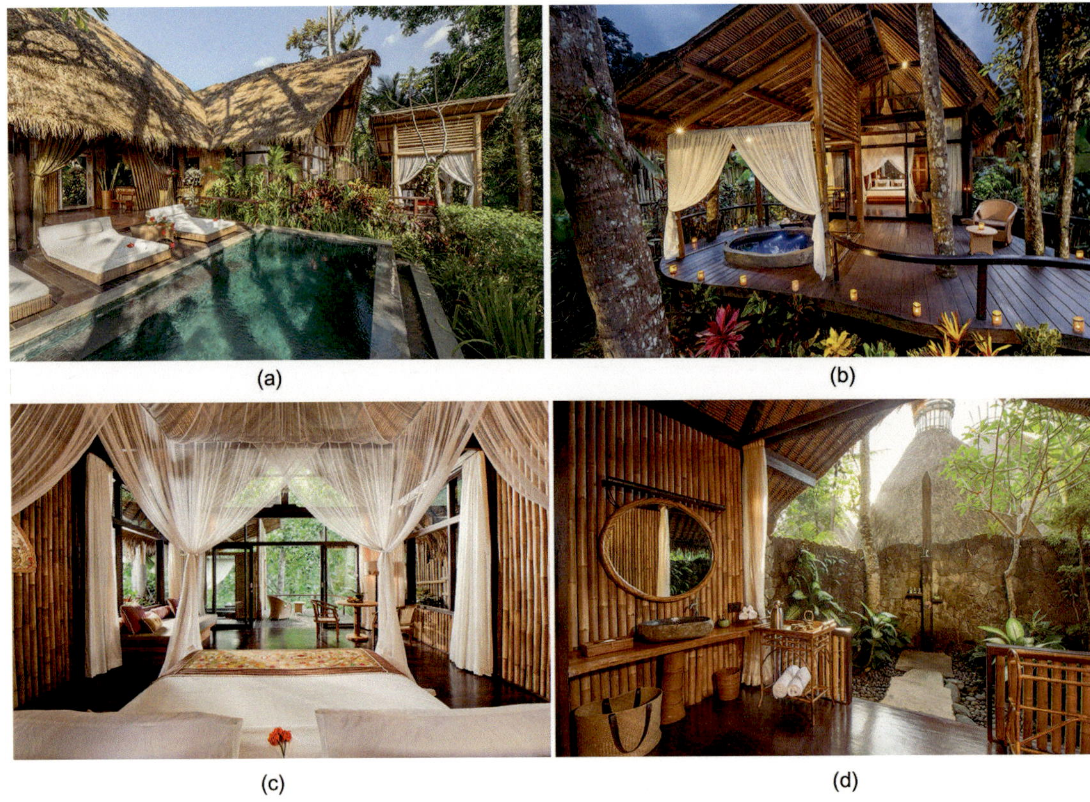

(a) (b) (c) (d)

8.9 Fivelements Sleeping Suites a) Pool Suite, b) Riverfront Suite, c) Suite Interior, d) Ensuite

(*Source: Fivelements*)

life itself. In fact, the Fivelements philosophy became the definition of a new eco-luxury that positively impacted seven dimensions of wellness: physical, emotional, mental, spiritual, social and environmental, all thoughtfully crafted from traditional building materials and guided by local wisdom to create an innovative, timeless architecture that promotes well-being.[3]

Fivelements Retreat Bali's innovative design merges the rich heritage of traditional Balinese architecture with contemporary eco-conscious elements. This synthesis not only enhances the aesthetic appeal but also cultivates a nurturing environment, seamlessly integrating natural materials, expansive open spaces, and verdant surroundings. The result is a sanctuary that not only inspires serenity and mindfulness but actively fosters holistic healing for those seeking profound well-being.[4]

Fivelements is an example of the future living on with nature in an environment that has comfort, style, and an intimate connection to the natural surroundings of Bali's nature and traditions.[5]

I loved my stay at Fivelements every time I can be there! It is really the perfect home away from home to just release and let go and ground.[6]

Most apparent, is the deep respect that Fivelements holds not only for the environment but also for the local people, their traditions, customs, and religion.[7]

Designed in accordance with eco-conscious principles, ancient Balinese architectonic guidelines, and sacred geometry, Fivelements embraces an authentic approach to healing and wellness.[8]

WELLNESS PLANNING AND DESIGN STRATEGIES

There were several primary design determinants that included personal wellness, social harmony, sustainability with a net-positive impact, and regenerative design. At the entrance to the property is located a Balinese temple shrine marking sacred sensibilities to the property. The Ayung River encircles the retreat to the south and west forming a tranquil and beautiful boundary. A spot in the site was discovered as a positive energy vortex and the Sacred Space was consecrated to protect it and define it as a healing and meditation circle accessible to guests on their healing journey as a place for meditation, number 3 on the master plan, Figure 8.2b. Another place within the retreat is a healing fire ceremony site, known as the *Agni* (meaning fire) *Hotra* (meaning healing), number 4. Nearly all the Sleeping Suites, Wellness Suites and the restaurant are positioned facing the river with a five-to-ten-meter setback. This provides guests with direct access to the wild riverbank while maintaining a conservation zone and enhancing the cool, positive air that flows up from the river across the land.

The light design was carefully curated using warm white and orange lighting synchronized according to circadian rhythm and the natural lighting cycle. Low-lit Balinese lanterns with customized LEDs were designed and placed along the pathways with customized speakers hidden inside piping kundalini mantra music and nature instrumentals throughout the property and public spaces. Instrumentals with binaural beats in the lower beta frequencies (14–30Hz) were intentionally selected to reduce stress, enhance focus, creativity and mood, and aid with relaxation and sleep. Overall, the music selection and positioning along pathways and inside public spaces were designed to create a calm, positive, and nurturing soundscape, gently accompanying guests, visitors, and staff alike in a harmonious "journey to wellness" seamlessly transitioning between spaces.

The project focuses on reducing total energy consumption, water savings, and air-cooling efficiencies. Following a study on baseline consumption budgeting, the design team was able to achieve a 42% reduction of peak load from the baseline study through sourcing more efficient appliances, designing more efficient systems, and 95% reduction of lighting energy budget through a customized LED light system. This system, combined with the in-house audio system and telephones, was designed to offer remote access through the Internet, allowing energy use to be closely monitored. Water use and savings are also a major priority for Fivelements. Water pressure throughout the property is set at a maximum flow, all wastewater is treated according to international standards through the constructed wetlands, and then recycled for use as irrigation water. Rainwater is harvested and stored on site in catchment ponds. Cooling was another area where reductions were made. Through passive cooling architecture and planning, less than 30% of the project building footprint is air conditioned, and appropriately sized "inverter" AC systems and low energy sycamore fans were chosen to move and cool air using less energy. The site has been designed to provide access to the medicinal gardens healing herbs for use in the wellness cuisine and treatment preparations.

FIVELEMENTS SUMMARY

The Fivelements Retreat Bali offers an in-depth look at a purpose-built, tradition reinterpreted wellness architecture sited in a lush and beautiful rural setting. While it is not a representation of an everyday setting all over the world, it does express enhanced wellness design principles, forms, and functions. Highly present are the physical, emotional, mental, social, spiritual, and environmental benefits. Evident are strategies of human-oriented design, trails, and forest bathing, pedestrianization, meeting places and socialization, gardens and nutrition, abundant access to nature, limited night pollution, and the presence of thin places.

Wellness tourism is directly associated with maintaining and enhancing personal health and well-being. What is important about these destinations are the host of wellness health-forward programs as well as the purposeful environments designed to support these activities. Fivelements exemplifies both the programs and environments in abundant and impactful ways in support of wellness experiences. Although not as intentional or dramatic, many wellness principles and design elements can be applied to everyday situations. Direct visual and non-visual contact with nature and the elements, encouragement of indoor-outdoor living, use of natural and non-toxic materials, healthy cuisine, and inspiring sacred moments can be applied to normal living conditions. City expansion, new developments, and architectural projects can integrate wellness principles into the planning and design process.

This case study illustrates the eliciting qualities of wellness design inclusive of the cluster, retreat, or compound scale of application. Achieving high-level wellness requires the preventative aspects of disease, disability, and social breakdowns, and requires more than overcoming "*un-wellness*." High-level wellness includes maintaining balance, purposeful direction, and maximizing potentials that are easily accessible and can be woven into everyday life.[9] This includes support of the physical, mental, emotional, spiritual, social, financial, and environmental pillars of wellness. The environment, whether it is at the

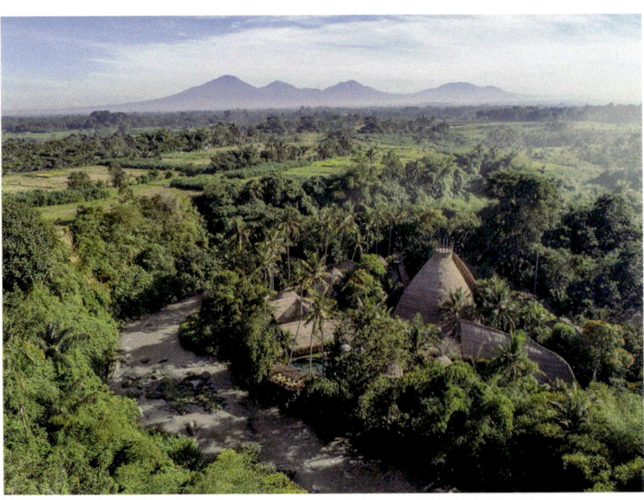

8.10
Fivelements Retreat Bali River Site
(*Source: Fivelements*)

architecture or community scale, is critical in eliciting positive wellness benefits and outcomes. Fivelements Retreat Bali is a compelling example of wellness retreat functions and architecture. Its lush grounds are an incredible backdrop to the plant-based wellness cuisine restaurant, the Balinese healing and wellness village, treatment rooms, outdoor healing baths, healing pools, and the eco-bamboo villas with terraces overlooking the Ayung River. This is a quintessential example of the seamless integration of outdoor and indoor wellness design. Table 8.1 lists the wellness strategies employed at Fivelements Retreat Bali.

Each of the wellness benefit pillars are present at Fivelements and serve as a principal function and high impact facilitator for the retreat. A listing of the Fivelements' wellness strategies follows:

1 Human-oriented retreat design – *master planning according to human proportion of the head, body, and feet, and human-centered wellness design committed to biophilia concepts, maintaining exceptional air quality, promoting a zero-waste mindset, measuring and minimizing resource use, and respecting the local community and traditions.*
2 Mixed use retreat functions – *provides diversity of nutritional/physical, mental, emotional, social, spiritual, environmental, and economic opportunities and benefits.*
3 Integrated wellness activities – *retreats and à la carte offerings, blending holistic wellness consultations, Balinese healing and wellness treatments, plant-powered nutrition and trainings, and transformative sacred arts sessions in rejuvenation, cleansing, and restorative programs as well as providing forest bathing opportunities by the river.*
4 Encouragement of physical activity – *both inside the property through an array of yoga, marital arts, and movement practices as well as in and around the property pathways.*
5 Trails and forest bathing opportunities – *provide easy access to restful seating, healing baths, and mindful walks along the Ayung River.*
6 Pedestrianization with no automobile traffic – *offering pathways throughout the property, river paths, small country roads through the traditional village and rice fields nearby.*
7 Multiple meeting places for socialization – *gardens, sacred spaces, restaurants, and multi-purpose buildings offering opportunities to connect for spiritual renewal, individual and group healing activities, and healthy dining spaces and terraces.*
8 Other shared elements – *seating areas in the restaurant, healing village, pool areas, ceremony spaces, medicinal gardens, gym, and other gardens and greenspaces.*
9 Encouraging indoor-outdoor spaces – *the entire site is designed in tropical indoor-outdoor style with covered terraces, balconies, healing bathhouses, and gardens.*
10 Promoting nudge designs – *where planning and architectural elements, such as bridges, stairs, corridors, outdoor spaces, and connecting paths, are encouraged through design.*

11 Access to organic gardens – *onsite medicinal herb gardens for use in treatments and cuisine and access to organic gardens nearby within a 0–20-kilometer radius.*
12 Access to healthy nutrition – *offering an innovative culinary journey through plant-based, regenerative cuisine at every meal, retreats, workshops, and trainings.*
13 Access to healing elements – *materials, treatments, and cuisine made from blending earth, water, fire, air, and ether, the five elements.*
14 Particular access to healing waters – *activation of the Ayung riverfront with nearly all buildings facing the river, leisure, and watsu healing pools and natural fishponds.*
15 Abundant access to nature – *on physical, visual, and non-visual levels.*
16 Large canopy roofs for shading – *in all private and public spaces, outdoor seating and relaxation with fresh air is encouraged while protected from UV rays.*
17 Abundant uses of natural light and ventilation – *cross-ventilation design for all structures, open air and glass to access and maximize natural light resources.*
18 Limited night light pollution – *utilization of low LED lighting and low lantern lighting for pathways.*
19 Integration of living color – *all buildings are open air or with glass to enhance the integration and access to the flora and fauna surrounding the property and along the river.*
20 Eurythmy of architectural forms – *encouraging balance of architecture proportions according to ancient wisdom and practices.*
21 Building with sustainability toward net-positive impact – *environmental awareness through workshops and trainings, social sustainability through encouraging ongoing dialogue with the local village as well as events with international guests, such as TEDx, social impact programs and partnerships, and minimizing construction impact and offsetting with positive action programs, such as replanting coral in the seas, supporting and participating in local community ceremonies, and supporting Friends of the Wildlife Foundation, among others.*
22 Use of local, natural, and non-toxic materials – *bamboo, alang alang thatch roofing, stones and recycled timber flooring, and rattan and locally sourced recycled wood used for many interior furnishings.*
23 Response to ecological flows – *planning with minimal disturbance to the pre-existing aesthetics and natural ecosystems and designating a 5–10-meter building setback to maintain the river form and flow and minimize erosion, plus many buildings face the river to enhance cooling and access to a natural, healing water source.*
24 Biophilic design – *biophilic principles employed throughout from acoustics, ventilation, orientation and geometry, materials, illumination, scents, and aesthetics.*
25 Passive cooling design – *employed on many buildings to move warm air out and enhance fresh air circulation.*
26 Utilization of natural and renewable resources – *locally sourced bamboo, alang alang thatched roofing and recycled timbers, and connection to wetlands for*

	FIVELEMENTS STRATEGIES							
1	Human-Oriented Retreat Design	X	X	X	X	X	X	X
2	Mix Use Retreat Functions	X	X	X		X	X	X
3	Integrated Wellness Activities	X	X	X	X	X	X	
4	Encouraging Physical Activity	X	X	X		X		
5	Trails and Forest Bathing	X	X	X	X	X		X
6	Pedestrianization & No Traffic	X	X	X	X	X	X	X
7	Meeting Places and Socialization	X	X	X	X	X	X	X
8	Other Shared Elements	X	X	X	X	X	X	X
9	Indoor-Outdoor Spaces	X	X	X	X	X		X
10	Nudge Design Strategies	X			X	X	X	X
11	Access to Organic Garden	X	X	X	X	X	X	X
12	Healthy Nutrition	X	X	X	X	X	X	X
13	Access to Healing Elements	X		X	X	X		X
14	Access to Healing Waters	X	X	X	X	X	X	X
15	Abundant Access to Nature	X	X	X	X	X	X	X
16	Large Canopy Roofs	X		X		X	X	X
17	Access to Abundant Natural Light	X	X	X	X	X	X	X
18	Limited Night Light Pollution	X	X	X	X	X	X	X
19	Integration of Living Color		X	X	X			
20	Eurythmy of Architctural Form	X	X	X	X			X
21	Building Sustainably	X	X		X		X	X
22	Use of Natural & Non-Toxic Materials	X	X	X			X	X
23	Response to Ecological Flows	X			X	X	X	X
24	Biophilic Design	X	X	X	X	X	X	X
25	Passive Cooling Dsign	X	X	X			X	X
26	Natural & Renewable Resources	X		X	X		X	X
27	Economic Benefits		X	X			X	X
28	Local Wisdom	X	X	X	X	X		X
29	Sacred Moments and Thin Places	X	X	X	X	X	X	X
	WELLNESS BENEFITS	Physical	Mental	Emotional	Spiritual	Social	Financial	Environmental

Table 8.1
Fivelements Retreat Wellness Design Strategies

landscape irrigation and onsite organic composting. A waste management and recycling system has also been designed.

27 Economic benefits – *increased land values, increased ROI from the accommodation rentals, restaurant, treatments and classes/sessions/retreats and events for healing and wellness, increased ROW with realized wellness outcomes for guests through life-changing program experiences and for employees and investors through their shared efforts living and supporting the vision and mission, positive wellness branding and brand equity, marketing and public relations, efficiency from energy reduction – LED customized lighting and water use especially.*

28 Local wisdom – *inspiring philosophies, planning, and building methods.*

29 Sacred moments and thin places – *created with nature on meandering pathways, the riverfront, and at meditation and prayer sites.*

As can be seen in Table 8.1, the Fivelements Retreat Bali wellness strategies are listed indicating the physical, mental, emotional, social, financial and environmental, and spiritual benefits.

Embodying the Balinese philosophy, Tri Hito Karana, Fivelements' architecture represents a balance between humans, the natural world, and the spiritual realm, and offers a profound connection to the island's heart and soul.[10]

NOTES

1. Idedhyana, Ida Bagus; Sueca, Ngakan Putu; Dwijendra, Ngakan Ketut Acwin; Wibawa, Ida Bagus Wira, *The Function and Typology of the Padmasana Tiga Architecture in Besakih Temple* (Bali Indonesia), Udayana University, *Journal of Social and Political Sciences*, Asian Institute of Research, pp. 291–299.
2. Wijaya, Made (White, Michael), *Architecture of Bali: A Sourcebook of Traditional and Modern Forms* (Singapore: Archipelago Press, 2002), p. 54.
3. Testimonial by Susie Ellis, Chairman and CEO, Global Wellness Institute.
4. Testimonial by Vivienne Tang, CEO, Destination Deluxe.
5. Posted of TripAdvisor about the Fivelements Retreat.
6. Testimonial by a visitor to Fivelements.
7. Testimonial by a visitor in 2010 to Fivelements.
8. Testimonial by a visitor in 2013 to Fivelements.
9. Dunn, Halbert L., *High Level Wellness* (Arlington, VA: Beatty, 1971), pp. 4–7.
10. Arthana, Ketut, Arte Architects & Associates, Bali, Indonesia (Accessed 30 January 2024).

Summary

It is clear that there are many benefits to wellness planning and design most of which are confirmed by evidence-based research and occur at both personal and planetary levels. Important to the effectiveness of the design strategies are the frequency (*how often*), duration (*how long*), accessibility (*how easy*), and quality (*how much or how intense*) of wellness experiences. How they promote preventative and wholistic activities, resiliency, positive lifestyle choices, and changes to the physical environment will ultimately be the greatest challenges. This entails addressing a multi-scalar approach to wellness across the entirety of the built environment from regions and cities to neighborhoods and buildings. Key to the success of a wellness future is the actualization of comprehensive approaches to preventative wellness design that encourage positive lifestyle choices. It is encouraging to know that this work is achievable. The many planning and design strategies, and the wellness benefits they elicit discussed throughout the chapters of this book, are concrete illustrations of this success. The case studies of Mado neighborhood and Fivelements Retreat Bali are excellent testaments to powerful wellness narratives and integrated design solutions. Following is a listing of wellness planning and design objectives:

1. **First** *is that wellness architecture and urban design solutions are wholistic and comprehensive.*
2. **Second** *is that wellness architecture and urban design solutions are realized across multiple scales of the built environment.*
3. **Third** *is that wellness architecture and urban design solutions are easily accessible and within reach.*
4. **Fourth** *is that architecture and urban design solutions have the ability to be experienced through everyday activities.*
5. **Fifth** *is that wellness architecture and urban design solutions strive for high impact elicitors of the seven pillars of wellness benefits as well as high-level wellness.*
6. **Sixth** *is that wellness architecture and urban design solutions are permanent and long lasting.*
7. **Seventh** *is that wellness architecture and urban design solutions encourage and help facilitate positive lifestyle choices.*

Suggested Reading

1. Allen, Summer (2018), *The Science of Awe,* https://ggsc.berkeley.edu/images/uploads/GGSC-JTF_White_Paper-Awe_FINAL.pdf
2. Balboni, Tracy A, Tyer J. VanderWheele, & Stephen Doan-Soares, *Spirituality in Serious Illness and Health,* https://jamanetwork.com/journals/jama/article-abstract/2794049
3. Baum, Fran & Matthew Fisher, *Critical Public Health,* https://www.tandfonline.com/doi/abs/10.1080/09581596.2010.503266
4. Buettner, Dan, *Blue Zones: 9 Lessons for Living Longer from the People Who've Lived the Longest* (National Geographic, 2012).
5. Coates, Gary, *Erik Asmussen, architect* (Stockholm, Sweden: Byggforlaget, 1997).
6. Dunn, Halbert, *High Level Wellness* (Pitman, New Jersey: Charles B. Slack Publisher, 1977).
7. Ehrenfeld, John R., *Sustainability by Design* (New Haven, CT: Yale University Press, 2008).
8. Global Wellness Institute, *What is Wellness?,* https://globalwellnessinstitute.org/what-is-wellness/
9. Global Wellness Institute, *Wellness Architecture and Design Initiative 2023 Trends,* https://globalwellnessinstitute.org/global-wellness-institute-blog/2023/08/07/wellness-architecture-design-initiative-2023-trends/
10. Heschong, Lisa, *Visual Delight in Architecture: Daylight, Vision, and View* (London, UK: Routledge, 2021).
11. Kaplan, R. & S. Kaplan, *The Experience of Nature: A Psychological Perspective* (Cambridge, MA: Cambridge University Press, 1989).
12. Kellert, Stephen R., *Biophilic Design: The Theory, Science and Practice of Bringing Buildings to Life* (Hoboken, NJ: Wiley & Sons, 2008).
13. Keltner, Dacher, *Awe: The New Science of Everyday Wonder and How it Can Transform Our Lives* (New York, NY: Penguin Press, 2023).
14. Kopec, Dac, *Person-Centered Health Care Design* (New York, NY: Routledge, 2021).
15. Louv, Richard, *Last Child in the Woods: Saving Our Children from Nature-Deficit Disorder* (Chapel Hill, NC: Algonquin Books, 2008).
16. Massy, Charles, *Call of the Reed Warbler: A New Agriculture, A New Earth* (White River Junction, VT: Chelsea Green Publishing, 2018).
17. McEwen, Bruce, *Stress and Your Body,* https://www.youtube.com/watch?v=0TUDwXPq67k
18. Olszewska-Guizzo, Agnieszka, *Neuroscience for Designing Green Spaces: Contemplative Landscapes* (London, UK: Routledge, 2023).
19. Positive Psychology, *What is Social Wellbeing? 12+ Activities for Social Wellness,* Accessed June 1, 2023), https://positivepsychology.com/social-wellbeing/
20. Roberts, Kay & Cheryl Aspy, *Development of a Serenity Scale,* https://www.researchgate.net/publication/15347724_Development_of_the_Serenity_Scale
21. Spiegel, Ross & Dru Meadows, *Green Building Materials: A Guide to Product Selection and Specification* (New York, NY: Wiley & Sons, 1999).

22. Swarbrick, Margaret, *Mapping Mental Health: Dr. Swarbrick & The Eight Wellness Dimensions,* https://alcoholstudies.rutgers.edu/mapping-mental-health-dr-swarbrick-the-eight-wellness-dimensions/
23. Travis, John, *Illness and Wellness Continuum, 1972,* https://www.houseofhealth.co.nz/wellness-continuum-blog-1-physical-health/
24. Tabb, Phillip, *Thin Place Design: Architecture of the Numinous,* https://www.annuity.org/personal-finance/financial-wellness/
25. Wilson, Alex, *Passive Survivability*, Accessed July 11, 2013, https://www.buildinggreen.com/op-ed/passive-survivability
26. VanderWeele, Tyler, *Spirituality Linked with Better Health Outcomes, Patient Care,* https://www.hsph.harvard.edu/news/press-releases/spirituality-better-health-outcomes-patient-care/
27. Zorn, Justin & Leigh Marz, *Golden: The Power of Silence in a World of Noise* (New York, NY: Harper Wave, 2022).

Index

Note: **Bold** page numbers refer to figures.